A CASE-BASED APPROACH TO **ECG** INTERPRETATION

A CASE-BASED APPROACH TO ECG INTERPRETATION

Kaye D. Nagell, RN, CEN

Former New York State Paramedic

Former New York State EMS Instructor/Coordinator for EMT–Paramedic Instruction

Ron Nagell

Tennessee EMT-Intermediate

Former New York State AEMT-3

New York State EMS Instructor/Coordinator for EMT–Advanced EMT Instruction

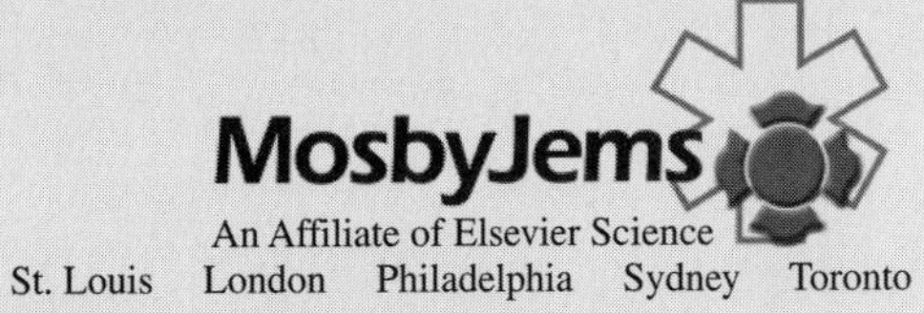

An Affiliate of Elsevier Science

St. Louis London Philadelphia Sydney Toronto

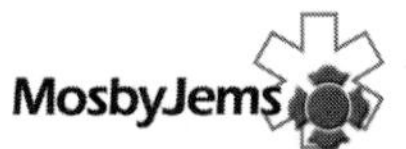

An Affiliate of Elsevier Science

11830 Westline Drive
St. Louis, Missouri 63146

A CASE-BASED APPROACH TO ECG INTERPRETATION ISBN 0-323-01968-4

NOTICE

Electrocardiography is an ever-changing field. Standard safety precautions must be followed but as new research and clinical experience broaden our knowledge, changes in treatment and drug therapy may become necessary or appropriate. Readers are advised to check the most current product information provided by the manufacturer of each drug to be administered to verify the recommended dose, the method and duration of administration, and contraindications. It is the responsibility of the licensed prescriber, relying on experience and knowledge of the patient, to determine dosages and the best treatment for each individual patient. Neither the publisher nor the author assumes any liability for any injury and/or damages to persons or property arising from this publication.

Library of Congress Cataloging-in-Publication Data

Nagell, Kaye D.
A case-based approach to ECG interpretation/Kaye D. Nagell and Ron Nagell.
p. cm.
Includes index.
ISBN 0-323-01968-4
1. Electrocardiography—Interpretation—Problems, exercises, etc. 2
Heart—Diseases—Diagnosis—Problems, exercises, etc. I. Nagell,
Ron. II. Title.
[DNLM: 1. Electrocardiography—Problems and Exercises. 2.
Heart—physiology—Problems and Exercises. WG 18.2 N147c 2003]
RC683.5.E5 N24 2003 2002067047

Acquisitions Editor: Claire Merrick
Developmental Editor: Laura Bayless
Publishing Services Manager: Deborah L. Vogel
Project Manager: Claire Kramer
Design Manager: Bill Drone
Cover Images: Index Stock Imagery

RT/QWV

Printed in the United States of America.

9 8 7 6 5 4 3 2 1

I would like to dedicate this book
in loving memory to my Mom and Dad.
Your love and support were always there.
Your love, character, and strength remain
with me on a day-to-day basis. You were the
best parents anyone could ever have.

Reviewers

The editors wish to acknowledge the reviewers of this book for their invaluable help in developing and fine-tuning the manuscript.

Robert D. Cook, NREMPT-P, PS, EMS-I, EMD
Iowa Central Community College
Ft. Dodge, Iowa

Julie Crawshaws, BSN, MICN
University of California, Los Angeles (UCLA)–Westwood, California
Long Beach Community College (LBCC)–Long Beach, California
St. Mary's Medical Center–Long Beach, California

Dennis Edgerly, EMT-P
HealthOne EMS
Englewood, Colorado

David S. Pecora, PA-C, NREMT-P, RN
Department of Emergency Medicine
West Virginia University
Morgantown, West Virginia

Dr. Anne Robenstein, DO
Cortland Memorial Hospital for Emergency Medicine Physicians
Cortland, New York

Preface

As both students and instructors of ECG interpretation, we have noted a distinct difficulty expressed by students in applying the academic knowledge gained from ECG instruction module and its actual application in field situations. Although nothing can replace actual practice in the field, the use of scenarios in conjunction with the academic interpretation of ECG strips gives students the skills necessary to begin to treat the patients as the ECG rhythm—before going out in the field. This gives the students a far better foundation than could otherwise be achieved.

DESCRIPTION

A Case-Based Approach to ECG Interpretation consists of 10 chapters designed to assist the health care provider in learning to interpret the ECG rhythms. Text, self-tests, practice ECG rhythms, scenarios with treatment needed, plus scenario-type questions are included. Chapter 10 is devoted completely to ECG practice rhythms with 200 practice strips. Chapter 9 is designed with 40 ACLS cases; the student is asked to interpret the ECG strip and to provide the correct ACLS treatment.

When I began using the scenarios as a regular teaching modality in conjunction with standard ECG texts, I found that students were more enthusiastic, more interested, and more responsive. Informal follow-ups showed that the students so instructed were able to integrate into the field faster and better than those instructed otherwise.

This book encompasses the entire picture: the heart, the problem, the ECG, and most important, the patient. We recognize that the unusual can and often does happen. The intent of the book is to train a student in the understanding and interpretation of ECG arrhythmias, not to be a glossary of medical technology. This book is meant to reaffirm that the patient care is so very important while at the same time teaching the student how to read ECGs. Explanations and procedures are simply explained whenever possible. With this concept the student may focus on what he or she wants, ECG interpretation. The student is not faced with attempting to learn a host of parallel information to reach this goal. Simplicity, in conjunction with the "building block" modality of presenting information, allows the student to rapidly grasp the content of each chapter—and with the knowledge just gained into the concept of "treating the patient—not the ECG." As a result the student enters each chapter with a greater understanding than could otherwise be achieved.

A Case-Based Approach to ECG Interpretation consists of 10 chapters, formulated to provide the health care professional (e.g., physicians, residents, interns, physician assistants, nurse practitioners, nurses, paramedics, EMTs, and other health care providers) with the necessary information, algorithms, scenarios, and review questions to understand and interpret normal ECGs and dangerous arrhythmias. It is designed to teach anyone the necessary information needed to learn, understand, and interpret normal ECG rhythms and ECG arrhythmias. A prerequisite for this book is a basic understanding of the anatomy of the circulatory system.

LEARNING PHILOSOPHY

Realizing that mastery can only be achieved by reinforcement, the initial chapters have been organized in a manner to give the broad-based spectrum of knowledge so necessary for the student if progression in ECG interpretation is to be accomplished. As the chapters advance, previous information is called on to understand the subject at hand. With this continual reinforcement, the student is able to achieve a rapid and accurate assessment of ECG interpretation. Such rapid assessment has become a vital part of prehospital and in-hospital treatment of cardiac problems, and it helps to reduce the number of serious cardiac events. We believe student learning is similar to building a house. First you must have a good foundation; the learning student must have general knowledge of anatomy and physiology to be able to understand how the circulatory system works before learning ECGs. A house is built one step at a time. If a step is left out, the remaining structure is in danger. It leaves a void, an incompleteness, about the structure. Have you ever taken a class and finished it with a feeling that "something was left out?"

FEATURES

• Consistent Format

The presentation of the material flows in a logical manner that continuously leads to placing the patient and the ECG rhythm together as one entity. The individual topic section is presented in a three-step concept—information, practice, and testing—ensuring a constant reinforcement and skill integration not readily accomplished with other modalities of similar presentation. This format presents the student with a continuing challenge and self-testing and assures confidence and mastery of the presented material before progressing on to the next chapter.

• ECG Practice Strips

Every topic section ends with a series of ECG strips that the student must identity (answers are in an appendix). The given strips will be relevant to the current chapter and will supply the student with an instant feedback as to proper assimilation of the presented information.

Most are actual patients who went to the emergency department or were ambulance calls. This feature promotes clarity of treatment not seen in other similar books. The scenario-type questions provide reinforcement of the chapter just learned.

• Real-Life Situation as Case Scenarios

The student is presented with original ECG strips from *actual* patient situations. The cases or scenarios are used in each chapter to reinforce that it is the patient being treated, not just the ECG rhythm. With experience in the field, the emergency department, plus the ICU, we strongly feel this book is a must for every student because it gives a complete picture. What happened to the patient? Did the ECG rhythm cause the scenario to occur, or did the scenario cause the ECG arrhythmia to occur? *A Case-Based Approach to ECG Interpretation* encourages students to think through the problem and treat the patient as well as the ECG rhythm. Having practiced this module in class, it was found to work extremely well. Treat the whole picture (patient) and build a house with a strong foundation.

• Self-Tests

At the end of each chapter is a short self-test to allow the student to evaluate his or her own progress and to find out if he or she is ready to advance to the next chapter. The self-tests included at the end of each chapter are placed so the student can do a reality check. "Where am I?" "Have I learned what I was supposed to from this chapter?" "Am I ready to build the next step, go on to the next chapter?" "Is my foundation strong enough to hold up through many storms, many crises?"

• "Think-It-Though" Approach

The topic–strips–case scenario sequence encourages students to constantly be thinking, "What caused this?" "How should I be caring for my patient?" "What treatment should my patient be receiving?" This book commands the student to realize that every arrhythmia is not necessarily cardiac related. It teaches the student to look beyond the circulatory system when assessing and evaluating their patient and to investigate other possibilities: Is the arrhythmia generated because of a neurologic problem? An orthopedic problem? A respiratory problem? If the problem is corrected, then hopefully the ECG arrhythmia will return to normal sinus rhythm. If not, what should be done next?

• Applied ECG Interpretation

The student must realize the ECG arrhythmia is only a part of the patient's illness. With this book and good class instruction the student will be able to lay a strong foundation that he or she will be able to use with confidence throughout his or her career. The main focus of this book continues to be ECG interpretation. This book is a *must have* for every student learning ECG interpretation and also those who are simply reviewing. This book, in conjunction with any cardiac textbook, would be of magnificent value when the student needs to understand the many cardiac disease states and multiple drugs/methods needed to treat such disease states. The students will then, and only then, be able to understand what causes, and what helps arrhythmias.

Acknowledgments

A very special thank you goes to two of the greatest nurses I've ever worked with, Mary Dolgin, RN, Cortland Memorial Emergency Department, Cortland, New York, and Lucy Ware, RN, Auburn Memorial Emergency Department, Auburn, New York. Thank you so much for the support and encouragement and friendship. You are two of the best ER nurses we have known, and it has been our pleasure to also have your friendship.

A thank you to Bonnie Huston, RN, and Colleen Hanley, RN, for all your help over the years.

I would also like to thank the following:

Victoria Thomas for her part in initiating this entire project and assisting me all the way. Thank you for just being there, for your guidance, help, encouragement, and support. Victoria, you are a very special person, and the publishing world is lucky to have you working with them. I will never forget those infamous words in our first conversation: "Why don't you write a book?"

Shirley Kuhn, who had ultimate faith in this project and never gave up. Thank you, Shirley.

Claire Merrick for the support given.

Laura Bayless, for the direction, guidance, and support given. You are a wonderful editor and so great to work with.

A special thank you to Claire Kramer, who helped so much, was always there to listen, and was so nice to work with.

Our wonderful family, Lorrie, Barbara, Mike, Shawn, and Scott. Thanks for your patience and for listening through the ups and downs of the entire project. You are the best!

The Four Town Ambulance Service. If it wasn't for you folks, I would never have gotten into emergency work. Keep up the good work; there aren't very many volunteer ambulance services left in our nation. A special thank you to all of our Practical Instructors: Robbie Perkins, EMT; Paul Connors, EMT; Steve Mulvaney, EMT; Shawn Dillon, AEMT-3; Joe Blair, AEMT-3; Sue O'Connor, EMT-I; and Audrey Sharpsteen, AEMT-3.

Contents

A CASE-BASED APPROACH TO **ECG** INTERPRETATION

1

Cardiac Anatomy and Physiology

OBJECTIVES

By the end of this chapter, the student will be able to do the following:

- **Know and understand the anatomy of the heart, its major structures, and its functions**
- **Identify the layers of the heart wall**
- **Identify the chambers of the heart, their location, and their function**
- **Identify the heart valves, their location, and their function**
- **Identify the coronary arteries**
- **Know and understand the coronary circulatory system**
- **Describe the contributing factors of cardiac output**
- **Calculate cardiac output**
- **Know and understand the autonomic nervous system**

OUTLINE

Cardiac Anatomy

Layers of the Heart

Chambers of the Heart

Valves of the Heart

Systole and Diastole

Coronary Arteries

Heart Rate and the Autonomic Nervous System

The Sympathetic Nervous System

The Parasympathetic Nervous System

Chapter 1 Self-Test

To understand electrocardiograms (ECGs), to read them, and to interpret arrhythmias, you must first have a good understanding of basic cardiac anatomy, physiology, and electrophysiology. It is imperative to know how the heart works before you learn how to treat it with appropriate drug and electrical therapy. Throughout this chapter and the book, you must be constantly alert to the concept that you are not treating just an arrhythmia, but a patient with an arrhythmia and that you are not treating a supraventricular tachycardia, but a patient with the problem of supraventricular tachycardia.

CARDIAC ANATOMY

The heart is located in the mediastinum (middle of the thorax), and two thirds of it is located to the left of the sternum. It lies just behind the sternum and of course between the lungs. The top portion (base) of the heart is located in the upper right side of the chest, just to the right of the sternum and below the second rib. The bottom of the heart (apex) lies just above and sometimes rests on the diaphragm. The heart is protected by the sternum and ribs anteriorly, and the spine and rib cage posteriorly.

The heart is a muscular organ and actually works as a mechanical pump, pumping blood to all parts of the body. The right side of the heart pumps unoxygenated blood through the pulmonary artery to the lungs where the blood picks up oxygen. The blood then returns through the pulmonary vein to the left side of the heart, which pumps oxygenated blood through the arterial system to the entire body and to the heart itself (Figure 1-1).

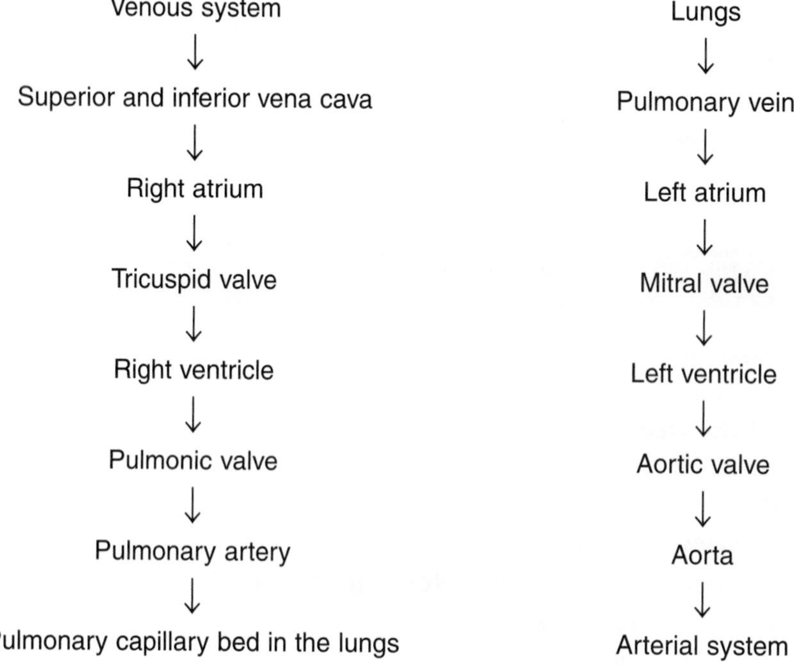

Figure 1-1 Circulatory system.

Layers of the Heart

The heart is enclosed by a thick, double-walled sac called the *pericardium.* The pericardium consists of two layers. The parietal pericardium (outer wall) is a fibrous sac, and the visceral pericardium (inner wall) is actually the outer surface of the heart itself. This visceral or inner layer is also known as the *epicardium.* Between these layers is a potential space, which has approximately 10 ml of a serous-type fluid. This fluid acts as a lubricant so that the layers slide together when the heart contracts and expands with each contraction. The pericardium has three functions:

- It reduces friction between the layers.
- It holds the heart securely in the mediastinum.
- It protects the heart from bacteria.

The heart wall is made up of three layers: the epicardium, the myocardium, and the endocardium (Figure 1-2). The epicardium is the outermost layer. It is also known as the visceral pericardium and is the inner wall of the pericardial sac. The myocardium is the thick, muscular middle layer. It contains cardiac muscle fibers that cause the heart to expand (fill) and contract (empty). The myocardium is the major working component of the heart and is also the place where most of the problems arise. The myocardium contains both the conduction system, which initiates the electrical impulses, and the coronary arteries, which nourish the heart. The myocardium has characteristics of both smooth and skeletal muscles. The myocardium is the muscular portion that causes the heart to contract. The endocardium is the innermost layer of the heart, made up of a smooth layer of connective tissue. It lines the chambers of the heart and covers the heart valves to protect them. The endocardium has a rich blood supply, which provides oxygen and nutrients to the chambers and valves. Coronary blood vessels travel through the three layers supplying them with arterial, oxygenated blood (Table 1-1).

Chambers of the Heart

The anatomy of the heart consists of four chambers: two atria and two ventricles. The atria are located on the top or superior part of the heart and are called the *right atrium* and *left atrium.*

TABLE 1-1 Layers of the Heart Wall

Layer	Description
Epicardium	Inner layer of the pericardium External layer of the heart wall Coronary arteries begin in this layer
Myocardium	Middle layer of the heart wall Thickest layer of the heart wall Contains contractile muscle fibers Contains the conduction system Coronary arteries travel through the myocardium and supply blood, oxygen, and nutrients to the myocardial cells
Endocardium	Innermost layer of the heart wall Made up of smooth connective tissue Lines the outside part of the chambers of the heart Covers the heart valves Provides pathway for blood supply to valves

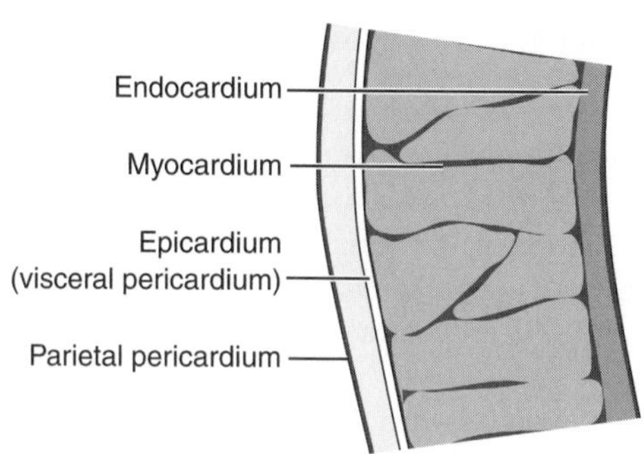

Figure 1-2 Layers of the heart.

The atria are thin-walled, low-pressured chambers. They are normally separated by the interatrial septum, which keeps the blood from going from one side to the other. The right atrium receives unoxygenated blood from the venous circulatory system via the superior and inferior vena cava and the coronary sinus. It then pumps the blood to the right ventricles. The left atrium receives oxygenated blood from the lungs via the pulmonary vein and pumps it directly to the left ventricle. The two lower heart chambers are the right and left ventricles. The right ventricle pumps unoxygenated blood through the pulmonary artery to the lungs to become oxygenated. The left ventricle pumps oxygenated blood through the aorta to the peripheral arterial system. The left ventricle is a high-pressured chamber because it pumps blood into the entire peripheral circulatory system. Of all four chambers the left ventricle works the hardest and is usually the first one to become weakened and damaged.

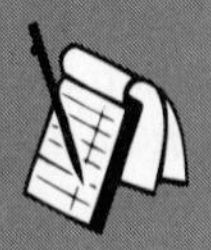

Note

Right and left refer to the patient's right or left side.

Valves of the Heart

It is important to know how the blood travels from one chamber to another. The blood exits each chamber through one-way valves, which prevent the blood from flowing backwards. This ensures that the blood keeps going in the proper direction. Each valve consists of cusps or leaflets that open when the chambers contract, allowing the blood to pass through, but then close to prevent a backflow. The valve between the right atrium and the right ventricle is called the ***tricuspid valve***. The valve between the left atrium and the left ventricle is called the ***mitral*** or ***bicuspid valve***. These valves are collectively known as the ***AV*** or ***atrioventricular valves***. The other two valves control the blood flow from the ventricles to the lungs and peripheral arterial system. These are known as ***semilunar valves***. The valve located between the right ventricle and the pulmonary artery is known as the ***pulmonic valve***. The valve located between the left ventricle and the aorta is known as the ***aortic valve*** (Figure 1-3).

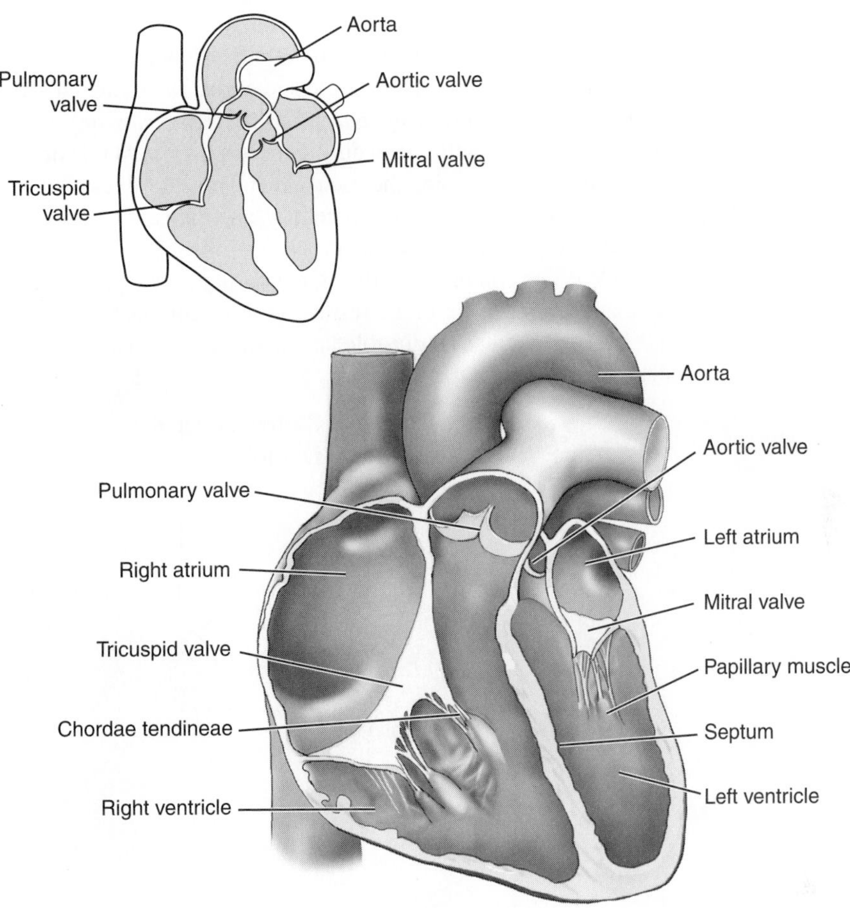

Figure 1-3 Heart valves.

Systole and Diastole

Expansion and contraction of the heart results in systole and diastole.

Diastole represents the passive or relaxation period of the cardiac cycle when the chambers are filling with blood. Note that both atrial and ventricular diastole occurs with each heartbeat; however, when the term diastole is used, it generally refers to ventricular diastole (Figures 1-4 and 1-5).

Systole represents the active or contracting period of the cardiac cycle when the chambers are contracting, sending blood to the pulmonary and systemic circulatory systems. Note that there are both atrial and ventricular periods of systole with each heartbeat. When the term systole is used, it generally refers to ventricular systole (see Figures 1-4 and 1-5).

- ***Atrial diastole** is a period of relaxation for the atria.* Blood enters from the superior vena cava, the inferior vena cava, and the coronary sinus. When the right atrium is filled, the tricuspid valve opens, allowing the blood to enter the right ventricle. At the same time the left atrium fills causing the mitral valve to open, and blood passes through into the left ventricle.
- ***Atrial systole** is a period when the atrial chambers are contracting.* The ventricles are approximately 70% filled passively, and the atria then contract, forcing the additional 30% of the blood to be forcefully ejected into the ventricles, filling them to capacity. This is known as "atrial kick." During this period of atrial systole the venous pressure rises and is greater than the atrial pressure. Blood does not flow into the atria at this time because of the rise in the venous pressure.

- ***Ventricular diastole*** *is a period of time when the ventricles are relaxing and filling*. The blood flows passively from the right and left atria into the right and left ventricles. The tricuspid and mitral valves are open while the pulmonic and aortic valves are closed.
- ***Ventricular systole*** *is a period of time when the ventricles are contracting*. The ventricles become completely filled with blood during the atrial kick. At this time the pressure in the atria and ventricles equalizes, causing the tricuspid and mitral valves to close. As these valves close the pulmonic and aortic valves open forcefully, and the ventricles contract, ejecting blood into the pulmonary and peripheral circulatory systems.

The cardiac cycle is one complete heartbeat, consisting of two phases for each chamber: diastole and systole. Each cardiac cycle in the resting adult usually lasts 0.08 second. The atrial systole lasts about 0.1 second with atrial diastole lasting 0.7 second. The ventricular diastole lasts about 0.5 second, and the ventricular systole lasts about 0.3 second.

Active phase = Systole or depolarization
Passive phase = Diastole or repolarization

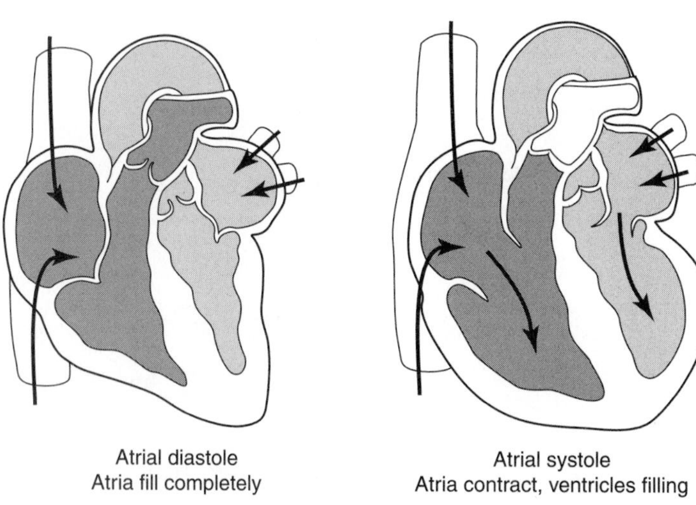
Atrial diastole
Atria fill completely
Atrial systole
Atria contract, ventricles filling

Figure 1-4 Atrial diastole and systole.

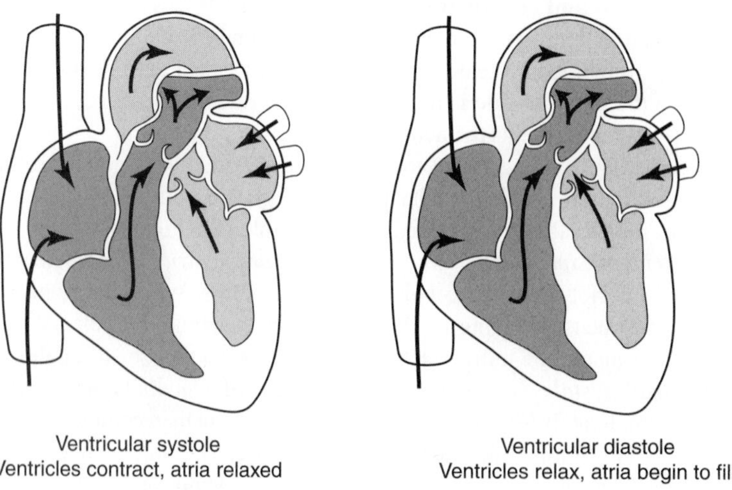
Ventricular systole
Ventricles contract, atria relaxed
Ventricular diastole
Ventricles relax, atria begin to fill

Figure 1-5 Ventricular diastole and systole.

Coronary Arteries

Blood is supplied to the three layers (endocardium, myocardium, and epicardium) by two main arteries, the right and left coronary arteries, which originate from the aorta just beyond the aortic arch. They further divide as shown in Tables 1-2, 1-3, and 1-4.

The filling of the cardiac chambers, mainly the ventricles and the coronary arteries, occurs during diastole. The heart muscle is stretched as the ventricles fill with blood. This causes what is known as *Starling's law of the heart*. According to Starling's law, the myocardial fibers contract

TABLE 1-2 Right Coronary Artery

Branch	Portion of Myocardium Supplied with Blood
Poster descending artery Right marginal or acute marginal artery	Right atrium Right ventricle–anterolateral wall Right ventricle–lateral wall Left ventricle–inferior wall Left ventricle–posterior wall (85%-90%) Posterior one third of interventricular septum

TABLE 1-3 Left Coronary Artery

Branch	Portion of Myocardium Supplied with Blood
Left anterior descending artery	Left ventricle–anterolateral wall, posterolateral wall, and posterior wall (10%-15%)
Left circumflex artery	Left atrium Right ventricle–anterior wall Interventricular septum–two thirds of interventricular septum

TABLE 1-4 Portions of the Conduction System Supplied with Blood

Supplied by the Right Coronary Artery	Supplied by the Left Coronary Artery
SA node (55% of population) AV node (90% of population) Posterior-inferior part of bundle of His Posterior one third of interventricular septum	SA node (45% of the population) AV node (10% of the population) Proximal portion of bundle of His Anterior two thirds of interventricular septum Most of right bundle branch Anterior-superior portion of left bundle branch Posterior-inferior portion of fascicle of left bundle branch

AV, Atrioventricular; *SA*, sinoatrial.

more forcefully when stretched. In accordance with this thought, when the ventricles are filled with larger-than-normal blood volumes (increased preload), they contract with greater-than-normal force to deliver the blood to the circulatory system. The amount of blood ejected with each ventricular contraction is known as ***stroke volume***.

An average heart beats approximately 70 times per minute and ejects approximately 70 ml of blood with each heartbeat or contraction. ***Cardiac output***, the amount of blood pumped by the heart each minute, is determined by multiplying the heart rate per minute by the stroke volume. If your patient has a heart rate of 82 beats per minute and a stroke volume of 70 ml, then his cardiac output is 5740 ml per minute.

Cardiac output = Heart rate × Stroke volume

Preload is the force exerted on the walls of the ventricles at the end of diastole. Thus the amount or volume of blood returning to the heart determines preload. ***Afterload*** is the resistance or arterial pressure against which the ventricles must pump to eject the blood. The less the resistance, the easier blood can be ejected.

HEART RATE AND THE AUTONOMIC NERVOUS SYSTEM

The heart is innervated by the autonomic nervous system, which plays a major role in heart rate and conduction. The autonomic nervous system is involuntary and regulates functions that are not under conscious control. It affects the heart rate, blood vessels, digestive tract, pancreas, liver, spleen, bladder, bronchi, and thyroid. Specifically, the autonomic nervous system is further divided into the ***sympathetic*** (adrenergic) and ***parasympathetic*** (cholinergic) nervous systems. Stated simply, the sympathetic system speeds up body functions, whereas the parasympathetic system slows down body functions. Each system produces the opposite effects when stimulated, mainly regulating stroke volume and heart rate. There is a constant interchange going on between the two nervous systems that keeps our body in complete harmony.

The Sympathetic Nervous System

The sympathetic nervous system (SNS) is responsible for the "fight or flight" response that enables the body to function under stress. When sympathetic (adrenergic) receptors are stimulated, it causes the release of the neurotransmitter *norepinephrine*, and receptors sites are activated. Then the SNS increases the heart rate (chronotropic) and plays a major role in conductivity and the force of contractions (inotropic) (Table 1-5). The results are an increase in cardiac output, an increase in blood pressure, and an increased heart rate.

TABLE 1-5 Effects of the Sympathetic Nervous System

Chronotropic Effect	Inotropic Effect
A change in heart rate	A change in myocardial contractility
Negative chronotropic effect refers to a decrease in the heart rate	*Negative* inotropic effect refers to a decrease in myocardial contractility
Positive chronotropic effect refers to an increase in the heart rate	*Positive* inotropic effect refers to an increase in myocardial contractility

TABLE 1-6 The Effects of Alpha and Beta Receptors and the Organs They Influence

	Alpha	Beta-1	Beta-2
Effects	Vasoconstriction Increased blood pressure	Increased heart rate Increased myocardial contractility	Bronchial dilation Vasodilation
Organs influenced	Heart (yes) Lungs (no) Vessels (yes)	Heart (yes) Lungs (no) Vessels (no)	Heart (no) Lungs (yes) Vessels (yes)

A *receptor* is a reactive site located on the surface of the cells. Receptors can combine with drug molecules to produce physiologic effects. Sympathetic receptors are divided into alpha, beta, and dopaminergic receptors. The effects of alpha and beta receptors and the organs they affect can be found in Table 1-6.

The Parasympathetic Nervous System

The parasympathetic nervous system (PNS) is an antagonist to the SNS and has the ability to regulate the restoration of body resources (rest, digest, and breed). The activation of the PNS results in a decrease in the heart rate, blood pressure, and cardiac output. The PNS, when stimulated, slows the firing rate of the sinoatrial (SA) node, slows conduction through the atrioventricular (AV) node, and decreases the strength of contractions. The following can stimulate the PNS:

- Straining to move the bowels
- Pressure of the carotid sinus
- The Valsalva maneuver
- A distended urinary bladder

Chapter 1 Self-Test

1. Multiple Choice: The heart is located:
   a. In the upper thorax
   b. In the lower thorax
   c. In the pleural cavity
   d. In the mediastinum or middle of the thorax

2. True or False: The top of the heart is the apex.

3. True or False: The heart is protected by the ribs anteriorly and the spine and rib cage posteriorly.

4. Multiple Choice: The right side of the heart:
   a. Pumps blood to all arteries to provide oxygen to tissues and organs
   b. Pumps unoxygenated blood to all veins
   c. Pumps blood to the left ventricle of the heart
   d. Pumps unoxygenated blood to the lungs where it picks up oxygen

5. Multiple Choice: The pericardium is the:
   a. Middle layer of the heart consisting of two layers, the parietal and visceral layers
   b. Innermost layer or lining of the heart consisting of two layers, the parietal and visceral layers
   c. Double-walled sac enclosing and protecting the heart
   d. Heart valve between the right atrium and the right ventricle

6. Multiple Choice: The heart wall is made up of three layers (from the most inner layer to the outer):
   a. Epicardium, pericardium, and myocardium
   b. Epicardium, myocardium, and endocardium
   c. Pericardium, endocardium, and myocardium
   d. Parietal, visceral, and endocardium

7. Trace the flow of blood through the heart beginning with the inferior and superior vena cava:

   Vena cava ____

   ____

   ____

   ____

   ____

   ____

   ____

8. True or False: The myocardium is a thick, fibrous layer of the heart, which has characteristics of both smooth and skeletal muscle.

9. Name the three functions of the pericardium:

 ____

 ____

 ____

10. Fill in the Blank: The thickest layer of the heart is the ____________ .

11. True of False: The coronary arteries are located in all three layers of the heart: the endocardium, the myocardium, and the epicardium.

12. Fill in the Blanks: The right coronary artery divides into which two main branches:

 ____________ and ____________ .

13. Fill in the Blanks: The left coronary artery divides into which two main branches:

 ____________ and ____________ .

14. Multiple Choice: Cardiac muscle fibers contract with greater force when stretched. This is known as:
 a. Diastole
 b. Starling's law
 c. Cardiac output
 d. Automaticity

15. True or False: The atria are thin-walled chambers under low pressure.

16. Fill in the Blanks: The ____________ and ____________ valves are located between the atria and the ventricles.

17. Fill in the Blanks: The four valves in the heart are called the

 ____

 ____

 ____

 ____

18. True or False: Beta-1 receptors decrease the heart rate, but increase contractility.

19. Multiple Choice: Diastole is the ____________ phase of the ventricle.
 a. Active
 b. Intermediate
 c. Contracting
 d. Passive

20. True or False: The passive phase of the coronary cycle is when the ventricles fill.

21. Fill in the Blank: When stimulated, the ________________ nervous system causes a decrease in blood pressure.

22. Fill in the Blank: Another name for the mitral valve is the ________________ valve.

23. Fill in the Blank: The neurotransmitter of the SNS releases ________________ .

24. Complete the formula:

    Cardiac output = ________________ × ________________ .

25. True or False: Preload is the force exerted on the walls of the ventricles at the end of diastole.

26. Fill in the Blanks: The heart is innervated by the ________________ and the

    ________________ nervous systems.

27. Multiple Choice: In which of the following chambers is the SA node located:
    a. Left atrium
    b. Right atrium
    c. Left ventricle
    d. Right ventricle

28. Multiple Choice: Which of the following is another name for the pulmonic and aortic valves:
    a. Semilunar valves
    b. Semipneumatic valves
    c. AV valves
    d. Atria-pulmonic valves

2

Electrophysiology

OBJECTIVES

By the end of this chapter, the student will be able to do the following:

- **Understand the primary characteristics of cardiac cells**
- **Describe normal cardiac conduction**
- **Know the sequence of the electrical conduction system**
- **Recognize the sites within the heart that may function as a pacemaker**
- **Recognize the intrinsic rates of the SA node, AV node/junction, Purkinje fibers**
- **Understand depolarization and repolarization**
- **Describe absolute and relative refractory periods**
- **Understand Einthoven's triangle**
- **Perform correct lead placement**
- **Understand ECG paper and its numerical values**
- **Determine and calculate heart rate**
- **Describe the function and location of the following: P wave, P-R interval, QRS complex, ST segment, T wave, and U wave**
- **Measure the durations of the P-R interval, QRS complex, and QT interval**
- **Identify and perform the seven steps in ECG analysis**

OUTLINE

OUTLINE—cont'd

Now that you have learned the anatomy and physiology of the heart, the next step is to learn how to read and interpret ECG strips. This is one of the most important skills you can be proficient in. If your patient, whether in-hospital or prehospital, manifests a fatal or dangerous rhythm that could place him or her in a life-threatening situation, you need to be able to identify and understand the rhythm. It is here, with the interpretation of arrhythmias, that you have the potential to save a life. Therefore this is one of the most important and challenging skills you can master.

This chapter covers how the heart's electrical activity is recorded on the ECG paper, what the various components mean, and how the waveforms are interpreted. Rhythm disturbances and conduction abnormalities are addressed, as well as how to measure the cardiac rates and intervals. You are shown how to analyze various ECG rhythms and put your findings together to reach a conclusion about the heart's electrical activity.

THE CARDIAC CONDUCTION SYSTEM

Through the special properties of the cardiac cells—automaticity, excitability, contractility, and conductivity—mechanical and electrical responses are produced. These responses result in the heart pumping blood to the lungs and the circulatory system. Electrical activity is centered around the depolarization and repolarization of the cardiac cells. The mechanical activity is the actual lengthening and shortening of the cardiac cells, which allows the atrial chambers and ventricular chambers to contract, to eject their blood supply, and to relax and refill.

The myocardium has two kinds of specialized cells: electrical and mechanical. An electrical impulse is initiated at the primary pacemaker site, the SA node. The electrical impulse is generated and then conducted throughout the heart with specialized conductive cells. While this electrical contraction travels through the heart, it activates the mechanical part of the cells. The mechanical part of the cells has muscle fibers, which contract and expand. It is this contracting action that empties the ventricles and pumps blood through the heart and the rest of the body. When the muscle fibers expand, the ventricles of the heart refill with blood.

The electrical activity of the heart is evaluated and assessed in the form of the ECG. The ECG gives a graphic display of electrical cardiac activity. The ECG can tell you if the heart is functioning normally. A heart in distress displays abnormal patterns known as *arrhythmias* or *dysrhythmias*.

The mechanical activity is evaluated and assessed with the patient's pulse, blood pressure, skin color, skin temperature, pulse oximetry, and level of consciousness. If the mechanical cells are not contracting properly, it is evident by the use of these assessment tools.

UNIQUE CHARACTERISTICS OF THE CARDIAC CONDUCTION SYSTEM CELLS

Automaticity is the ability of specialized cells in the conduction system to initiate an electrical impulse spontaneously. These cells are located in the SA node, the AV node, the Purkinje fibers, the bundle of His, and the bundle branches.

Conductivity is the ability to transmit an impulse from one cardiac cell to another.

Excitability is the ability of cardiac cells to respond to an electrical impulse.

Contractility is the ability of the cardiac cells to contract after receiving an electrical stimulus, such as an electrical impulse.

Cardiac cells have both mechanical and electrical properties. Both conductivity and contractility are mechanical properties, whereas excitability and automaticity share electrical properties (Table 2-1).

THE CARDIAC CONDUCTION PATHWAY

The myocardium, the major muscle of the heart, has the ability to generate and conduct electrical impulses. These electrical impulses cause the depolarization-repolarization cycle and in turn cause the atria and ventricles to contract and expand, pumping blood to the coronary arteries and the peripheral circulatory system. The main pacemaker site where the electrical impulses are generated is usually the SA node, which is located in the right atrium. The SA node produces an electrical impulse that travels through the heart's conduction system, as follows:

- SA node (normally the pacemaker)
- Interatrial pathways
- AV node
- AV junction
- Bundle of His
- Right and left bundle branches and fascicles
- Purkinje fibers of ventricles

Normally the electrical impulse begins at the SA node in the superior aspect of the right atrium and travels down the atrium to the AV node. Just below the AV node it goes to the AV junction, which is the junction between the atria and the ventricles. After the impulse reaches the AV junction, it actually slows a little to allow time for the atria to contract. Once the atria have contracted, the impulse then travels through the bundle of His, then follows the right and left bundle branches, and continues into the smallest branches, the Purkinje fibers (Figure 2-1).

TABLE 2-1 Cell Characteristics

Name	Property	Characteristic
Conductivity	Mechanical	Conducts electrical impulses from one cell to another
Contractility	Mechanical	Cardiac cells have the ability to contract or shorten
Automaticity	Electrical	Ability of cells within the cardiac conduction system to initiate electrical impulses
Excitability	Electrical	Cardiac cells have the ability to respond to an external stimulus to the heart

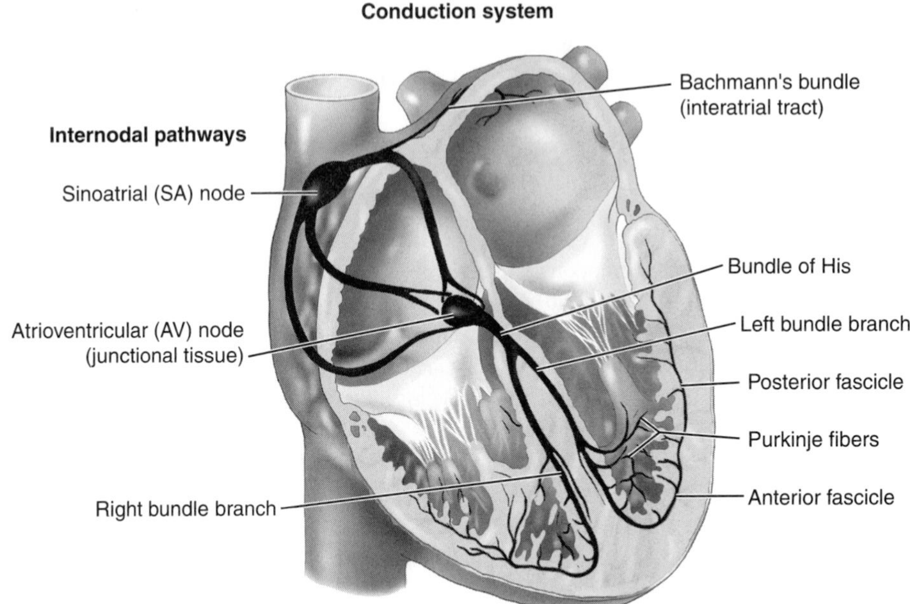

Figure 2-1 Pathway of electrical conduction system.

Pacemaker Sites

The heart contains three main pacemaker sites. The main pacemaker site of the heart is the SA node, located in the upper right atrium. This site fires or discharges at a rate of 60 to 100 times per minute (Table 2-2). If the SA node fails, the AV node or junction takes over but at a slower rate. The AV node is located just above the junction between the atria and the ventricles and fires at a rate of 40 to 60 times per minute. If both the SA node and the AV node fail, the bundle if His, the bundle branches, or the Purkinje system takes over firing at a rate of 20 to 40 times a minute. The ability that allows a cardiac cell to spontaneously initiate an electrical impulse is called *automaticity*. It provides the cell with the ability to receive and carry out the given function on an automatic basis. The ability that enables a polarized, resting cell to depolarize in response to the electrical stimulus is called *excitability* (e.g., if the SA node is diseased and does not initiate an electrical impulse, then the other pacemaker sites in the heart automatically take over, initiating the impulse and responding to them).

TABLE 2-2 Discharge Rates for Pacemaker Sites

Pacemaker Site	Discharge Rate (times per minute)
SA node	60-100
AV node/AV junction	40-60
His/Purkinje system	20-40

AV, Atrioventricular, *SA,* sinoatrial.

All of the components of the conduction system have the property of conductivity and automaticity, which initiate and conduct electrical impulses. This automatic firing of the pacemaker sites is known as *automaticity*. Other cells in the heart act as pacemakers if the main pacemaker, the SA node, is dysfunctional. You will note that the pacemaker sites previously listed have different intrinsic rates. As you travel down through the heart, the pacemaker-firing rate slows: the SA node is 60 to 100, the AV node/AV junction is 40 to 60, and the ventricles or Purkinje fibers are 20 to 40 times per minute.

The Depolarization-Repolarization Cycle

Depolarization describes the electrical and electrolyte change that occurs as an impulse is spread throughout the myocardial tissue. Depolarization is the movement of positive and negative ions across the cell membrane, which makes the inside of the cell more positive than the outside. With the entry of sodium (Na^+) ions the inside of the cell becomes more positive and increases the ability to respond to a stimulus. This exchange of the electrolytes, sodium, potassium, and calcium in myocardial cells produces electrical activity. This electrical activity or stimulus creates waveforms on the ECG, which we see as P waves, QRS complexes, and T waves.

The *resting membrane potential* is the time when the cardiac cells are in the resting state. The cells are said to be polarized, and no electrical activity is occurring at this time. The electrical potential of a cell membrane at rest is at –90 millivolts (mV).

It is important to understand that the heart has both electrical and mechanical events. Depolarization is not to be confused with contraction. The heart has two kinds of cardiac cells: the specialized cells and the working cells. The "working cells" contain thin myofibrils, which consist of protein filaments. These protein filaments are known as *myosin* and *actin* and have the ability of contracting when stimulated. These are fast-acting cells and allow a rapid influx of Na^+ ions. They shorten, or contract, when stimulated and return to their regular length after the stimulus. It is important to understand that you may have depolarization (electrical stimulus) and not have a contraction (mechanical) as seen in pulseless electrical activity (PEA). The specialized cells usually found in the SA node and the AV node have a slow response. They do not contain myofibrils and cannot contract. They have slower Na^+ ion and calcium (Ca^+) ion channels (Figure 2-2).

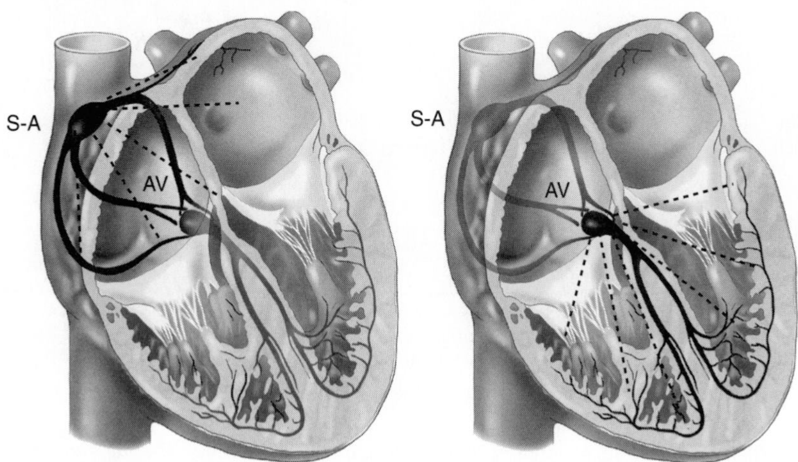

Figure 2-2 Atria and ventricles contracting. *AV*, Atrioventricular; *S-A*, sinoatrial.

The process normally begins with an initiated stimulus from the SA node, which causes an electrical impulse to spread across the atria to the ventricles. This electrical charge results in the depolarization, which travels through the layers from the endocardium, the innermost layer of the heart, to the myocardium, and then to the epicardium. The electrical impulse travels to the AV node in approximately 0.03 seconds. There is an interatrial tract, known as *Bachmann's bundle*, a branch of specialized fibers, that extends from the SA node across the atria and aids specifically in sending impulses across to the left atrium. On the ECG, the P wave represents atrial depolarization *(atrial systole)*. The atrial chambers are contracting or emptying. The QRS complex represents ventricular depolarization *(ventricular systole)*. The ventricles are contracting or emptying. Atrial diastole, or repolarization, is the period of relaxation during which the atrial chambers again begin to refill. Ventricular systole occurs as atrial diastole begins. This wave usually hides the electrical representation of atrial repolarization.

The P-R interval is the length of time it takes the impulse to travel from the SA node to the AV junction and is normally 0.12 to 0.20 seconds. Next, the impulse travels from the AV node to the AV junction, to the bundle of His, to the bundle branches and their fascicles, to the Purkinje fibers, and to the ventricles (Figure 2-3). The ventricles contracting are represented by the QRS complex on the ECG. The normal QRS complex is 0.10 second or less (Box 2-1).

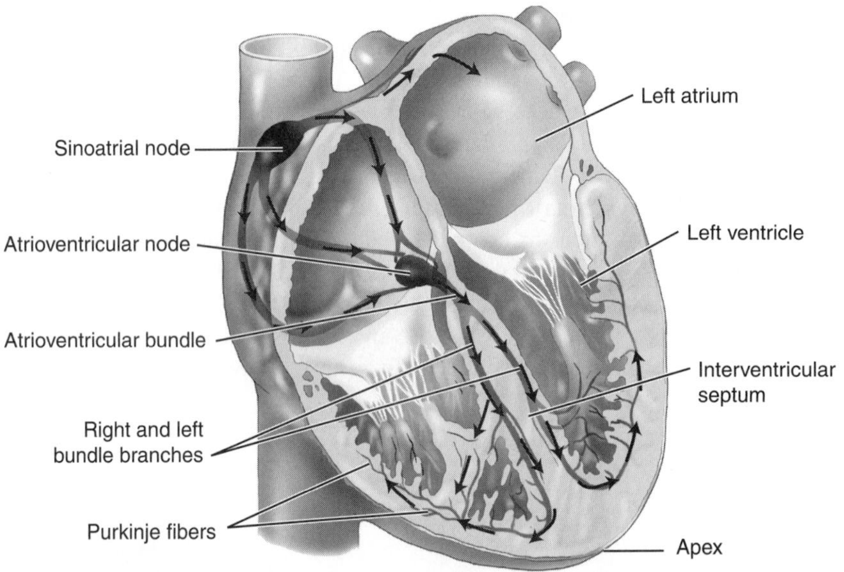

Figure 2-3 Electrical conduction system.

Box 2-1 Waveform Summary

- *P wave* represents atrial depolarization *(atrial systole)*.
- *P-R interval* represents the interval of time between atrial depolarization and ventricular depolarization.
- *QRS complex* represents ventricular depolarization *(ventricular systole)*. Ventricular systole occurs as atrial repolarization *(atrial diastole)* begins.
- *Q-T interval* represents the length of time for ventricular depolarization and ventricular repolarization.
- *T wave* represents ventricular repolarization *(ventricular diastole)*.

During *depolarization* the cardiac cell receives the stimulus sent from a pacemaker site, such as the SA node. The cell, which is at the moment resting and polarized, begins to change. It then becomes permeable to the charged Na^+ ions on the outside of the cell, allowing them to begin to flow inside. As the sodium rapidly enters, the potential resting membrane, which is –90 mV, drops until it is at 0 mV. At 0 mV the concentration on the inside of the cell equals that on the outside. During this time potassium slowly leaves the cell. During this influx of Na^+ ions, calcium also enters the cells but at a slower rate. This complete process of reversing the polarized cells resting state is known as *depolarization*.

During *repolarization* the sodium is pumped out of the polarized cell, potassium moves back in, and the calcium channels close. The cell is in a negative state or resting phase. At this time the chambers relax and refill with blood. During this time of repolarization the heart does not usually respond to a stimulus (Figure 2-4).

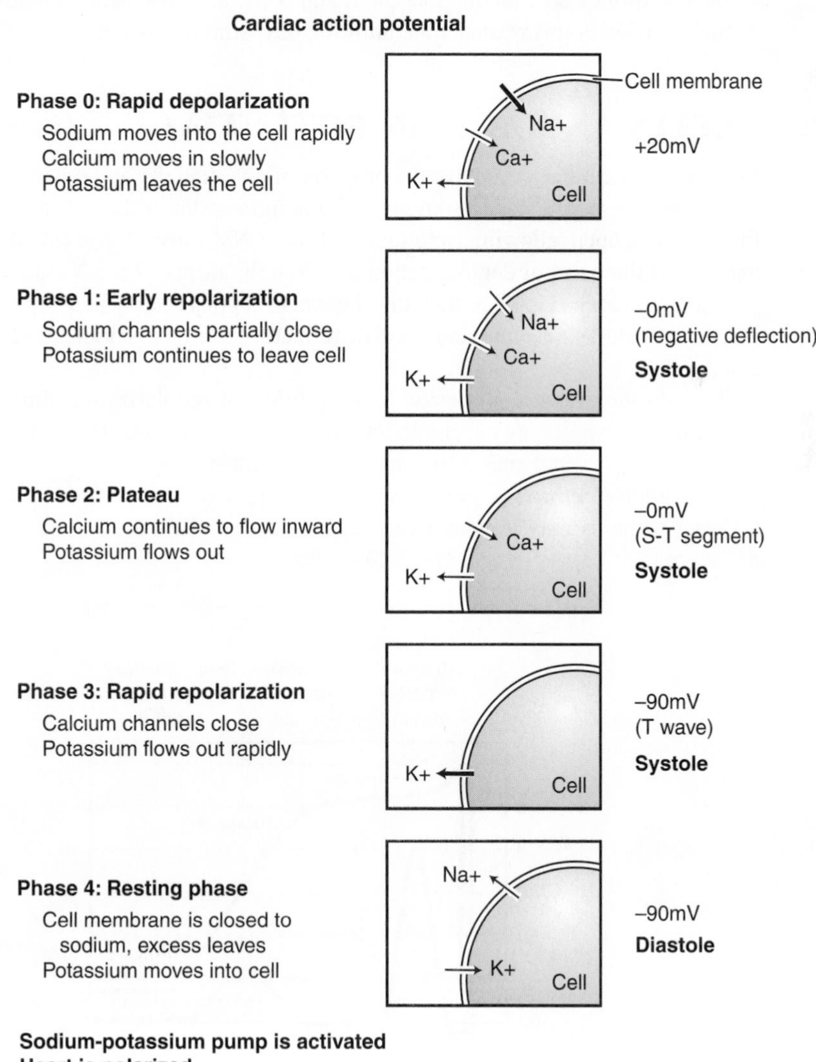
Cardiac action potential
Phase 0: Rapid depolarization
Sodium moves into the cell rapidly
Calcium moves in slowly
Potassium leaves the cell
Cell membrane
Na+
Ca+
K+
Cell
+20mV
Phase 1: Early repolarization
Sodium channels partially close
Potassium continues to leave cell
Na+
Ca+
K+
Cell
–0mV
(negative deflection)
Systole
Phase 2: Plateau
Calcium continues to flow inward
Potassium flows out
Ca+
K+
Cell
–0mV
(S-T segment)
Systole
Phase 3: Rapid repolarization
Calcium channels close
Potassium flows out rapidly
K+
Cell
–90mV
(T wave)
Systole
Phase 4: Resting phase
Cell membrane is closed to
sodium, excess leaves
Potassium moves into cell
Na+
K+
Cell
–90mV
Diastole
Sodium-potassium pump is activated
Heart is polarized

Figure 2-4 Sodium-potassium exchange.

Depolarization occurs in the first phase, phase 0, and the action potential is initiated. Originally the cell was negatively charged at –90 mV. During phase 0, sodium enters the cell making it more positive, +20 to +30 mV. After phase 0, the cell membrane is closed to Na^+ ions.

1. Phase 1 is early repolarization; the cell is impermeable to sodium.
2. Phase 2 is the plateau phase or slow repolarization. The cell is positively charged by the influx of Ca^+ ions. During this stage the cardiac cell is in the *absolute refractory period* and cannot be stimulated.
3. Phase 3 is the repolarization phase: potassium flows outward, returning the cell to its negative state. This is known as the *relative refractory period*, and the cell can be stimulated.
4. In phase 4, the resting membrane potential has returned to its resting phase; at this time you still have an excess of Na^+ ions on the inside of the cell and an excess of potassium (K^+) ions on the outside of the cell. It is at this time the "sodium-potassium pump" is activated. This activation results in a rapid exchange of Na^+ and K^+ ions, the sodium quickly moves to the outside of the cell, and the potassium enters the cell. The heart is polarized during this phase and remains in this resting state until the next stimulus is sent.

CARDIAC CELLS AND ACTION POTENTIAL

Why do some cardiac cells have the property of automaticity and others do not? All cells usually do not become permeable to sodium until the intracardiac voltage is at –60 mV. At this time the fast channels open, allowing for a rapid influx of Na^+ ions. This is called the *threshold potential* and begins the onset of depolarization and then the influx of the Na^+ ions (Figure 2-5).

The *refractory period* is the time between depolarization and repolarization. This can be further defined as absolute and relative refractory periods. The heart rests briefly without any activity.

The *absolute refractory period* is the portion of repolarization time when no stimulus, no matter how strong it may be, can initiate a cardiac contraction. This period begins at the onset of the QRS complex and ends at the apex of the T wave.

The *relative refractory period* is the latter part of this period during repolarization when a strong stimulus may initiate a cardiac contraction. This usually occurs on the downslope of a T wave.

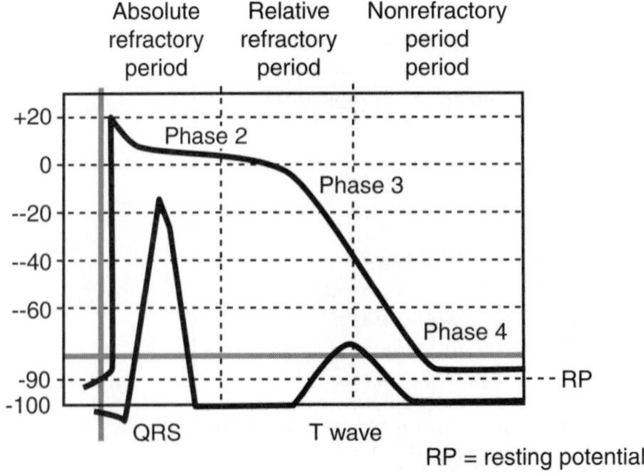

Figure 2-5 Action potential.

COMMON CAUSES OF DYSRHYTHMIAS

Dysrhythmias, also known as arrhythmias, may occur for several reasons. These include escape beats, enhanced automaticity, circus reentry, damage to the conduction system, electrical disturbances, ischemia, and myocardial infarction (MI).

Escape beats occur when the heart's pacemaker, the SA node, fails to initiate depolarization. These escape beats are compensatory mechanisms that originate lower in the cardiac conduction system at the AV node or ventricles to maintain cardiac output.

Enhanced automaticity occurs when cardiac cells without the property of automaticity begin to fire an impulse. These impulses are referred to as *ectopic beats* because they originate outside the normal conduction pathway. Enhanced automaticity may be caused by hypoxia, metabolic alkalosis, hypokalemia or hypocalcemia, and drugs such as atropine and digitalis. Enhanced automaticity occurs when cells lose stability in phase 4 of the action potential curve. Associated arrhythmias include the following:

- Atrial tachycardia
- Wandering atrial pacemaker
- Atrial fibrillation
- Atrial flutter
- Junctional tachycardia
- Premature atrial, junctional, or ventricular beats
- Supraventricular tachycardia
- Accelerated junctional rhythm
- Accelerated idioventricular rhythm
- Ventricular tachycardia
- Ventricular flutter
- Ventricular fibrillation

Circus reentry occurs when an impulse travels slowly or sluggishly through the AV node (Figure 2-6). This may be caused when cardiac tissue is activated two or more times by the same impulse. The impulse is initiated at the SA node and travels in multiple directions across the atria and downward to the AV node/AV junction. If one impulse is blocked or delayed in one area while the others keep on traveling down the heart's conduction pathway, the impulse may then enter cardiac cells that have already been depolarized. The impulse may also occur when refractory periods of neighboring cells occur at different times. The *impulse returns to stimulate previously depolarized tissue that has not had a chance to repolarize*. This can be serious because it can initiate ectopic beats and tachycardia or even precipitate fibrillation.

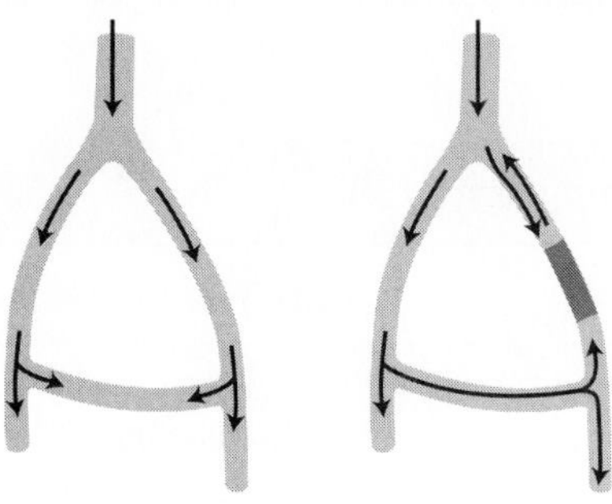

Figure 2-6 Circus reentry.

Conduction disturbances arise when the system is impaired; these disturbances may be temporary or permanent. Such impairments to the heart may be caused by trauma, cardiac surgery, ischemia of the myocardium, an MI, electrolyte disturbances, toxicity, or congenital heart disease.

THE ECG ITSELF

The heart's electrical activity is transcribed onto graph paper by means of the ECG machine. The electrocardiogram represents this electrical activity of the heart with positive and negative waveforms on the ECG paper. Each lead has both a positive and a negative pole. When the electrical current travels along toward a positive pole, the waveform is an upward deflection on the ECG paper, and when the current travels toward a negative pole, the deflection is downward. Leads I, II, and III provide you with a view of the heart's electrical activity between two points (or poles). Between the two poles, + and –, lies an imaginary line of sight representing the lead's *axis*.

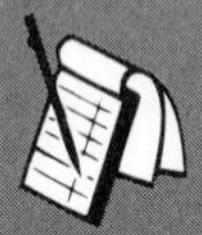

Note

When there are no electrical impulses present, a flat baseline or isoelectric line is produced on the ECG paper.

Lead Placement

Electrodes are placed as follows: right arm lead (white lead), left arm lead (black lead), and left leg lead (red lead). The left leg lead may also be placed on the upper left side of the abdomen. These three leads are bipolar and are also collectively known as *lead I*, *lead II*, and *lead III*. An axis reflects the direction of electrical activity of the heart showing the view from the positive end of the pole toward the negative pole. The axis of lead I extends from shoulder to shoulder with the right shoulder (arm) lead being negative and the left shoulder (arm) lead being positive. The axis of lead II runs from the negative right arm to the positive left leg. The axis of lead III goes from the negative left arm to the positive left leg (Table 2-3). These comprise the bipolar leads, which are also known as *Einthoven's triangle* (Figure 2-7). Einthoven's triangle is the axis of these three leads forming an equilateral triangle with the heart being the center. These are the leads we commonly use to monitor the patient's ECG rhythm.

TABLE 2-3 Lead Placement

Lead I	Lead II	Lead III
+ Positive left clavicle	+ Positive at lowest rib, midclavicular line	+ Positive at lowest left rib, midclavicular line
– Negative right clavicle	– Negative right clavicle	– Negative below left clavicle
G = ground at lowest palpable left rib at midclavicular line	G = ground below left clavicle	G = ground at right clavicle

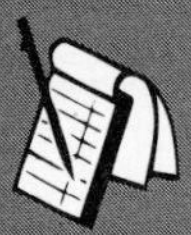

Note

If the leg lead is placed on the abdomen, the baseline rhythm on the monitor may be affected by the patient's respirations.

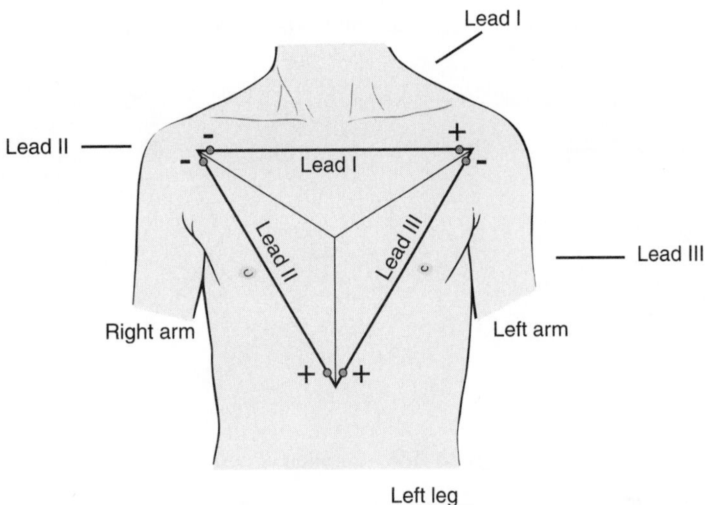

Figure 2-7 Lead placement.

When the current travels along the axis toward the positive pole, the ECG wave deflection is upward. When the current travels toward the negative pole, the ECG deflection is down or below the baseline. When the current travels perpendicular to the lead, the wave may go in both directions (biphasic) (Figure 2-8).

With a 12-lead ECG you receive 12 different views of the heart; its axis and information are from 12 different leads of the heart. It usually takes a 12-lead ECG to determine if there has been any ischemia or injury to the heart muscle or if the patient has had or is having an MI.

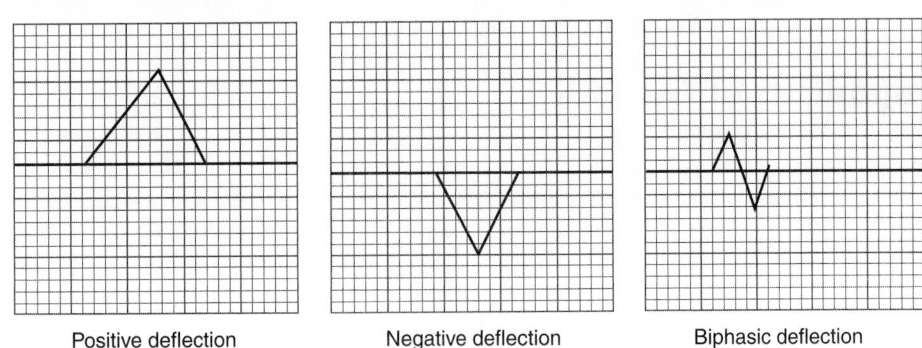

Figure 2-8 Positive and negative deflections.

Applying the Electrodes

Applying the electrodes with the correct technique helps to provide accurate monitoring and a better picture of what the heart is doing.

- First, prepare the patient's skin by removing any excessive hair around the electrode site.
- Then clean the skin with alcohol to remove any skin oil.
- Third, if the patient has diaphoresis, you may use special electrodes or apply tincture of benzoin to help the electrodes adhere and not loosen.

Once you open the packet of electrodes, make sure they are not dried out and have an ample amount of gel on them. Then apply the leads to the appropriate places, ensuring a good contact with the skin (Figure 2-9). The arm leads are best applied just below the clavicles.

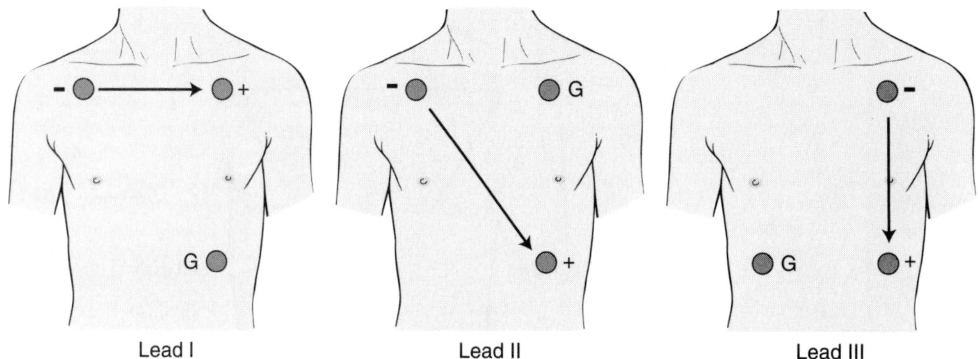

Figure 2-9 Location of positive, negative, and ground poles.

ECG interference or what we call *artifact* is a distorted ECG rhythm. Artifact can easily be mistaken for some of the serious arrhythmias. Artifact may be caused by the following:

- Muscle tremors, shivering
- Patient movement
- The placement of electrodes over bony prominences
- Skinfolds, breast tissue, and scar tissue
- Loose electrodes
- Broken ECG cable wires
- 60-cycle interference
- Seizures or Parkinson's disease

You may find the baseline moves or wanders if the electrodes are placed directly over the ribs because of respiratory movement of the chest. Poor skin contact of the electrodes may cause artifact and thus an improper reading of the ECG rhythm.

Components of the ECG

ECG Paper

The electrocardiograph records the heart's electrical activity, with a heated stylus on heat-sensitive paper (Figure 2-10). The standard grid paper is run at 25 mm/sec. On the ECG paper the horizontal lines represent *time*. The vertical lines represent *voltage* or *amplitude*.

Vertically, each small box is equal to 1 mm in size or 0.1 mV in voltage. Horizontally, each small box represents 0.04 second, and each large box (made up of five small boxes) represents 0.20 second. Then in turn, five large boxes equal 1 second; thus 30 large boxes equal 6 seconds. Most of the time you will calculate in 6-second strips to determine the rate of the rhythm.

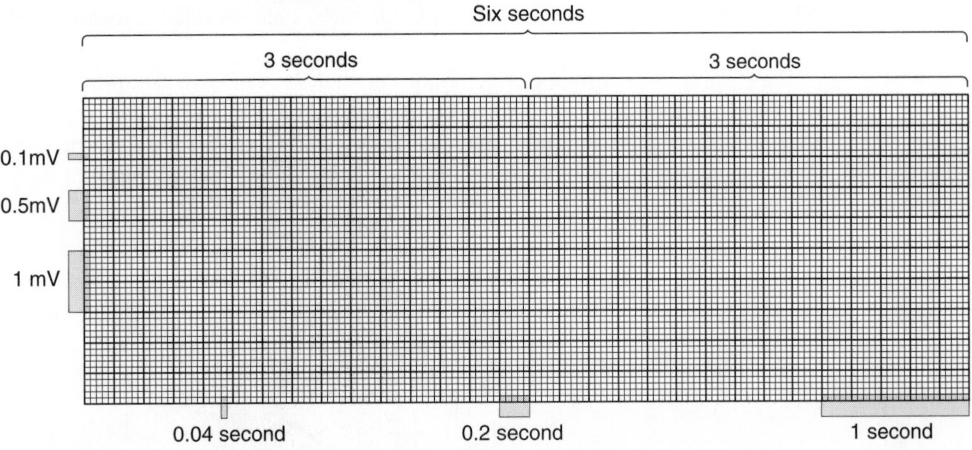

Figure 2-10 Components of the electrocardiogram (ECG).

ECG Waveforms

The heart's electrical activity produces several waveforms while the electrical wave travels down the electrical conduction system. The waveforms are the P wave, the QRS complex, and the T wave (Figure 2-11). The baseline is also known as the *isoelectric line* on the ECG strip. Positive waves are deflections that are above the isoelectric line, whereas negative waves are deflections that are below the isoelectric line. An equiphasic, also known as biphasic, wave occurs both above and below the isoelectric line, usually in equal portions.

The P wave represents atrial depolarization. Normally an electrical impulse is initiated at the SA node and travels across and down through the atria to the AV node.

P Waves. The following are characteristics of P waves:

- The P wave represents atrial depolarization.
- Atrial depolarization is the spread of an electrical impulse from the SA node through the atria.
- Normal P waves are rounded (upright) in leads I, II, aV_F, V_2, V_3, V_4, V_5, and V_6.
- P waves may be positive, negative, or biphasic in leads III, aV_L, and V_1.
- Normal P waves precede a QRS complex.
- Duration is 0.06 to 0.11 second.

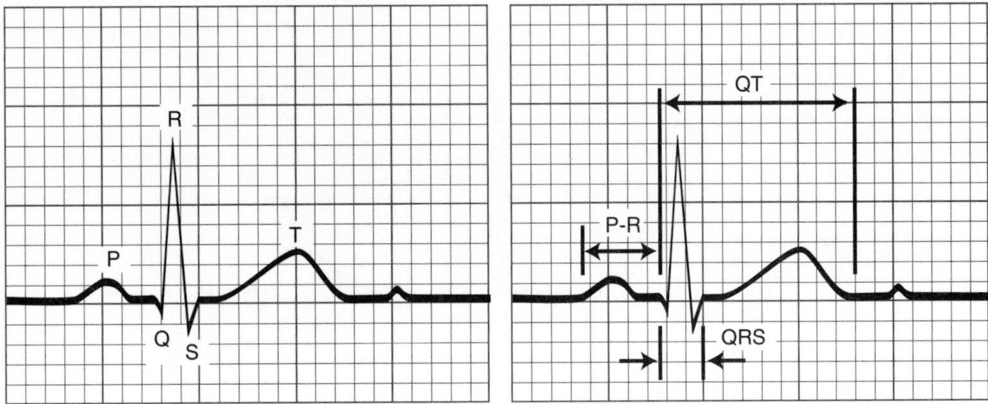

Figure 2-11 P-QRS-T waves.

When you evaluate the P waves, look for three characteristics: location, configuration, and deflection.

If a P wave with normal characteristics precedes every QRS complex, the electrical impulses are being conducted from the SA node in the right atrium (Figure 2-12). If all of the P waves do not look alike, then the impulse may be coming from elsewhere in the atria and not the SA node. If the pacemaker site is in the atria, then the P waves are upright, but if at the AV junction, they may be inverted in lead II.

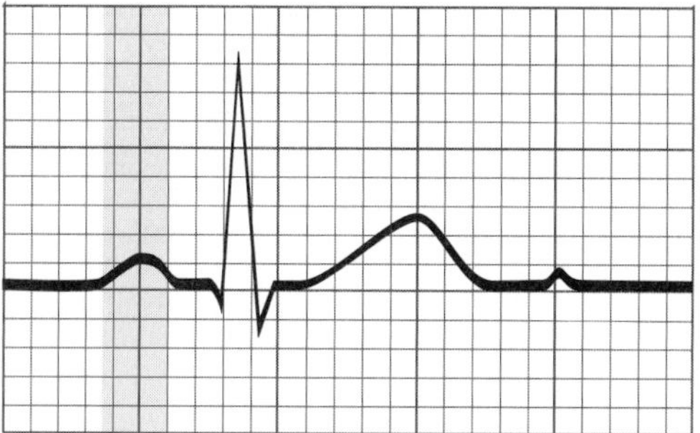

Figure 2-12 P wave.

The following are some medical problems that may cause abnormal P waves:

- *Right atrial hypertrophy, right atrial dilatation*—P waves are peaked, and tall (e.g., chronic obstructive pulmonary disease [COPD], congestive heart failure [CHF] and valvular disease)
- *Left atrial hypertrophy*—P waves are broad and notched.
- *Wandering atrial pacemaker*—P waves may be of various shapes and sizes.
- *Third-degree heart block*—P waves are present but have no relationship to the QRS complex. The atria and ventricles are pacing independently of each other.

P-R Intervals. The P-R interval represents the electrical activity in the conduction system from the beginning of atrial depolarization to the beginning of ventricular depolarization. Basically, it is the amount of time (in seconds) it takes for the impulse to travel from the SA node, through the atria, through the AV node and AV junction, to the bundle branches (Figure 2-13). Normal characteristics of the P-R interval include the following:

- The P-R interval is the time from the beginning of the P wave to the beginning of the QRS complex.

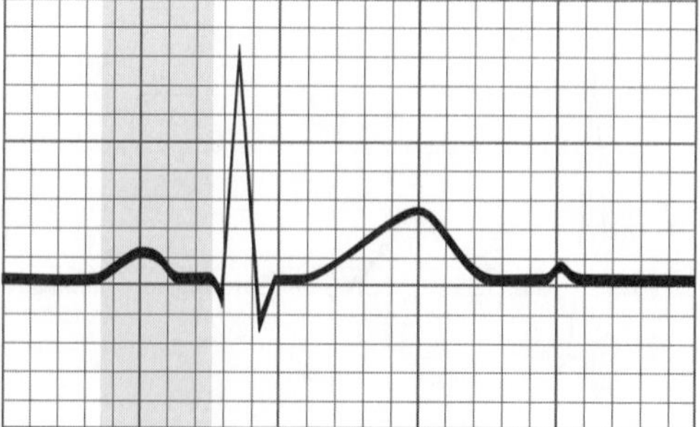

Figure 2-13 P-R interval.

- Normal duration of a P-R interval is 0.12 to 0.20 second.
- A normal P-R interval indicates that the electrical impulse is being conducted and travels through the atria, AV node, AV junction, bundle of His, bundle branches, and Purkinje fibers.

Variations of the P-R interval may have the following attributes:

- A short P-R interval may indicate that the impulse is coming from the atria or a pacer site close to the AV node or AV junction.
- A prolonged P-R interval usually indicates that the impulse has been delayed while it passes through the AV node and junction; this is usually indicative of a first-degree heart block, second-degree type I AV block, and digitalis toxicity.

QRS Complexes. The QRS complex follows the P wave on the ECG and represents ventricular depolarization and atrial repolarization. In a normal QRS complex, the Q wave is the first negative deflection after the P wave. The R wave is the first positive deflection after the Q wave, and the S wave is the first negative deflection after the R wave. A QRS complex begins where the first wave begins to deviate from the baseline and ends where the S wave begins to level out on the baseline (Figure 2-14). The following are characteristics of the QRS complex:

- Represents ventricular depolarization
- Follows P-R interval
- Normal duration is 0.06 to 0.10 second
- Normal duration is measured from the beginning of the Q wave (where it begins to deviate from the baseline) to the end of the S wave (where the S wave returns to the isoelectric line or baseline)
- Q wave = Negative deflection
- R wave = Positive deflection
- S wave = Negative deflection, after the R wave

Variations of the QRS complex include the following:

- A widened QRS complex (more than 0.10 second) may indicate slowed conduction through the ventricles or that the impulse originated in the ventricles.
- A missing QRS complex means that the ventricles did not depolarize; it can also be indicative of an AV block.

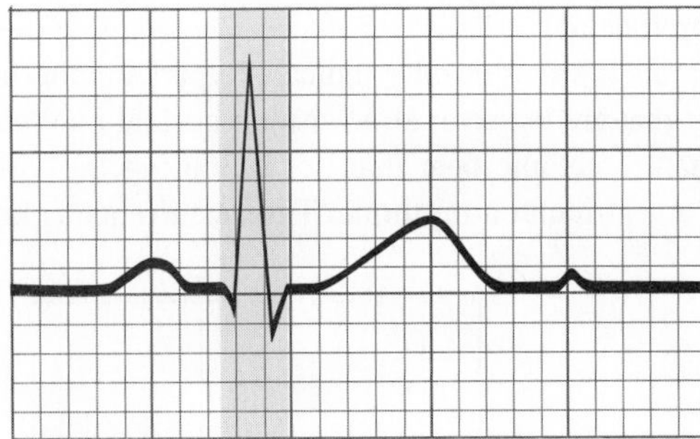

Figure 2-14 QRS complex.

ST Segments. The ST segment marks the beginning of ventricular repolarization; the ventricles have contracted and are now beginning to refill. This is also known as the *absolute refractory period*, which is a time when the heart cannot be stimulated. Also note that the point of the end of the QRS complex and the beginning of the ST segment is known as the *J point* (Figure 2-15). Characteristics of the ST segment are the following:

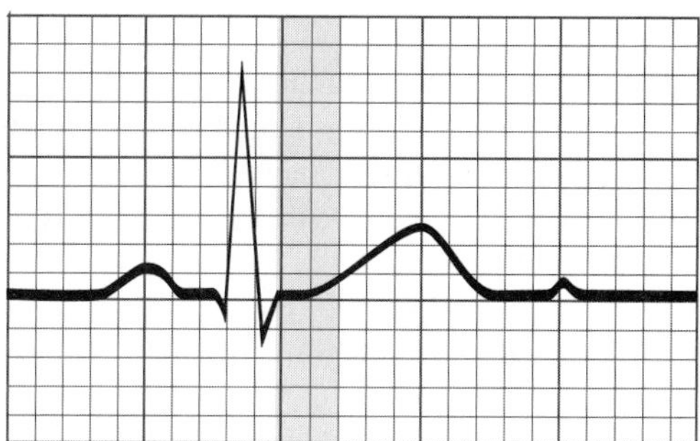

Figure 2-15 ST segment.

- The ST segment extends from the end of the QRS complex to the beginning of the T wave.
- A normal ST segment is flat on the isoelectric line or baseline. A 1-mm depression or elevation also falls under the category of a normal ST segment.
- An elevated or depressed ST segment may be indicative of an MI. Depression of more than 1 mm in the ST segment indicates possible myocardial ischemia. Also, an elevation greater than 1 mm in the precordial leads indicates possible myocardial damage or injury.

T Waves. The T wave represents ventricular repolarization and occurs during the last part of ventricular systole. The absolute refractory period is usually still present at the beginning of the T wave. When the cardiac cycle is in the relative refractory period, the ventricles are refilling and usually do not respond to any stimulus. However, if the stimulus is strong enough, it can initiate an impulse. An impulse initiated during the T wave can be dangerous and can cause a ventricular fibrillation arrhythmia.

The T wave normally begins with a gradual slope from the ST segment and is identified as the point where the slope becomes gradually steeper. The end of the T wave is the point where it returns to the baseline. The T wave always follows the QRS complex (Figure 2-16).

- The normal T wave is positive (upright) in lead II and slightly asymmetrical.
- Usually the T wave is not more than 5 mm (limb leads) or 10 mm (precordial leads) in height.
- Inverted or negative deflecting T waves are suggestive of myocardial ischemia or a ventricular conduction delay.
- Peaked, tall T waves usually indicate hyperkalemia (high potassium).
- T waves that are larger or smaller than normal may indicate an electrolyte imbalance.
- A premature ectopic beat that occurs during the vulnerable relative refractory period may initiate a ventricular arrhythmia. This occurrence is known as *R on T phenomenon*.

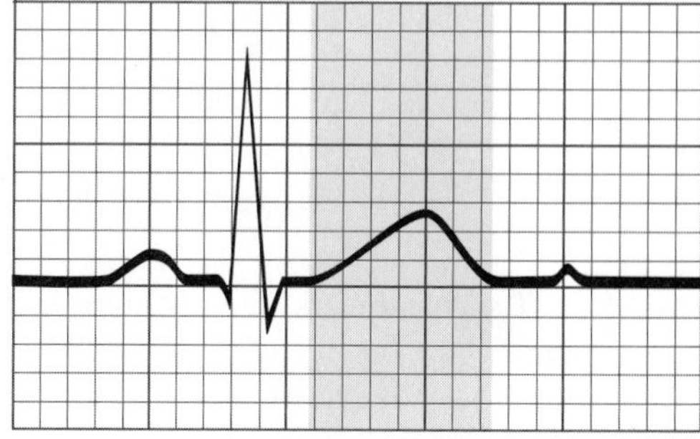

Figure 2-16 T wave.

Q-T Intervals. The Q-T interval represents both ventricular depolarization and repolarization (refractory period of the ventricles). It measures from the beginning of the Q wave to the end of the T wave on the isoelectric line. If the Q wave is not present, then the measurement begins with the R wave. The usual measurement of the Q-T interval is 0.36 to 0.44 second (Figure 2-17).

- A prolonged Q-T interval may indicate a prolonged ventricular repolarization, which means the relative refractory period is going to be longer. This may be caused by some of the cardiac drugs, including antiarrhythmics, or may indicate a decrease in calcium (hypocalcemia), an acute MI, myocarditis or pericarditis, and left ventricular hypertrophy.
- A shortened Q-T interval may indicate a high calcium level (hypercalcemia) and may be seen in patients taking digitalis medications.
- Normal duration for the Q-T interval is 0.36 to 0.44 second.

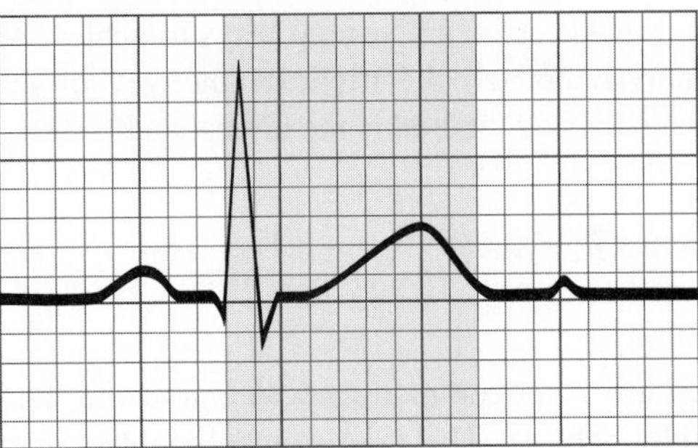

Figure 2-17 Q-T interval.

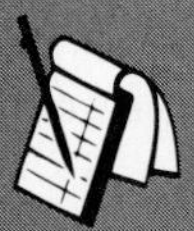

Note

The QT interval may vary with the patient's heart rate, age, and gender.

U Waves. U waves are not always present on a 12-lead ECG or on an ECG rhythm strip, unless the heart rate is slow. If present, the U wave is the first gradual or abrupt slope after the end of the T wave. A U wave, if present, follows the T wave and occurs before the P wave. However, a large U wave may be easily mistaken for a P wave, especially if the P wave is absent (e.g., junctional rhythm) (Figure 2-18).

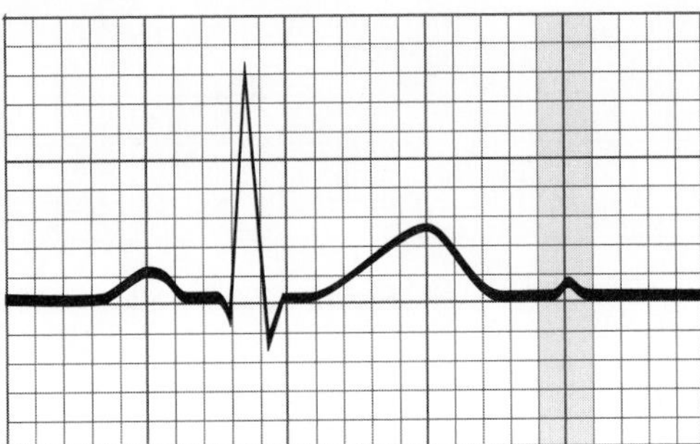

Figure 2-18 U waves.

- U waves are usually rounded and symmetrical when present.
- U waves are smaller than the preceding T wave.
- Prominent U waves may indicate hypokalemia.
- Prominent U waves may also indicate the effect of an excessive amount of digoxin on the conduction system.
- If the T wave and the U wave are inverted, suspect cardiac ischemia.

ANALYZING YOUR ECGs

Now you can recognize the basic waveforms, know what they represent, and understand how the heart uses its conduction system to contract and refill. The next step is to be able to read and analyze the ECG rhythms and to interpret them correctly. For this to be done, the heart rate must first be determined. There are several ways to achieve this: for example, the 6-second method, the R-R interval method, the triplicate method, or the use of a heart rate calculator ruler. Although the 6-second method is the easiest and fastest, it also is the least reliable.

Evaluate the Heart Rate

The 6-Second Method

The simplest and most common method is to count the number of R-R intervals in a 6-second strip and multiply by 10. This gives you the number of beats per minute, if the rhythm is regular (Figure 2-19). First identify a 6-second strip on the ECG paper. This is done by locating the 3-second markers (15 large boxes). Most ECG paper is divided into 1- and 3-second intervals. If there are, for example, $8\,^1/_2$ R-R intervals, then the rate is 85. If the rate is extremely slow, use a 12-second strip and multiply by 5 instead of 10.

If the rhythm is irregular, then count the number of complete QRS complexes in a 6-second strip and multiply by 10. This gives you an *approximate* number of beats per minute.

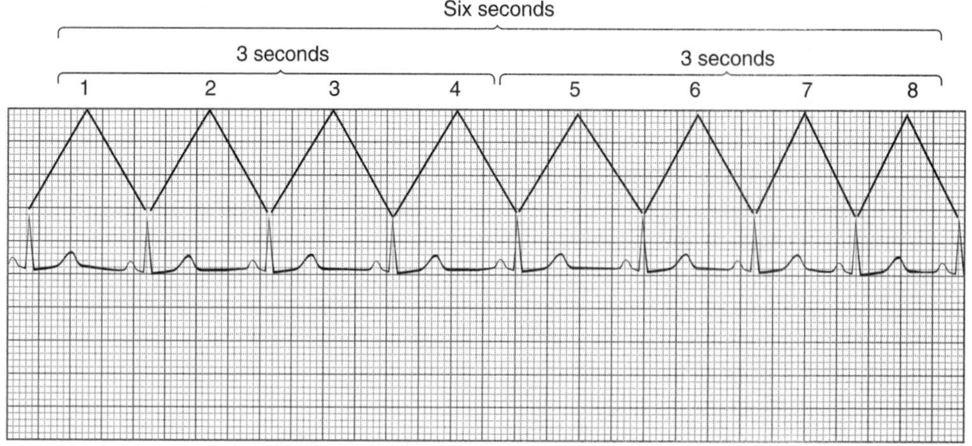

Figure 2-19 Six-second method.

The Sequence Method

The second method is the "300, 150, 100, 75, 60, 50" (Figure 2-20). Locate an R wave on a *heavy, black line* of a large box (0.20 second) on the ECG paper. Label the consecutive heavy, black lines as follows: 300, 150, 100, 75, 60, and 50. Identify where the next R wave falls in respect to the numbered heavy black lines. If the next R wave falls halfway between two heavy black lines (e.g., between the ones you have labeled 70 and 60), you would have a rate of 65. Below 60, you know you have a bradycardia and will treat according to the rhythm and how the patient looks. The first rule of thumb is to *treat the patient*, not the monitor.

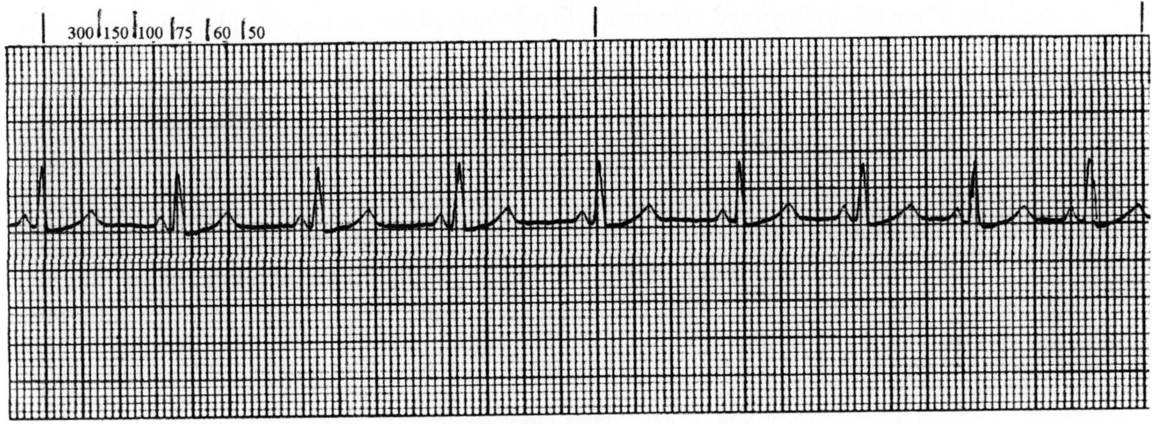

Figure 2-20 Sequence method.

The Large Box Method

This method is similar to the sequence method. Locate two consecutive R waves. Count the number of large boxes between the R waves and divide into 300. This method may also be used to calculate the P waves or atrial rate. Locate two consecutive P waves, count the number of large boxes between them, and divide into 300 (Figure 2-21).

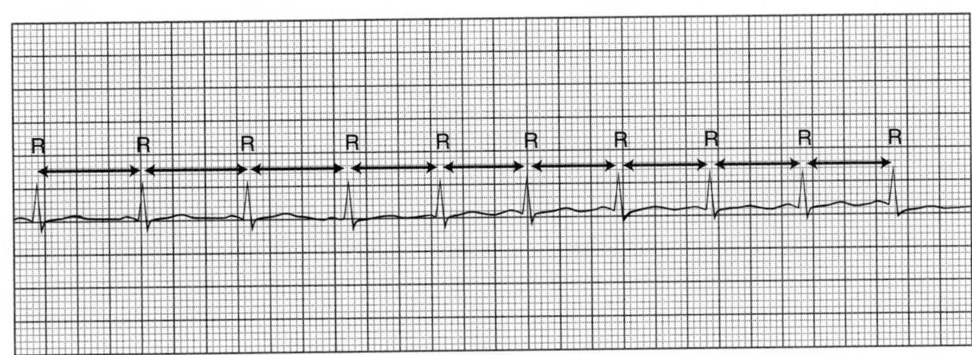

300 ÷ 3.1 (large box) = 96.7 or a heart rate of 97

Figure 2-21 Large box method.

The Small Box Method

The small box method helps you to estimate not only ventricular rates, but also atrial rates. There are 1500 small boxes (0.04 second each) in a 1-minute strip. For the *ventricular* rate, count the number of small boxes between two R waves and divide into 1500. To estimate an *atrial* rate, count the number of small boxes between two P waves and divide into 1500. For example, if there are

16 small boxes, divide 16 into 1500, which equals 93.75 or a rate of 94. However, let's say you have a strip with some of the R-R intervals with 16 small boxes and some with 15 small boxes. Divide 15.5 into 1500, which equals 96.7, and round off to receive a rate of 97 beats per minute.

The Heart Rate Calculator Ruler Method

A new way to calculate ECGs is with the *Heart Rate Calculator* developed by Robert J. Huszar, MD. Place the arrow of the ruler on the first ECG complex on the left side of your strip. The third complex from the arrow is the rate per minute. This method is most accurate when used on a regular rhythm. Premature beats, if possible, should not be included. The ruler also has the markings to measure in "seconds" and also in centimeters. This ruler is found inside the front cover of this book. Thank you, Dr. Huszar.

Determine the Rhythm

To determine the heart rhythm, use your calipers and place the ECG on a flat surface. Place one point of the calipers on the peak of an R wave, then adjust the caliper legs so the other point is on the peak of the next R wave. Now, move the calipers (without adjusting the distance between the caliper legs) and place the first point on the peak of the second R wave. Then note if the other caliper leg is on the third R wave. Continue to measure succeeding R-R intervals in the same manner. If all cardiac cycle intervals are the same, the rhythm is regular. If the intervals vary, the rhythm is irregular. Next you should note if there is just an occasional irregular beat, if there is a pattern of irregular beats, or if the beats are "irregularly irregular." When the beats are irregularly irregular, there is no pattern between the R-R intervals. Also, you need to consider if the P waves are consistent (e.g., in size, shape, and duration) and if the P-P intervals are regular. Then check to make sure that all P-R intervals are equal. If not, then determine the relationship to the QRS complexes. Are they regular, or is the rhythm regularly irregular versus irregularly irregular (no pattern at all)? Now let's put this all together.

Step 1

Determine the rate. Determine the number of beats per minute by one of the methods previously listed. This determines the electrical activity produced, whereas the patient's pulse indicates if the heart is actually contracting (mechanical activity).

Step 2

Determine the regularity of the rhythm. Compare the atrial and ventricular rates. Are they regular? If the rhythm is irregular, is there a pattern to the irregularity, or is it irregularly irregular?

Step 3

Evaluate the P waves. First, are there P waves present? Are they regular? Is there a P wave before every QRS complex in lead II? Are the P waves all the same in shape and size? Are the P waves upright or inverted? If upright and rounded in lead II, the P waves are usually originating from the SA node, and this indicates a sinus rhythm.

Step 4

Evaluate the P-R interval. Does it measure within the normal scope of 0.12 to 0.20 second? A normal P-R interval indicates the electrical impulse originated in the SA node or atrium. A P-R interval longer than 0.20 second indicates a delay in conduction through the AV node, AV junction, or bundle of His. Is the P-R interval constant, or does it vary in duration?

Step 5

Evaluate the QRS complex. Are the QRS complexes all alike in duration and shape? Do they measure less than 0.10 second in duration? If they measure 0.10 second or less, they are normal. If their measurement is greater than 0.10 second, they are considered abnormal (wide and bizarre).

Step 6

Is there a P wave before every QRS complex? Using one of the methods previously listed, count the number of P waves in a 6-second strip and determine the atrial rate per minute. The atrial rate may be greater than the ventricular rate, especially if there is ventricular ectopy or if heart blocks are present.

Is there a QRS complex after every P wave? Again, another necessary component. You may have a P wave before every QRS complex, but not a QRS complex after every P wave. For example, you may have two or three P waves for each QRS complex. You already counted the number of QRS complexes in step 1 to determine the ventricular rate per minute.

Step 7

Evaluate the T wave. Are they T waves of normal configuration, and are they upright? Are the T waves elevated or depressed from the isoelectric line? Inverted, elevated, or depressed T waves may indicate myocardial ischemia or injury.

Chapter 2 Self-Test

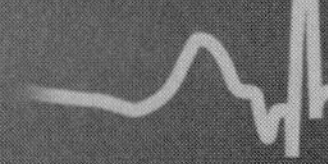

1. Multiple Choice: When the heart produces a mechanical response, it:
   a. Causes depolarization
   b. Produces repolarization
   c. Pumps blood to the lungs and circulatory system
   d. None of the above

2. Multiple Choice: When both depolarization and mechanical action take place, the heart:
   a. Contracts and the chambers empty
   b. Contracts and the chambers fill
   c. Relaxes and the chambers empty
   d. Relaxes and the chambers fill

3. Circle the Correct Answer: When repolarization occurs and the cell returns to its normal resting state, it becomes *positively/negatively* charged.

4. True or False: During the refractory periods, the heart rests, and the ventricles relax and fill and become ready for the next stimulus.

5. Circle the Correct Answer: It is *mechanical/electrical* impulses that cause the depolarization-repolarization cycle.

6. Trace the conduction pathway beginning with the SA node:

   SA node ____

   ____

   ____

   ____

   ____

   ____

   ____

7. True or False: The normal rate for the SA node is 40 to 60 times a minute.

8. True or False: The AV node/AV junction is a secondary pacemaker site and has an intrinsic rate of 20 to 40 beats per minute.

9. True or False: Automaticity is the ability of specialized cells to initiate an electrical impulse spontaneously.

10. True or False: Excitability is the ability of the cardiac cells to shorten, causing a cardiac contraction in response to an electrical stimulus.

11. Fill in the Blank: The ability that causes cardiac cells to contract or shorten is ____________ ____________________ .

12. Multiple Choice: The ability of the pacemaker cells to initiate electrical impulses is called:
    a. Automaticity
    b. Contractility
    c. Excitability
    d. Conductivity

13. Place either an *M* or an *E* next to each of the following characteristics in the space provided according to whether it has as a mechanical property or an electrical property.

    a. ____________________ Conductivity

    b. ____________________ Contractility

    c. ____________________ Automaticity

    d. ____________________ Excitability

14. Multiple Choice: Which of the following is true about the movement of positive and negative ions during depolarization?
    a. Sodium moves into the cell slowly, while potassium leaves the cell rapidly.
    b. Both sodium and potassium move out of the cell as calcium moves in.
    c. Sodium moves into the cell rapidly, while calcium moves in slowly and potassium begins to leave the cell.
    d. None of the above

15. True or False: When the inside of a cardiac cell is positively charged, the charge stimulates the cardiac muscle to contract.

16. True or False: During repolarization, the sodium moves outside the cell, potassium moves back in, and the calcium channels close.

17. Fill in the Blanks: The "resting membrane potential" is when the inside of the cell is ____________________ charged and the outside is ____________________ charged.

18. True or False: The resting membrane potential measures about –90 mV and is known as diastole.

19. True or False: The absolute refractory period is the stage when cardiac cells cannot respond to a stimulus.

20. True or False: During the relative refractory period, the cardiac cell may contract prematurely if the stimulus is strong enough.

21. Multiple Choice: Which of the following has a rate ranging between 60 and 100 beats per minute?
    a. SA node
    b. AV node
    c. AV junction
    d. Purkinje fibers

22. True or False: Circus reentry occurs when an impulse travels too rapidly through the myocardial tissue.

23. Fill in the Blank: Because the ECG leads I, II, and III form a particular shape, they are also known as:

    ____

24. Multiple Choice: The axis of lead II runs:
    a. From the right arm to the left arm
    b. From the left arm to the right arm
    c. From the right arm to the left leg
    d. From the left arm to the right leg

25. Fill in the Blank: When the ECG's electrical current flows along the axis toward the positive pole, the deflection is ______________ on the ECG paper.

26. True or False: With a 12-lead ECG you receive 12 different views of the heart.

27. List three common causes of ECG interference:

    ____

    ____

    ____

28. Fill in the Blanks: On the ECG paper the horizontal lines represent ______________ , whereas the vertical lines represent ______________ .

29. Multiple Choice: Each small box on the ECG paper measures:
    a. 0.20 second
    b. 0.04 second
    c. 2.0 seconds
    d. 0.1 mV

30. Fill in the Blank: Thirty large boxes on the ECG paper equals ______________ seconds.

31. Circle the Correct Answer: The P wave represents atrial *depolarization/repolarization*.

32. Multiple Choice: The electrical activity that extends from the beginning of atrial depolarization to the beginning of ventricular depolarization is a:
    a. QRS segment
    b. P wave
    c. P-R interval
    d. Q-T interval

33. Fill in the Blank: Normal P-R interval duration is ________________ seconds.

34. Multiple Choice: The QRS segment's normal duration is:
    a. 0.12 to 0.20 second
    b. 0.04 to 0.20 second
    c. 0.04 to 0.10 second
    d. 0.10 to 0.20 second

35. Fill in the Blank: Ventricular ________________ is represented on the ECG by the T wave.

36. List the seven steps for determining an ECG rhythm:

    ____

    ____

    ____

    ____

    ____

    ____

    ____

37. Match the following abilities with their cell characteristics

    ________________________________ Automaticity

    ________________________________ Conductivity

    ________________________________ Excitability

    ________________________________ Contractility

    a. Cardiac cells have the ability to respond to an outside stimulus
    b. Transmits electrical impulses from one cell to another
    c. Causes cardiac cells to contract or shorten
    d. Ability to initiate electrical impulses in the pacemaker cells

38. Multiple Choice: You have an ECG rhythm strip with five large boxes between each of the peaks of two consecutive R waves, and the rhythm appears regular. The heart rate is how many beats per minute?
   a. 50
   b. 100
   c. 80
   d. 60

39. Multiple Choice: When P waves are inverted in lead II on the ECG, it usually indicates the pacemaker site is:
   a. In the bundle of His
   b. At or below the AV node
   c. In the AV junction
   d. All of the above

3

Sinus Rhythms

OBJECTIVES

By the end of this chapter, the student will be able to do the following:

- **Describe the ECG characteristics of a normal sinus rhythm**
- **Describe the characteristics of the following sinus dysrhythmias:**
  - **Sinus bradycardia**
  - **Sinus tachycardia**
  - **Sinus arrhythmia**
  - **Sinus arrest**
  - **Sick sinus syndrome**
- **Know and understand the possible causes, signs and symptoms, and emergency treatment for each of the following dysrhythmias that originate in the SA node:**
  - **Sinus bradycardia**
  - **Sinus tachycardia**
  - **Sinus arrhythmia**
  - **Sinus arrest**
  - **Sick sinus syndrome**

OUTLINE

OUTLINE—cont'd

When the cardiac conduction system functions normally, the sinoatrial (SA) node is the primary pacemaker, located in the upper right atrium. It has the fastest automatic firing rate of all the normal pacemaker sites in the heart. What causes the SA node to have such increased automaticity? First, the cells in the SA node have the least negative charge during the resting phase of the depolarization-repolarization cycle. Second, depolarization actually begins during the resting phase. Thus the sinus node having the least negative charge takes the initiative and begins its automatic firing rate. Changes in either one of these characteristics may lead to disturbances in the functioning of the SA node, causing sinus dysrhythmias. This chapter teaches you to identify sinus rhythms and dysrhythmias and correlates these ECG interpretations with clinical signs and symptoms your patient may be experiencing. In addition it provides the emergency treatment and appropriate interventions. Remember, *always treat the patient, not just the ECG on the monitor.*

These rhythms should demonstrate normal, upright, rounded P waves, regular QRS complexes, and normal T waves. The difference between the rhythms is the rate of each (Box 3-1).

NORMAL SINUS RHYTHM

The normal pacemaker of the heart has an intrinsic firing rate of 60 to 100 beats per minute (Figure 3-1). Sinus rhythms are characterized by regular atrial and ventricular rates again at a rate of 60 to 100 beats per minute. P waves are upright, rounded, and normal in appearance. There is a P wave before every QRS complex. The P-R interval measures 0.12 to 0.20 second. The QRS complexes are normal in shape and size, measuring less than 0.10 second in duration (Box 3-2).

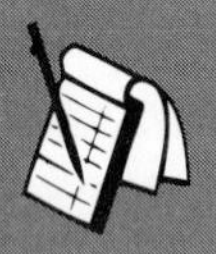

Note

For the sake of simplicity the rates and descriptions in this chapter pertain to lead II.

Box 3-1 Sinus Rhythms

Normal sinus rhythm: 60 to 100 beats per minute
Sinus tachycardia: 101 to 180 beats per minute
Sinus bradycardia: <60 beats per minute

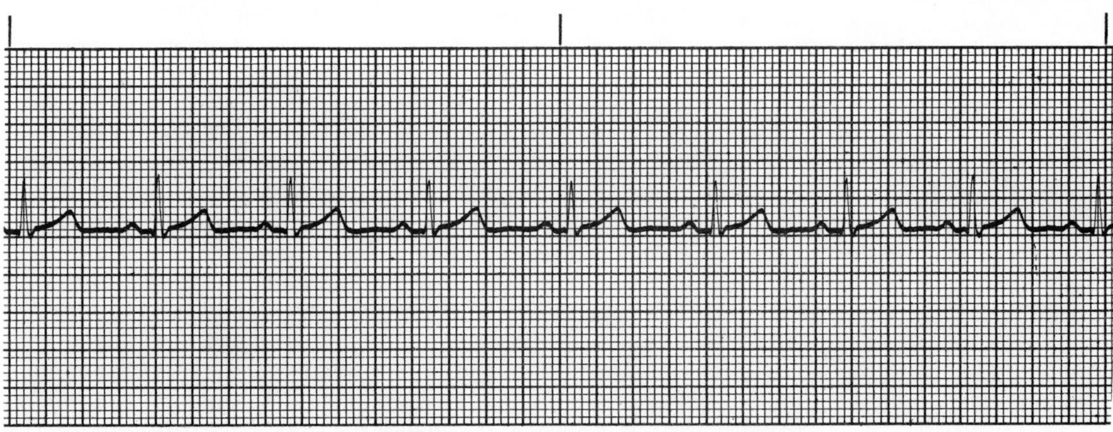

Figure 3-1 Normal sinus rhythm.

Box 3-2 Normal Sinus Rhythm

Rate: 60 to 100 beats per minute
Rhythm: Atrial rate is regular; ventricular rate is regular
P waves: Upright, rounded, normal shape and uniform in appearance
P-R interval: 0.12 to 0.20 second
QRS complex: Duration is <0.10 second

SINUS RHYTHMS

Sinus Bradycardia

When the SA node fires at a rate of less than 60 beats per minute, it is called *sinus bradycardia* (Figure 3-2). This rhythm is characterized by having a regular cardiac rhythm, which originates in the SA node and follows the normal pathway of electrical conduction through the atria and the ventricles. The P waves are normal in size and configuration. A P wave precedes each QRS complex and a QRS complex follows each P wave. The P-R interval is within normal limits, and the QRS complex is of normal duration and configuration (Box 3-3).

Sinus bradycardia may be seen in athletes because their hearts are well conditioned and are able to maintain stroke volume with a reduced amount of effort. It is also seen in healthy adults with no signs of cardiac compromise.

Causes

Causes of sinus bradycardia include the following:

- Disease of SA node
- An MI, which produces vagal tone, with or without hypotension
- Vagal stimulation or parasympathetic stimulation
- Increased intracranial pressure
- Hyperkalemia

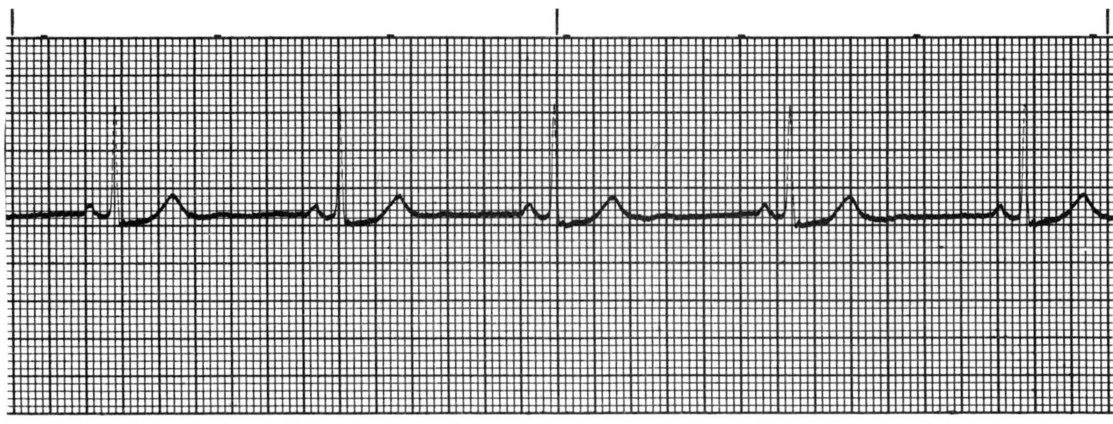

Figure 3-2 Sinus bradycardia.

Box 3-3 Sinus Bradycardia

Rate: <60 beats per minute
Rhythm: Atrial regular, ventricular regular
P waves: Are uniform in appearance: upright, rounded, and normal shape and size; there is a P wave before every QRS complex
P-R interval: Normal duration with a 0.12 to 0.20 second
QRS complex: Is normal configuration and duration; <0.10 second; there is a QRS complex after every P wave

- Digitalis, propranolol, quinidine, morphine, beta blockers, and calcium channel blockers
- Hypothermia

Sinus bradycardia also occurs normally during sleep.

Treatment

Treat the patient, not the monitor! If the patient is symptom free, then treatment is unnecessary. On the other hand, if the patient is showing signs and symptoms of cardiac compromise (e.g., chest pain, an MI, hypotension, pulmonary congestion, CHF, shortness of breath, weakness, dizziness, or syncope), then *treat* the patient. The first drug of choice is oxygen, then atropine IV push. After atropine the next choice of treatment is transcutaneous pacing. If the blood pressure remains low, consider a dopamine drip titrated to effect. Other drugs that may be used per guidelines of advanced cardiac life support (ACLS) are an epinephrine drip and possibly an isoproterenol drip.

Cardiac compromise with bradycardia may be caused by the following:

- Drugs such as beta blockers, anticholinesterase, digitalis, and morphine
- MI, which may increase the vagal tone
- Patients with hyperkalemia, patients with intracranial pressure
- Vagal stimulation (e.g., vomiting, having a bowel movement, or any acts that cause vagal stimulation)
- Patients with sick sinus syndrome
- Athletes, because their hearts are well conditioned, allowing them to maintain the stroke volume with reduced effort

Sinus Tachycardia

When the SA node discharges (fires) at a rate greater than 100 beats per minute, it is called *sinus tachycardia* (Figure 3-3). The range is 101 to 180 beats per minute; any rate greater than 180 is considered to be supraventricular tachycardia and does not originate from the SA node. Both atrial and ventricular rhythms are regular. The P waves are normal in size and configuration. A P wave precedes each QRS complex, and a QRS complex follows each P wave. The P-R interval is within normal limits of 0.12 to 0.20 second (Box 3-4). Sinus tachycardia usually occurs because of the normal demand of the body for increased oxygen. When the body calls for an increase in oxygen, the heart rate speeds up to create more cardiac output.

Causes

Some of the more common causes may include the following:

- Exercise
- Fever
- Hypoxia
- Hypovolemia (shock)
- Stimulation of sympathetic nervous system
- Fright
- Stress
- Anxiety
- MI
- Pump failure
- Anemia
- Caffeine, nicotine, or alcohol
- Drugs (atropine or epinephrine)
- Pain

Usually with sinus tachycardia, the patient is asymptomatic. However, as the rate reaches the upper limits of tachycardia, remember that the diastolic period is shortened, thus allowing for less ventricular filling time. The end result is that cardiac output may start to decline. This usually occurs with rates greater than 140 beats per minute. Treatment should be directed at the under-

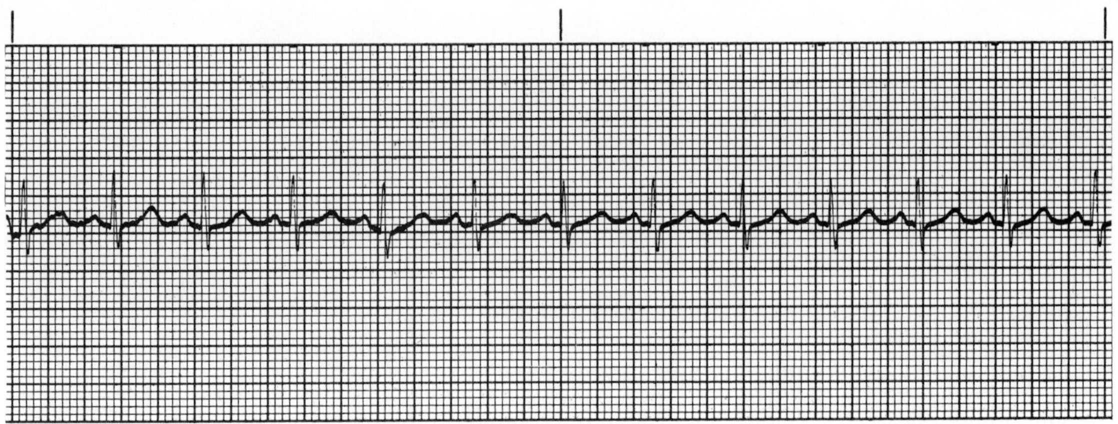

Figure 3-3 Sinus tachycardia.

Box 3-4 Sinus Tachycardia

Rate: 101 to 180 beats per minute
Rhythm: Both atrial and ventricular rates are regular
P waves: Upright, normal shape and configuration; uniform in appearance; P wave before every QRS complex
P-R interval: Normal duration, 0.12 to 0.20 second
QRS complex: Normal configuration; <0.10-second duration; QRS complex after every P wave

lying cause if the patient has symptoms. The patient may be hypotensive and experience altered mental status, dizziness, syncope, chest pain, difficulty breathing, or any other signs of cardiac compromise depending on the underlying problem.

Treatment

Again, treat the patient, not the monitor. If the patient is experiencing dizziness or light-headedness, you probably need only oxygen for treatment. Always ensure an open airway and evaluate breathing, circulatory status, and level of consciousness. First determine if the patient's symptoms are from the fast heart rate, or, if the patient is having chest pain or dyspnea, treat the situation as a potential AMI. When the rate is fast, the diastolic time is decreased, resulting in a decrease in the amount of blood to fill the arteries. If there are signs and symptoms of hypovolemia, treat with intravenous (IV) fluids. With sinus tachycardia, treatment is usually aimed at the underlying cause, not the rhythm. *A full evaluation of your patient is always necessary.*

Sinus Arrhythmia

A sinus arrhythmia is a normal variant that occurs with respirations and the changes of intrathoracic pressure (Figure 3-4). The respiratory cycle causes the R-R intervals to shorten with inspiration and to lengthen with expiration. This is a rhythm most commonly seen in young people and older adults. When associated with a bradycardiac rate, it is called a *bradydysrhythmia*, and when associated with a tachycardiac rate, its known as a *tachydysrhythmia* (Box 3-5). Because this is a normal finding, treatment is not needed.

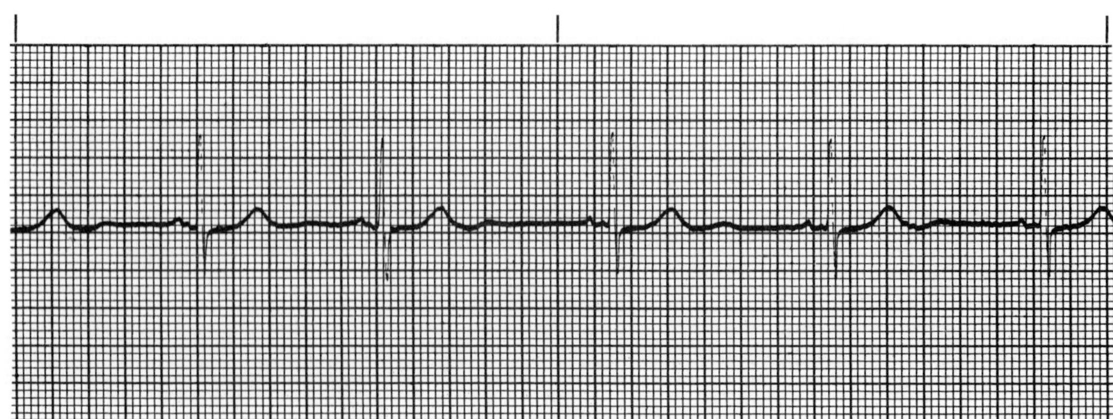

Figure 3-4 Sinus arrhythmia.

Box 3-5 Sinus Arrhythmia

Rate: Usually 60 to 100 beats per minute, both atrial and ventricular rates are normal but vary
Rhythm: Irregular; the atrial rate and ventricular rates are irregular, the P-P interval and the R-R intervals become shorter with inspiration and longer with expiration
P wave: Upright, and normal in size and configuration; there is a P wave before every QRS complex
P-R interval: Normal with a duration of 0.12 to 0.20 second
QRS complex: Normal in configuration; <0.10-second duration; there is a QRS complex after every P wave
Note: Using the 300, 150, 100 rate method may be difficult without a short run of regular beats

Sinus Arrest

Sinus arrest is failure of the SA node to initiate an impulse resulting in the absence of a P wave, QRS complex, and T wave. Sinus arrest is also known as a *sinus pause* or *cardiac standstill* (Figure 3-5). Usually, with the exception of missing complex, the ECG will be normal (Box 3-6).

Causes

The following are causes of sinus arrest:

- Drugs such as digitalis, quinidine, or salicylates
- Ischemia of the SA node
- Excessive vagal tone
- Carotid sinus massage

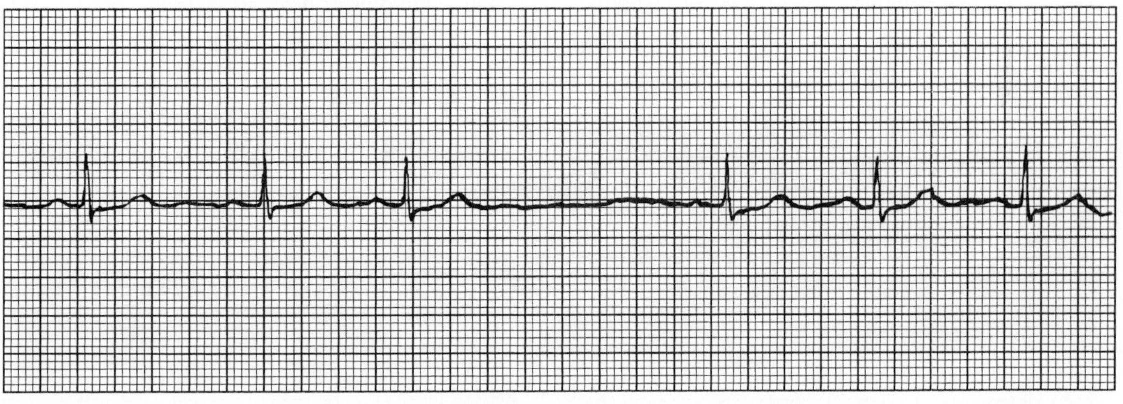

Figure 3-5 Sinus arrest.

Box 3-6 Sinus Arrest

Rate: Usually within normal limits, both atrial and ventricular
Rhythm: Both atrial and ventricular are regular except for the missing complex
P waves: Upright, uniform in appearance, normal shape and size; there is a P wave before every QRS complex
P-R interval: Normal with a duration 0.12 to 0.20 second when present
QRS complex: Is of normal configuration and duration when present, <0.10 second

- Rheumatic heart disease
- Myocarditis
- MI
- Coronary artery disease
- Degenerative fibrotic disease

Treatment

If the patient is symptom free, monitor and observe the patient. Drug therapy is not needed. Usually symptoms are precipitated by the bradycardia, which may cause weakness, dizziness, light-headedness, or syncope. Then apply oxygen, initiate IV access, and give a 0.5- to 1.0-mg atropine IV push. This can be given every 5 minutes until the arrhythmia resolves or you reach a maximum total dose of 0.03 to 0.04 mg/kg. If the sinus arrest still does not resolve, consider transcutaneous pacing or a temporary pacemaker.

Sick Sinus Syndrome

The sick sinus syndrome refers to several sinus dysrhythmias that are also known as *tachy-brady syndrome, brady-tachy syndrome*, and *Stokes-Adams syndrome*. The syndrome may be initiated by the autonomic nervous system or may be intrinsic. It is either a sinus node dysfunction or the failure of an escape pacemaker. The most common patterns seen are normal sinus rhythm alternating with a supraventricular tachycardia or a normal sinus rhythm alternating with a sinus bradycardia (Figure 3-6 and Box 3-7). This rhythm is seen most commonly in older adult patients and most usually is associated with atherosclerosis. It can be very serious with patients who already have underlying heart problems. With these patients you may see the following signs and symptoms: normal, slow, or fast pulse; signs and symptoms of decreased cardiac output such as syncope, hypotension, dizziness, and altered mental status; fatigue; and palpitations.

Causes

The following are causes of sick sinus syndrome:

- Cardiomyopathy
- Collagen disease
- Inferior or lateral wall MI
- Progressive muscular dystrophy
- Ischemic heart disease
- SA node trauma

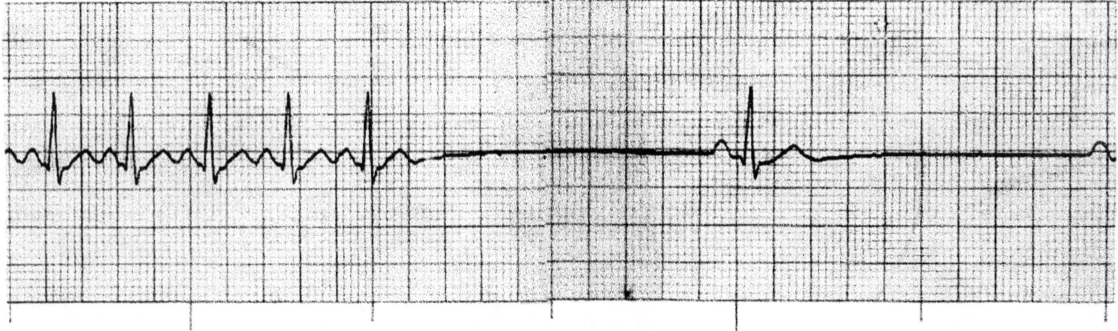

Figure 3-6 Sick sinus syndrome.

Box 3-7 Sick Sinus Syndrome

Rate: May be slow, fast, or alternating, depending on the rhythm presented
Rhythm: Atrial and ventricular rates are irregular because of sinus pauses and abrupt changes
P wave: Varies according to the prevailing rhythm; may be of normal size and configuration or may be absent; when P waves are present, there is usually one before each QRS complex
P-R interval: Is usually within normal limits, 0.12 to 0.20 second, but varies with rhythm changes
QRS complex: Again, varies with rhythm changes, but is usually of normal size and configuration, <0.10 second; there is usually a QRS complex after each P wave

Treatment

Treatment usually includes basic medical care, such as oxygen, IV access, monitor, then atropine 0.5- to 1-mg IV if a slow rhythm presents. If hemodynamic stability is being compromised, be prepared for a temporary pacemaker.

Chapter 3 Self-Test

1. Fill in the Blank: The ____________________ is the primary pacemaker of the heart with a rate of ____________________ to ____________________ beats per minute.

2. Fill in the Blank: If a normal sinus rhythm has 64 QRS complexes per minute, it has ____________________ P waves per minute.

3. Circle the Correct Answer: The SA node has the *least negative/most negative* charge during the resting phase of the depolarization-repolarization cycle.

4. True or False: Sinus bradycardia has a faster rate than normal sinus rhythm ranging from 101 to 160 beats per minute.

5. True or False: In a sinus bradycardia rhythm the pacer site originates below the AV node/AV junction producing a slower rhythm of 40 to 60 beats per minute.

6. Multiple Choice: Sinus bradycardia:
   a. Is caused by ventricular disease
   b. Can be normal for a person or is very serious and requires immediate treatment
   c. Produces vagal stimulation
   d. Is an irregular rhythm

7. Match the terms in the first column with the lettered terms in the second column:

   ____________________ 60 to 100 beats per minute
   ____________________ Less than 60 beats per minute
   ____________________ 101 to 180 beats per minute
   ____________________ Sinus arrhythmia
   ____________________ Sick sinus syndrome

   a. Is a normal variant that occurs with respirations and the changes of intrathoracic pressure
   b. Sinus tachycardia
   c. Is failure of the SA node to initiate an impulse resulting in the absence of P waves, QRS complexes, and T waves
   d. Normal sinus rhythm
   e. Sinus bradycardia

8. True or False: Sinus tachycardia has a regular rhythm with normal P waves, P-R intervals, and QRS complexes.

9. Fill in the Blank: Name four common causes of sinus bradycardia:

    ____

    ____

    ____

    ____

10. Fill in the Blank: Sinus arrest is failure of the ______________ node to initiate an impulse resulting in absence of a P wave, QRS complex, and T wave.

11. Multiple Choice: Because of the slower rhythm, the P-R interval of a sinus bradycardia is:
    a. Less than 0.12 second
    b. Greater than 0.12 second
    c. 0.08 to 0.20 second
    d. 0.12 to 0.20 second

12. True or False: Usually with sinus tachycardia the patient is asymptomatic.

13. Multiple Choice: Sinus tachycardia usually has an intrinsic rate of:
    a. 80 to 120 beats per minute
    b. 101 to 140 beats per minute
    c. 101 to 180 beats per minute
    d. 90 to 150 beats per minute

14. Multiple Choice: Sinus arrest occurs when the SA node fails to initiate an impulse resulting in:
    a. Absence of a P wave
    b. Absence of the QRS complex
    c. Absence of the QRS complex and T wave
    d. Absence of the P wave, QRS complex, and T wave

15. True or False: A sinus arrest is a regular rhythm with equal R-R intervals.

16. Multiple Choice: A sick sinus syndrome may also be known as:
    a. Tachy-brady syndrome
    b. Brady-tachy syndrome
    c. Sinus arrhythmia
    d. All of the above

ECG Practice Strips

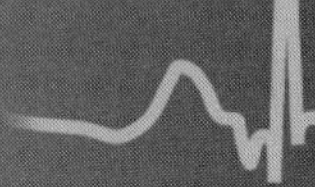

Please calculate the following 15 ECG practice strips:

- Determine the rate.
- Is the rhythm regular or irregular?
- Measure the P-R interval.
- Measure the QRS complex duration.
- Check to see if there is a P wave *before* every QRS complex.
- Check to see if there is a QRS complex *after* every P wave.
- Then give your interpretation of the rhythm.
- All strips are lead II unless otherwise noted.

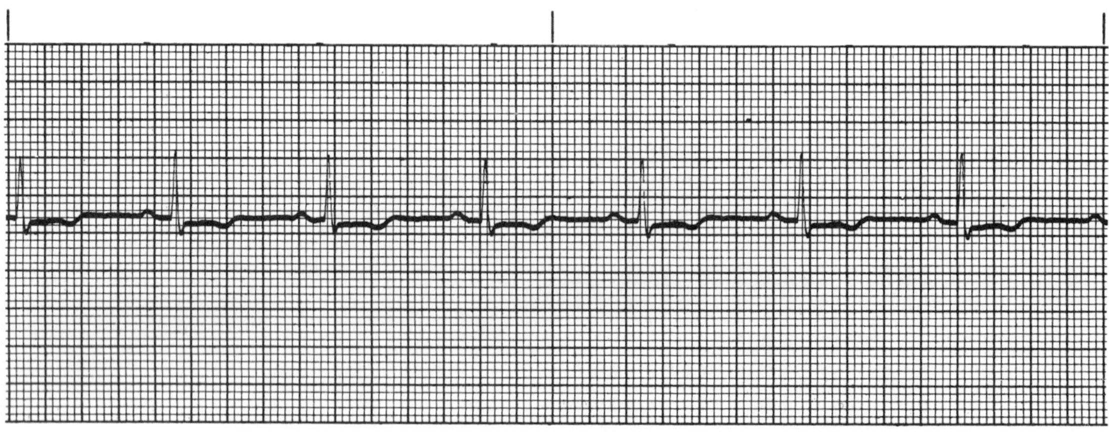

Practice Figure 3-1

Rate: ____________ Rhythm: ____________ P-R interval: ____________ QRS complex: ____________

Is there a P wave before every QRS complex? ____________

Is there a QRS complex after every P wave? ____________

Interpretation: ____________

____

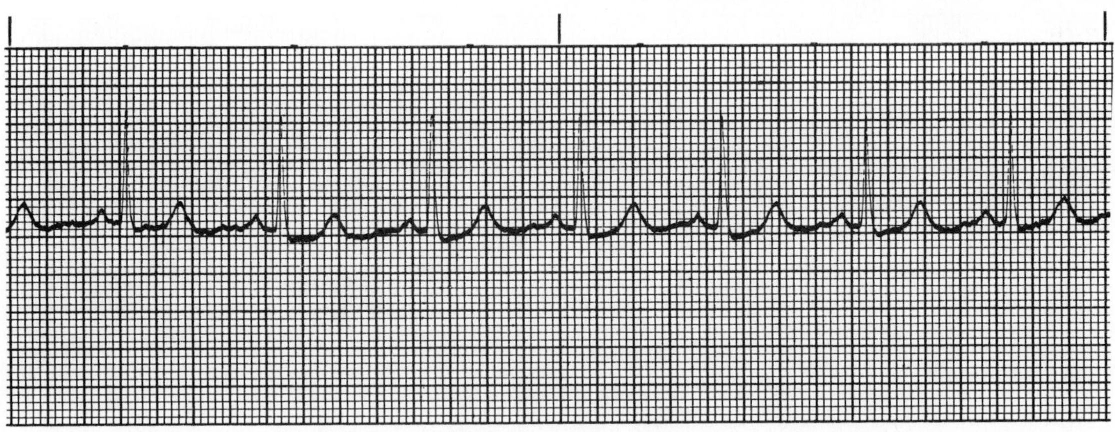

Practice Figure 3-2

Rate: ____________ Rhythm: ____________ P-R interval: ____________ QRS complex: ____________

Is there a P wave before every QRS complex? ____________

Is there a QRS complex after every P wave? ____________

Interpretation: ____________

Practice Figure 3-3

Rate: ____________ Rhythm: ____________ P-R interval: ____________ QRS complex: ____________

Is there a P wave before every QRS complex? ____________

Is there a QRS complex after every P wave? ____________

Interpretation: ____________

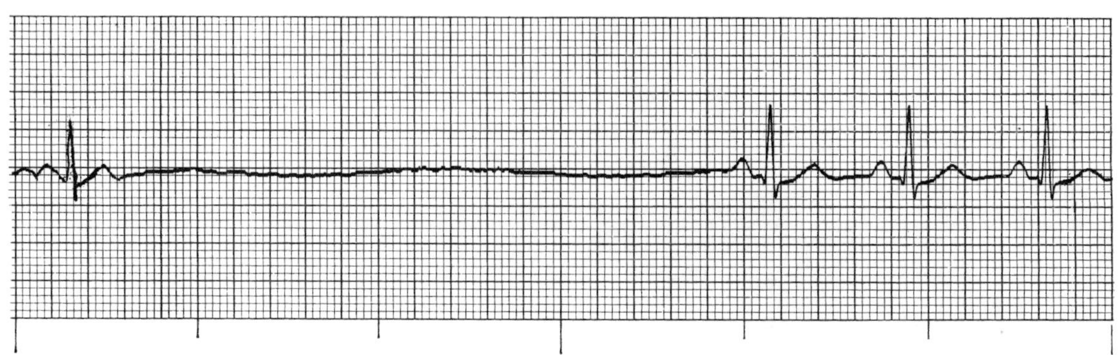

Practice Figure 3-4

Rate: ____________ Rhythm: ____________ P-R interval: ____________ QRS complex: ____________

Is there a P wave before every QRS complex? ____________

Is there a QRS complex after every P wave? ____________

Interpretation: ____________

____

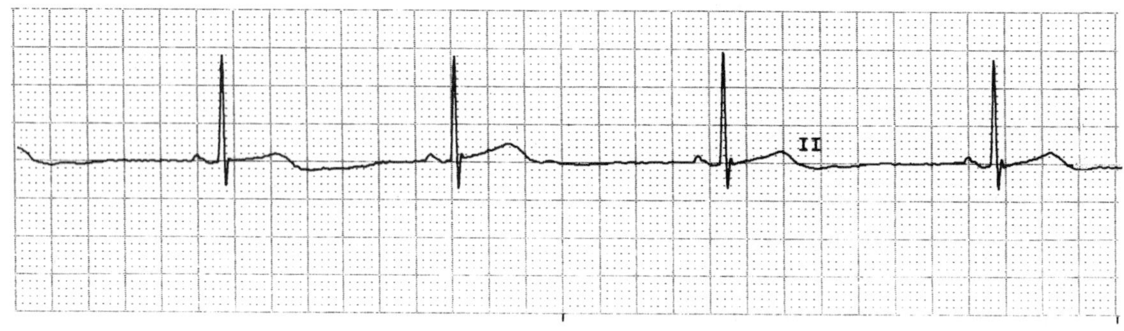

Practice Figure 3-5

Rate: ____________ Rhythm: ____________ P-R interval: ____________ QRS complex: ____________

Is there a P wave before every QRS complex? ____________

Is there a QRS complex after every P wave? ____________

Interpretation: ____________

____

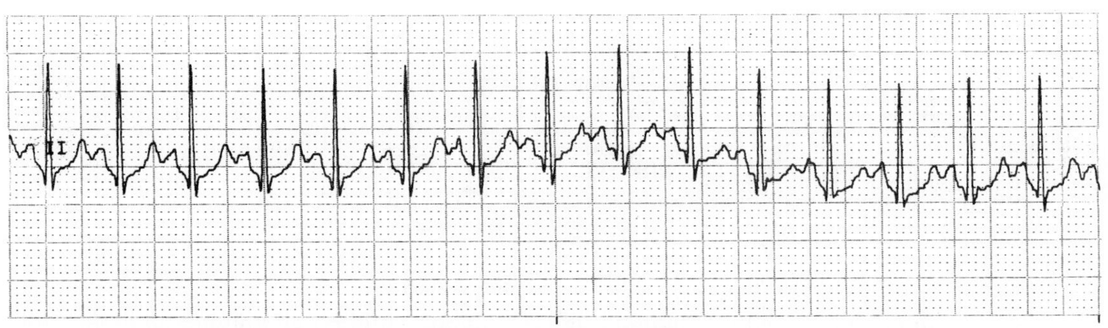

Practice Figure 3-6

Rate: ____________ Rhythm: ____________ P-R interval: ____________ QRS complex: ____________

Is there a P wave before every QRS complex? ____________

Is there a QRS complex after every P wave? ____________

Interpretation: ____________

____

Practice Figure 3-7

Rate: ____________ Rhythm: ____________ P-R interval: ____________ QRS complex: ____________

Is there a P wave before every QRS complex? ____________

Is there a QRS complex after every P wave? ____________

Interpretation: ____________

____

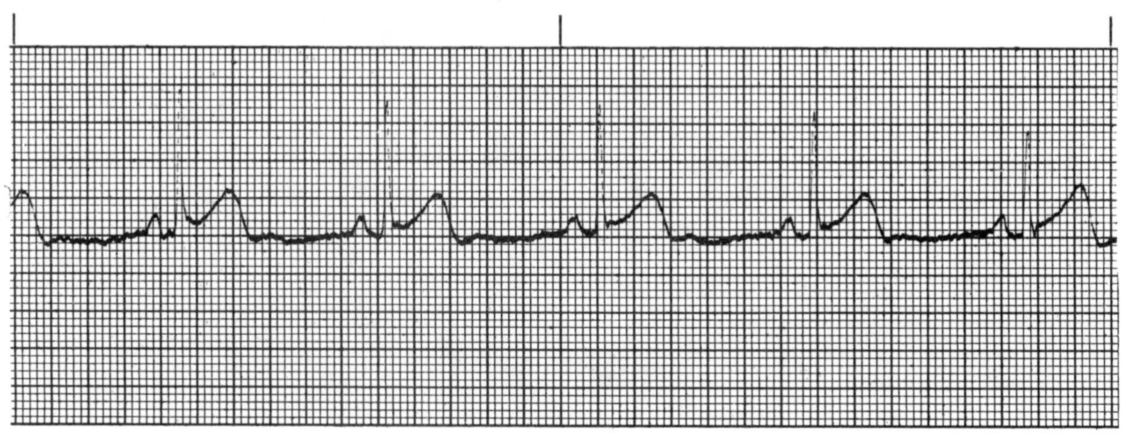

Practice Figure 3-8

Rate: ____________ Rhythm: ____________ P-R interval: ____________ QRS complex: ____________

Is there a P wave before every QRS complex? ____________

Is there a QRS complex after every P wave? ____________

Interpretation: ____________

____

Practice Figure 3-9

Rate: ____________ Rhythm: ____________ P-R interval: ____________ QRS complex: ____________

Is there a P wave before every QRS complex? ____________

Is there a QRS complex after every P wave? ____________

Interpretation: ____________

____

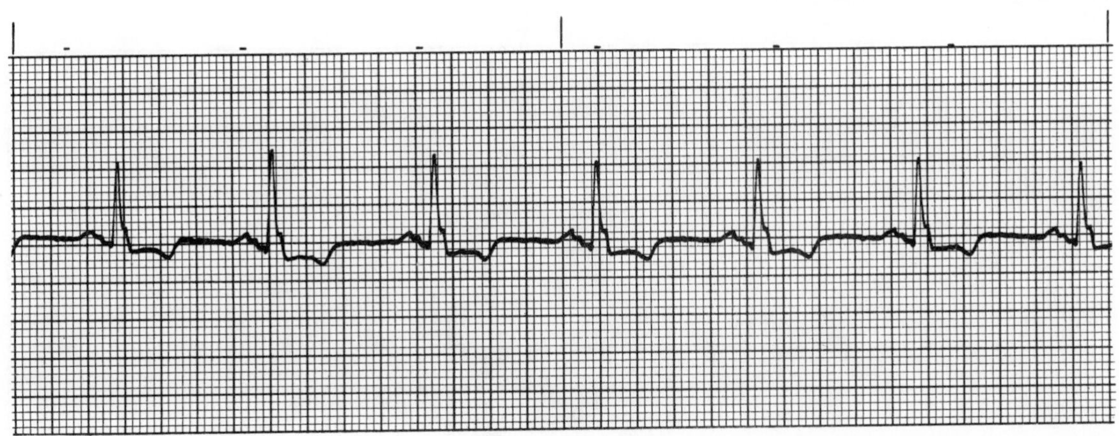

Practice Figure 3-10

Rate: ____________ Rhythm: ____________ P-R interval: ____________ QRS complex: ____________

Is there a P wave before every QRS complex? ____________

Is there a QRS complex after every P wave? ____________

Interpretation: ____________

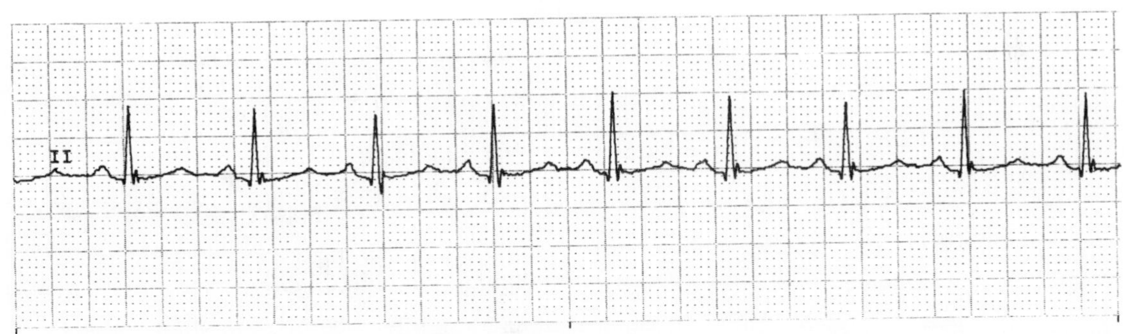

Practice Figure 3-11

Rate: ____________ Rhythm: ____________ P-R interval: ____________ QRS complex: ____________

Is there a P wave before every QRS complex? ____________

Is there a QRS complex after every P wave? ____________

Interpretation: ____________

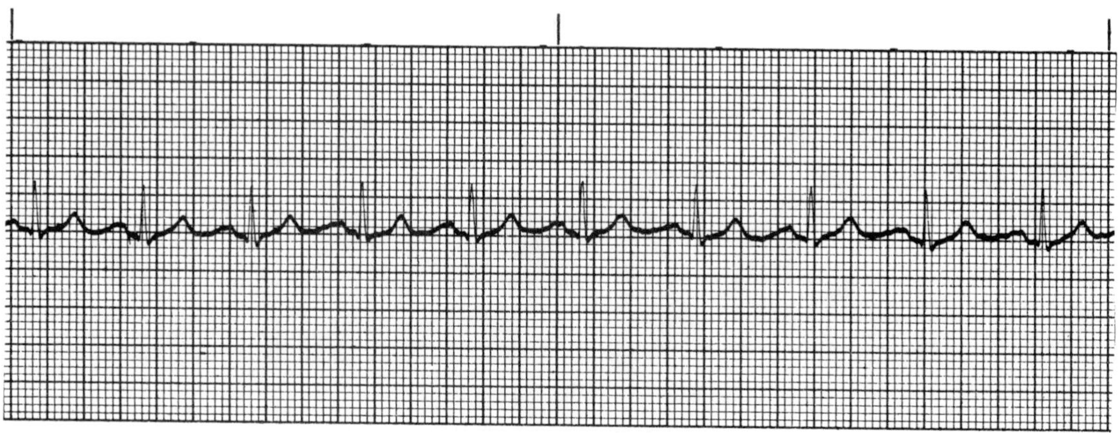

Practice Figure 3-12

Rate: __________ Rhythm: __________ P-R interval: __________ QRS complex: __________

Is there a P wave before every QRS complex? ______________________________

Is there a QRS complex after every P wave? ______________________________

Interpretation: ______________________________

____

Practice Figure 3-13

Rate: __________ Rhythm: __________ P-R interval: __________ QRS complex: __________

Is there a P wave before every QRS complex? ______________________________

Is there a QRS complex after every P wave? ______________________________

Interpretation: ______________________________

____

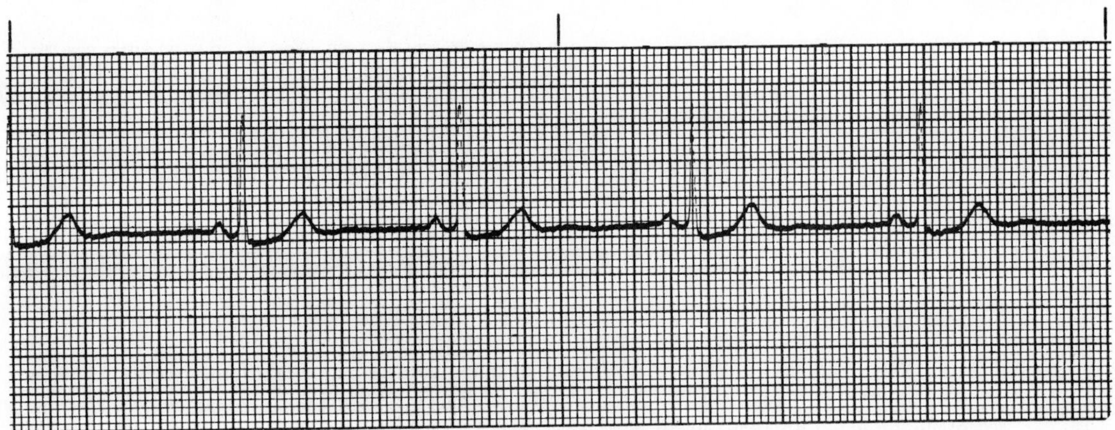

Practice Figure 3-14

Rate: ____________ Rhythm: ____________ P-R interval: ____________ QRS complex: ____________

Is there a P wave before every QRS complex? ____________

Is there a QRS complex after every P wave? ____________

Interpretation: ____________

____

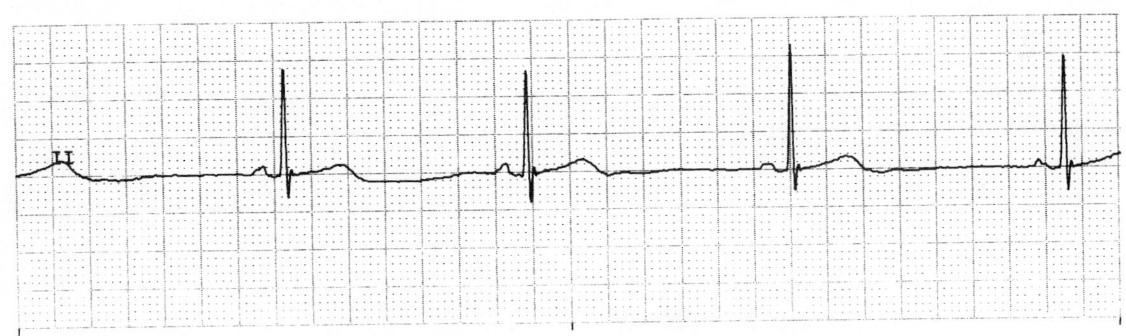

Practice Figure 3-15

Rate: ____________ Rhythm: ____________ P-R interval: ____________ QRS complex: ____________

Is there a P wave before every QRS complex? ____________

Is there a QRS complex after every P wave? ____________

Interpretation: ____________

____

Case Scenarios

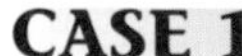

CASE 1

Scenario:

A 47-year-old man complains of midsternal chest pain, which is radiating to his left arm. He rates the pain as 7 on the 1 to 10 scale and describes it as heaviness. He states he was watching television when it began, and it was accompanied with diaphoresis. He denies nausea, shortness of breath, or weakness. There is nothing in his medical history, and he takes no medications. His vital signs are stable with BP, 126/70; P, 75; R, 24; and Sao_2 = 99%. His ECG rhythm is as follows:

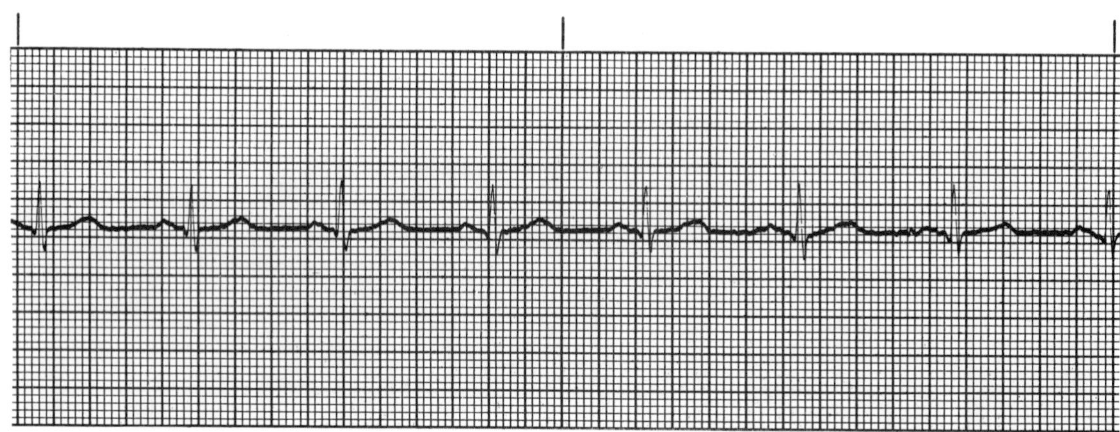

Identify the Rhythm

What is the rate? ______________ What is the rhythm (regular or irregular)? ______________

Is there a P wave before every QRS complex? ______________ Is there a QRS complex after every P wave? ______________

What is the P-R interval? ______________ QRS complex duration? ______________

Interpretation:

____

____

Case 1 Self-Test

In the spaces below give your treatment for the Primary Survey and Secondary Survey, plus the continued care under Oxygen-IV-Monitor-Fluids and Vital Signs. How would you care for this patient and what orders would you expect from the physician? At the bottom list your potential diagnosis or impression of the patient's problem.

Primary Survey

A.

B.

C.

D.

Secondary Survey

A.

B.

C.

D.

Oxygen-IV-Monitor-Fluids: ______________________________

____

Vital Signs: ______________________________

____

Your Impression: ______________________________

____

CASE 2

Scenario

A 50-year-old man is complaining of not feeling well for the past 2 to 3 days. He has been feeling tired, weak, and dizzy. He also states he has had a sore throat and left ear pain. There is nothing in his medical history, and he is not taking any medications. He tells you he does exercise by jogging 2 to 3 miles, 5 days a week. Vital signs are BP, 110/70; P, 52; R, 20; and Sao_2 = 98% and his lungs are clear. He is alert and oriented ×4. Skin is pink, warm, and dry. You see the following on the monitor:

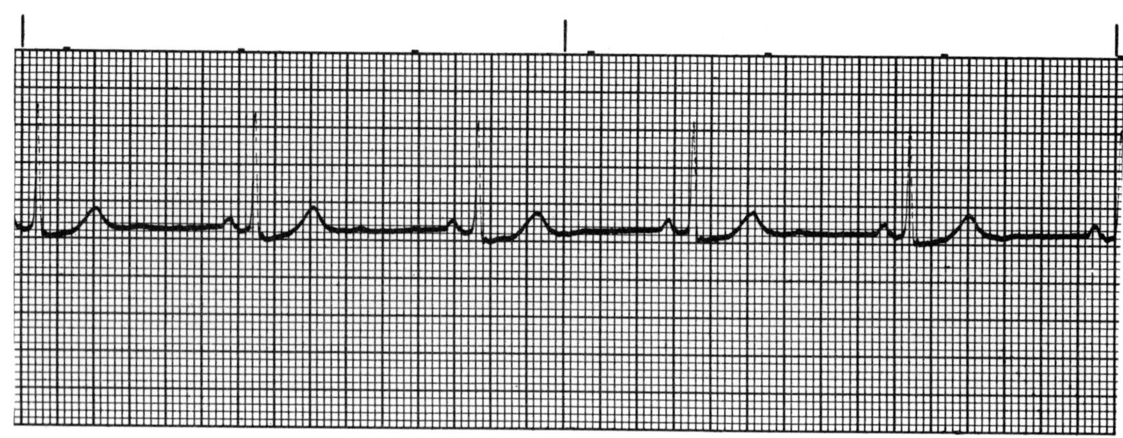

Identify the Rhythm

What is the rate? ____________ What is the rhythm (regular or irregular)? ____________

Is there a P wave before every QRS complex? ____________ Is there a QRS complex after every P wave? ____________

What is the P-R interval? ____________ QRS complex duration? ____________

Interpretation:

____

____

Case 2 Self-Test

In the spaces below give your treatment for the Primary Survey and Secondary Survey, plus the continued care under Oxygen-IV-Monitor-Fluids and Vital Signs. How would you care for this patient and what orders would you expect from the physician? At the bottom list your potential diagnosis or impression of the patient's problem.

Primary Survey

A.

B.

C.

D.

Secondary Survey

A.

B.

C.

D.

Oxygen-IV-Monitor-Fluids: ______________________________

____

Vital Signs: ______________________________

____

Your Impression: ______________________________

____

CASE 3

Scenario (Actual EMS Call)

A 67-year-old man complains of left-sided chest pain. The onset was 2 hours ago. The pain is radiating to the left shoulder and arm and is accompanied with diaphoresis and nausea. He rates the pain as 6 on the 1 to 10 scale. The pain is described as a heaviness-type feeling on his chest. Vital signs are stable with BP, 110/72; P, 72; R, 18; and Sao_2 = 97%. He denies any dyspnea, and his lungs are clear. There is nothing in his medical history, and he is not taking any medications. After beginning your transport to the hospital, you notice the following on the monitor:

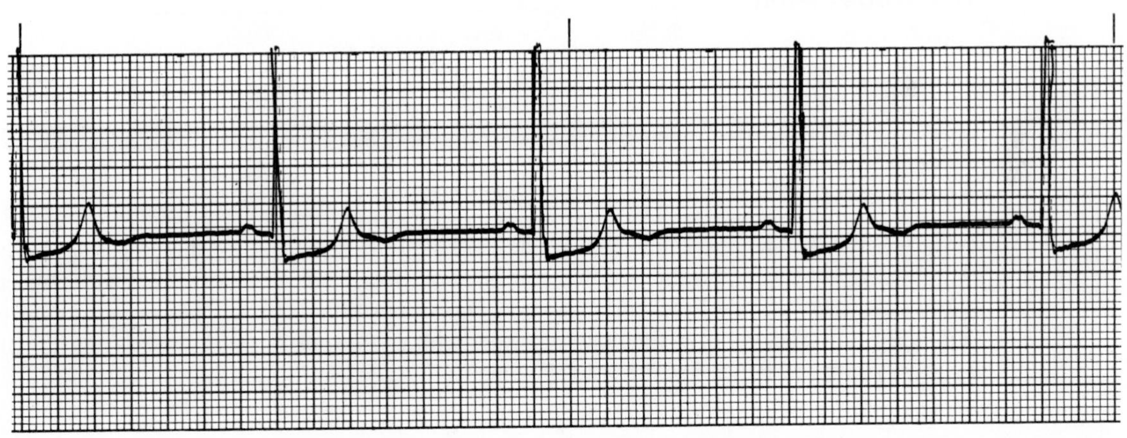

Identify the Rhythm

What is the rate? ____________ What is the rhythm (regular or irregular)? ____________

Is there a P wave before every QRS complex? ____________ Is there a QRS complex after every P wave? ____________

What is the P-R interval? ____________ QRS complex duration? ____________

Interpretation:

____

____

Case 3 Self-Test

In the spaces below give your treatment for the Primary Survey and Secondary Survey, plus the continued care under Oxygen-IV-Monitor-Fluids and Vital Signs. How would you care for this patient and what orders would you expect from the physician? At the bottom list your potential diagnosis or impression of the patient's problem.

Primary Survey

A.

B.

C.

D.

Secondary Survey

A.

B.

C.

D.

Oxygen-IV-Monitor-Fluids: ____________________

____

Vital Signs: ____________________

____

Your Impression: ____________________

____

CASE 4

Scenario

A 60-year-old woman is complaining of nausea, vomiting, and fever for the past 2 days. She states she is keeping some fluids down, but no food. Her medical history consists of hypertension. Her medication is hydrochlorothiazide. On examination she is alert and oriented ×4. Her skin is flush, warm, and dry. The lungs are clear with an Sao_2 of 97%. The vital signs are BP, 140/84; P, 136; and R, 22. She has the following ECG strip:

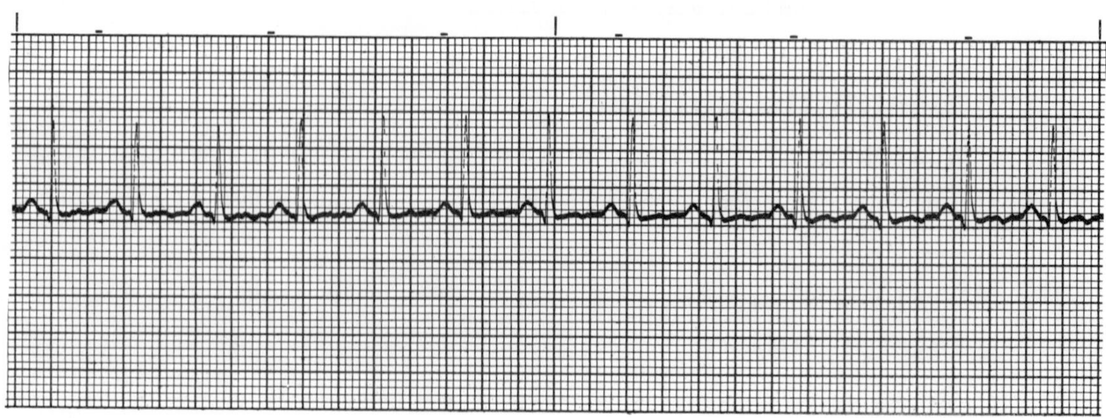

Identify the Rhythm

What is the rate? ______ What is the rhythm (regular or irregular)? ______

Is there a P wave before every QRS complex? ______ Is there a QRS complex after every P wave? ______

What is the P-R interval? ______ QRS complex duration? ______

Interpretation:

______

______

Case 4 Self-Test

In the spaces below give your treatment for the Primary Survey and Secondary Survey, plus the continued care under Oxygen-IV-Monitor-Fluids and Vital Signs. How would you care for this patient and what orders would you expect from the physician? At the bottom list your potential diagnosis or impression of the patient's problem.

Primary Survey

A.

B.

C.

D.

Secondary Survey

A.

B.

C.

D.

Oxygen-IV-Monitor-Fluids: ______

______

Vital Signs: ______

______

Your Impression: ______

______

CASE 5

Scenario

You are examining a 46-year-old man who is complaining of intermittent episodes of weakness for the past 4 to 5 days. Today he had an episode of syncope, which lasted 1 to 2 minutes. At present he is alert and oriented ×4. His skin is pink, warm, and dry. The lung sounds are clear, and the Sao_2 = 99%. His vital signs are BP, 128/76; P, 55; and R, 20. The following is his ECG rhythm:

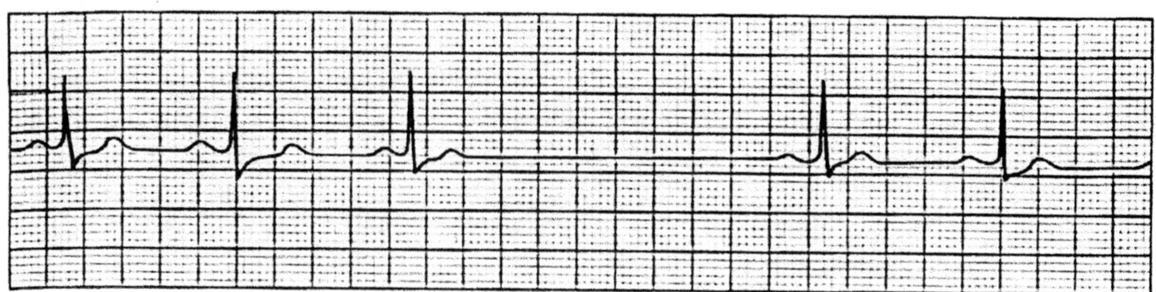

Identify the Rhythm

What is the rate? ____________ What is the rhythm (regular or irregular)? ____________

Is there a P wave before every QRS complex? ____________ Is there a QRS complex after every P wave? ____________

What is the P-R interval? ______________ QRS complex duration? ____________

Interpretation:

____

____

Case 5 Self-Test

In the spaces below give your treatment for the Primary Survey and Secondary Survey, plus the continued care under Oxygen-IV-Monitor-Fluids and Vital Signs. How would you care for this patient and what orders would you expect from the physician? At the bottom list your potential diagnosis or impression of the patient's problem.

Primary Survey

A.

B.

C.

D.

Secondary Survey

A.

B.

C.

D.

Oxygen-IV-Monitor-Fluids: ____

____

Vital Signs: ____

____

Your Impression: ____

____

4

Atrial Rhythms

OBJECTIVES

By the end of this chapter, the student will be able to do the following:

- **Specify the characteristics for the following atrial rhythms:**
  - **Supraventricular tachycardia**
    - **SVT**
    - **Paroxysmal supraventricular tachycardia (PSVT)**
    - **Atrial tachycardia**
    - **Narrow complex tachycardia**
  - **Wandering atrial pacemaker**
  - **Premature atrial complexes**
  - **Atrial flutter**
  - **Atrial fibrillation**
  - **Wolff-Parkinson-White (WPW) syndrome**
- **Know and understand the signs, symptoms, causes, and treatment of the following rhythms:**
  - **Supraventricular tachycardia**
  - **SVT**
  - **PSVT**
  - **Atrial tachycardia**
  - **Narrow complex tachycardia**
  - **Wandering atrial pacemaker**
  - **Premature atrial complexes**
  - **Atrial flutter**
  - **Atrial fibrillation**
  - **WPW syndrome**
- **Define and understand the following terms:**
  - **Wandering atrial pacemaker**

OBJECTIVES—cont'd

- PSVT
- "Controlled" fibrillation/flutter
- "Uncontrolled" fibrillation/flutter
- Bigeminy
- Quadrigeminy
- Trigeminy

- Describe the association of strokes and atrial fibrillation
- Understand when to use counter shock in atrial rhythms
- Explain compensatory and noncompensatory pauses

OUTLINE

Atrial Rhythms

Premature Atrial Contractions

Atrial Tachycardia/Narrow-Complex Tachycardias

Atrial Flutter

Atrial Fibrillation

Wandering Atrial Pacemaker

Wolff-Parkinson-White Syndrome

Chapter 4 Self-Test

ECG Practice Strips

Case Scenarios

This chapter allows you to understand what causes atrial rhythms, what signs and symptoms you should look for, and how emergency treatment is applied. Always evaluate the patient first before treating. Always treat the patient, not the monitor.

The atria are the two upper chambers of the heart, which are thin-walled, low-pressure chambers. They receive blood from the lungs and the systemic circulation. The two atria are separated by an interatrial septum. During the depolarization-repolarization period about two thirds of the blood supply moves passively from the atria into the ventricles. The other one third of the atrial blood supply is pushed into the ventricles by atrial contraction. This additional push or contribution of blood is called "the atrial kick."

Most of the common atrial dysrhythmias result from impulses that originate in the atrial tissue (Box 4-1). This is important because it affects ventricular filling time and decreases the atrial kick. Most atrial arrhythmias result from altered automaticity. This causes ectopic sites (those outside the normal conduction system) to initiate impulses spontaneously, fire quickly, and produce rapid atrial rates. Not all of these atrial impulses are conducted to the ventricles because of the normal delay mechanism at the AV node.

Box 4-1 Reasons for Atrial Dysrhythmias

Automaticity

Abnormal impulses are triggered by the increasing automaticity of atrial fibers. This may happen because of the following:
- Extracellular factors such as hypoxia, digitalis toxicity, or hypocalcemia
- SA node function is decreased, a result of hypokalemia or increased vagal tone

"Circus Reentry"

Mechanisms develop when impulse conduction is one-way and slow. Normal conduction is multidirectional throughout the heart. This may occur because of the following:
- MI causing a lengthening of the fibers. When fibers are short, conduction occurs quickly. However, when conduction is slowed because of the lengthening of the fibers, circus reentry occurs.
- Also caused by coronary artery disease and tachydysrhythmias

After Depolarization

During phase 3 of the action potential, the movement through the normally slow sodium and calcium channels increases. This may result from the following:
- Hypoxia, injury
- Hypokalemia
- Hypothermia
- Cardiac glycoside toxicity

MI, Myocardial infarction.

ATRIAL RHYTHMS

Premature Atrial Contractions

A premature atrial contraction (PAC) is a beat that occurs outside the SA node and usually is caused by the enhanced automaticity in the atrial tissue or an irritable focus in the atria that overrides the SA node pacemaker (Figure 4-1). A premature beat is one that occurs earlier than the next expected beat. The site of origin (atrial, junctional, or ventricular) usually identifies premature beats. Because the PAC comes before the next expected sinus beat, the rhythm is irregular. PACs may occur in groups of twos (bigeminy) and usually are followed by a pause. At times the PACs are nonconducted, so no QRS complex follows the P wave (Box 4-2).

Causes

Causes of PACs include the following:
- Ingestion of caffeine
- Ingestion of alcohol
- Stress
- Hypoxia
- Hypokalemia
- Digoxin toxicity
- Theophylline therapy
- Pulmonary disease
- Heart disease

PACs may occur in healthy individuals.

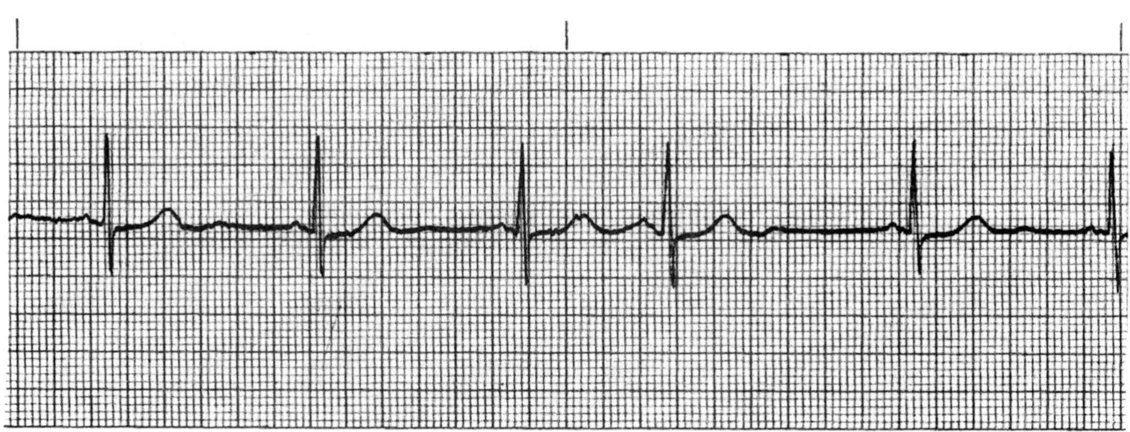

Figure 4-1 Premature atrial contractions.

Box 4-2 Premature Atrial Contractions

Rate: Usually normal, but also depends on the underlying rhythm
Rhythm: Irregular as a result of the PACs; underlying rhythm may be regular
P waves: Usually upright, but premature and abnormal shape in comparison with the underlying rhythm; the P wave also may be buried in the T wave and not visible
P-R interval: Usually within normal limits, 0.12 to 0.20 second; may be prolonged depending on the location of the ectopic focus
QRS complex: Usually of normal configuration and duration, but may be prolonged; if there is a P wave and no QRS complex, it is a nonconducted PAC; the impulse presents to the ventricles at the absolute refractory period; these may be confused with sinus arrest; QRS complexes do not always follow the P wave

PAC, Premature atrial contraction.

Compensatory and Noncompensatory Pauses

When the rhythm on the ECG monitor is irregular, it is necessary to determine if the ectopic beat is coming from the atria or the ventricles. The R-R interval may be full or incomplete. If the sum of the R-R interval with the pause or irregular beat (from the R wave before the irregular beat to the R wave after the irregular beat) *is equal to* the sum of two normal R-R intervals of the underlying rhythm, then it is a *complete or compensatory pause*. If the sum of the R-R interval with the irregular beat or pause *is not equal* to the sum of two normal R-R intervals of the underlying rhythm, then it is a *noncompensatory pause*. To determine which pause is occurring, first determine, or measure, what the normal R-R interval is in the underlying rhythm that you are calculating. Then measure or calculate the pause or irregular R-R interval. Basically, the compensation or no compensation depends on whether the SA node is polarized by the irregular premature contraction. When the SA node is not depolarized by the early contraction, you will find a complete compensatory pause. When the SA node is depolarized by the early contraction, you will find an incomplete or noncompensatory pause.

The first normal R-R interval of underlying rhythm equals 18 small boxes, or 0.72 seconds; the second normal R-R interval equals 18 small boxes, or 0.72 seconds. The two combined equal

36 small boxes, or 1.44 seconds. If the R-R interval from the beat preceding to the beat following the irregular beat equals 1.44 seconds, it is termed *compensatory*. However, if the R-R interval measuring from the preceding beat to the beat following the irregular beat measures less then 1.44, it is *noncompensatory*.

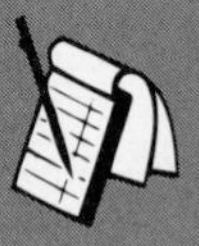

Note

A noncompensatory pause often follows a PAC and a compensatory pause usually follows a premature ventricular complex (PVC). The only exception to this is an interpolated PVC.

Treatment

Patients with symptomatic PACs may complain of occasional palpitations. Always observe your patient for any or all signs of decreased cardiac output, such as hypotension, syncope, and blurred vision accompanied with an altered level of consciousness. Rarely do patients with PACs complain of chest pain.

Most patients do not have symptoms and do not need intervention. However, those who are showing signs of cardiac compromise and have more than six PACs per minute may be treated with drugs that prolong the atrial refractory period. To identify PACs, you also need to know if there is a noncompensatory pause. If treatment is needed, the drug therapy may include digoxin, quinidine, or procainamide.

Atrial Tachycardia or Narrow-Complex Tachycardias

Atrial tachycardia or narrow-complex tachycardias (above the ventricles) are tachyarrhythmias with a rate of 150 to 250 beats per minute or simply any tachyarrhythmia with a rate greater than 150 (Figure 4-2). The impulse originates in the atrial tissue, above the bifurcation of the bundle of His, and may be precipitated by a premature atrial complex. They are also called *supraventricular tachycardias* (SVTs). The SVT rhythm also has a narrow QRS complex and a rate greater than 150 beats per minute. The rate is so fast that you cannot see the P waves, but because it has a narrow QRS complex you know it is originating above the ventricles. An atrial tachycardia also has a narrow QRS complex and is rapid. However, you usually can make out the P waves, so you know it is originating in the atria (Box 4-3).

Paroxysmal atrial tachycardia is a rapid rhythm that starts and stops suddenly. If you do not see the onset of the tachycardia, then it is simply an atrial or supraventricular, not paroxysmal, tachycardia. The rapid atrial rate often overrides the SA node and becomes the dominant pacemaker. The QRS complexes of atrial tachycardia are usually narrow. Because the word *paroxysm* means "sudden," a paroxysmal rhythm is one that begins or stops suddenly.

Causes

The cause of atrial tachycardia in young healthy persons is usually excessive caffeine, other stimulants, marijuana, hypokalemia, or physical or psychologic stress (Box 4-4). However, in a person with underlying cardiac problems, the main cause is that because the heart rate is so fast,

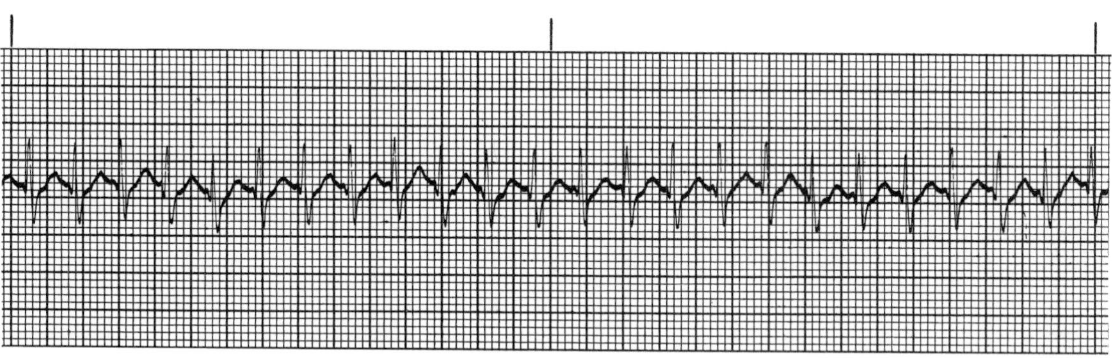

Figure 4-2 Narrow complex tachycardias.

Box 4-3 Narrow Complex or Atrial Tachycardias

Rate: 150 to 250 beats per minute
Rhythm: Regular, both atrial and ventricular
P wave: Configuration varies, may be flattened, notched, pointed or biphasic; P waves may be present at the lower rates (150 to 160 beats per minute), but not visible at rates more than 200 beats per minute; when P waves are present, there is a P wave before every QRS complex
P-R interval: Most usually are not measurable because P wave is difficult to distinguish from the preceding T wave
QRS complex: Configuration is normal, with a narrow complex, <0.10 second; the R-R is regular; at faster atrial rates, conduction may become aberrant

the ventricles simply do not have enough time to fill and empty adequately. Thus the cardiac output decreases, which in turn causes a decrease in perfusion to the entire system, and the patient experiences symptoms such as light-headedness, dizziness, nausea, diaphoresis, syncope, and even chest pain.

A young person with stable tachycardia may complain of a racing heart and palpitations. However, vital signs remain stable, and no altered level of consciousness occurs. The unstable patient may complain of or show signs and symptoms of any of the following:

- Shock
- Decreased level of consciousness
- Hypotension
- Chest pain
- Shortness of breath
- CHF
- AMI

Treatment

Treatment depends on the patient's signs and symptoms. If the patient is stable but has symptoms, start with oxygen therapy, monitor, IV access, and vagal maneuvers. Such vagal maneuvers include carotid sinus massage, coughing, bearing down, breath holding, stimulation of the gag reflex, or eyeball pressure application. You may use carotid massage as long as the patient does not have

Box 4-4 Causes of Atrial Tachycardia

Hypertension
Excessive caffeine
Physical stress
Myocardial infarction
Wolff-Parkinson-White syndrome
Rheumatic heart disease
Respiratory failure
Cardiomyopathy
Excessive stimulants
Psychologic stress
Congenital heart disease
Coronary artery disease
Mitral valve prolapse
Digitalis toxicity

a history of coronary artery disease. When these measures produce vagal stimulation, the result is slowing of the SA and AV node impulses; hopefully, the SA node will take over as the dominant pacemaker.

Drugs used to control atrial tachycardias are adenosine, digoxin, propranolol, and diltiazem. If the drugs are ineffective, then synchronized cardioversion (electrical therapy) is next in the line of treatment. Synchronized cardioversion allows for the countershock to be delivered on the peak of the QRS complex (R wave deflection). It programs the shock so it is not delivered on the T wave, which is the vulnerable part of the refractory period. See Algorithm 4-1; if there is a wide QRS complex, see Algorithm 2.

Another method to use is atrial overdrive pacing. The pacing interferes with the conduction circuit, allowing for the SA node to take over as the main pacemaker.

Atrial Flutter

Atrial flutter occurs when the atria discharge at a rate of 250 to 400 beats per minute; the ventricles are usually discharging at a rate of 60 to 100 beats per minute (Figure 4-3). Atrial flutter results from circus reentry, which originates in one atrial focus. Because of the rapid waveform, it resembles a sawtooth form or picket fence and is called *flutter waves*. Atrial flutter is considered controlled if the ventricular rate remains below 100 beats per minute. It is due to varying degrees of AV block, which allow for the ventricular rate to be one fourth to one half of the atrial rate. The ventricles are protected from the fast atrial rates by having the AV node block the impulses. When the ventricular rates are too slow (less than 40 to 50 beats per minute) or too fast (greater than 150 to 160 beats per minute), then cardiac output declines. Atrial flutter can result in hypotension, syncope, shortness of breath, CHF, chest pain, angina, or an MI (Box 4-5).

Causes

Underlying cardiac problems usually cause atrial flutter. Some of the disease states that cause atrial flutter are ischemic heart disease, valvular disease, cor pulmonale, inferior-wall MI, pulmonary embolism, hypoxia, and digitalis or quinidine toxicity.

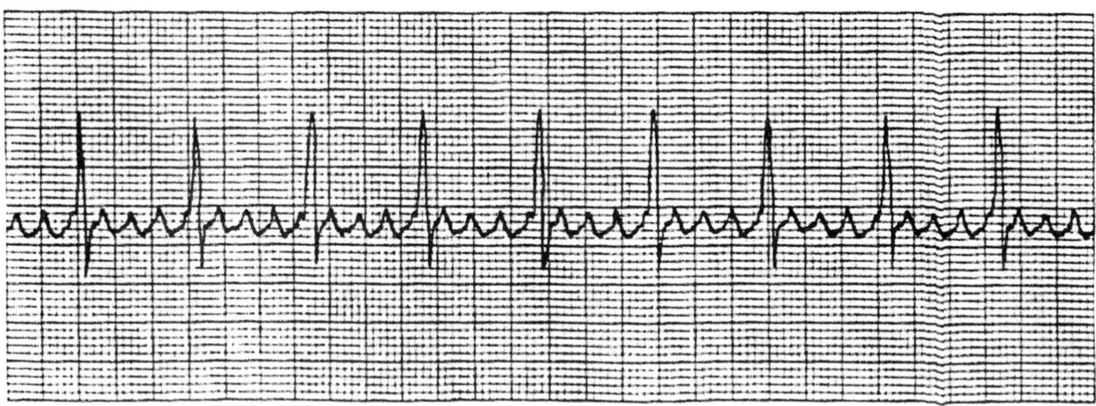

Figure 4-3 Atrial flutter.

Box 4-5 Atrial Flutter

Rate: Atrial rate is usually 250 to 400 beats per minute; ventricular rate depends on the degree of the AV block; it is usually 60 to 100 beats per minute and may go as high as 150 beats per minute; there is an atrial/ventricular ratio of 2:1, 3:1, 4:1, etc.
Rhythm: Atrial—regular; ventricular—may be irregular
P wave: There are no identifiable P waves, instead sawtooth waves called *flutter waves*
P-R Interval: Not measurable
QRS complex: Normal duration unless the flutter waves are buried in the QRS complex

Signs and symptoms of compromise usually are not seen if the pulse rate and rhythm are normal. Problems arise when the ventricular rate or pulse is high. The usual signs and symptoms will probably be seen, such as shortness of breath, a decreased level of consciousness, hypotension, and chest pain.

Treatment

Treatment for atrial flutter is amiodarone, procainamide, diltiazem, digoxin, ibutilide, or other beta blockers. If hemodynamic compromise is present, then anticipate immediate direct current (DC) cardioversion.

Atrial Fibrillation

Atrial fibrillation occurs when the atria produce impulses from multiple sites in the atrium, causing an atrial rate of 350 to 600 beats per minute (Figure 4-4). In essence the atria are not really contracting, they are simply quivering (like a bowl of Jell-O), producing what are known as *f waves* or *fibrillatory waves*. This produces an erratic baseline that almost looks like artifact. The result is ineffective atrial contractions. Most of these atrial impulses are blocked at the AV node, allowing only a limited number to pass through to the ventricles. If the ventricular rate is rapid, it is difficult to distinguish it from an atrial tachycardia. The one difference is that atrial tachycardia is regular when slowed down with discernable P waves, whereas the atrial fibrillation is irregular when slowed down with no discernable P waves. At the fast rates, above 140 to 150 beats per minute Algorithm 4-1, the R-R interval may appear regular, but when measured it is not (Box 4-6).

Two different forms of atrial fibrillation exist: "controlled" and "uncontrolled." In controlled atrial fibrillation, the ventricular rate is less than 100 beats per minute; thus the patient will probably be without symptoms. In uncontrolled atrial fibrillation, the rate is greater than 100 beats per minute, which decreases the diastolic filling time and diminishes cardiac output. The faster rates cause a further decline in cardiac output, causing symptoms such as hypotension, syncope, and CHF (Algorithm 4-1).

Causes

Causes of atrial fibrillation include the following:

- Hypertension
- Ischemic heart disease
- AMI
- Rheumatic heart disease
- Cardiac valve disorders
- Coronary artery disease
- Pulmonary embolism
- COPD
- Pericarditis
- CHF
- Hypoxia
- Digitalis or quinidine toxicity

Signs and symptoms of atrial fibrillation depend on whether the ventricular rate is normal or rapid. If symptoms are present, the patient may experience signs of any of the following: palpitations, skipped beats, syncope, weakness, dizziness, shortness of breath, decreased level of consciousness, and chest pressure or pain.

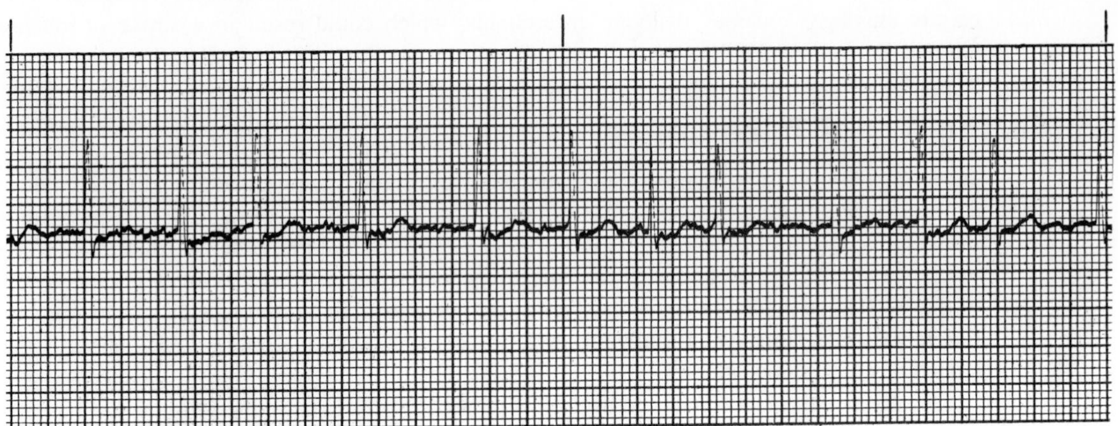

Figure 4-4 Atrial fibrillation.

Box 4-6 Atrial Fibrillation

Rate: Atrial rate is usually greater than 350 impulses per minute (350 to 600 per minute); ventricular is less than 150 per minute; under 100 is considered controlled
Rhythm: Atrial and ventricular are grossly irregular, often called *irregularly irregular*
P wave: Absent, not identifiable as P waves, instead fibrillatory waves (f waves) are present; they present a chaotic, erratic, wavy pattern
P-R interval: Not able to measure
QRS complex: Duration and configuration are usual, <0.10 second, but may be widened if an intraventricular deficit exists

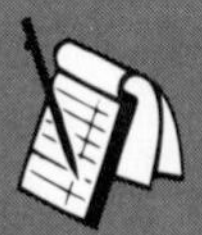

Note

You should probably take both a radial and apical pulse because there may be a difference between the two. Some of the beats may be so weak that they do not produce a palpable radial pulse. Obviously the pulse rate will be irregular because of the irregular rhythm.

Treatment

If the patient is stable with a fast ventricular rate, the treatment is aimed at drug therapy to control the ventricular rate and hopefully convert the patient to a normal sinus rhythm The drug of choice is adenosine. If this does not convert the rhythm, other possible drug treatments include beta blockers (esmolol, atenolol, and metoprolol) and calcium channel blockers (diltiazem and verapamil). Also included are amiodarone, digoxin, and procainamide.

If the patient is unstable, treatment measures such as the Valsalva maneuver, carotid sinus massage, gag reflex stimulation, or synchronized cardioversion are used. When using carotid massage, make sure you check for carotid bruits. If a bruit is detected and you perform the carotid massage, you may dislodge an embolus, which could result in a stroke or cerebral emboli.

Wandering Atrial Pacemaker

When impulses are sent from various pacemaker sites in the SA node and atria, they are known as *wandering atrial pacemaker* (WAP) (Figure 4-5). The impulse constantly shifts its point of origin in the atrium. Because the impulses are not coming from the same pacemaker site, the P waves vary in shape, size, and direction. They may be upright, inverted, or absent. For a diagnosis of the WAP to be made, the focus must come from at least three different sites, producing three different P waves (Box 4-7). Usually this rhythm occurs in young children or older adults, although sometimes it occurs in athletes.

Usually no treatment is required because the patient has no symptoms. Treatment, if required, would be based on the underlying cause. If the WAP is prolonged, it may indicate an underlying cardiac problem.

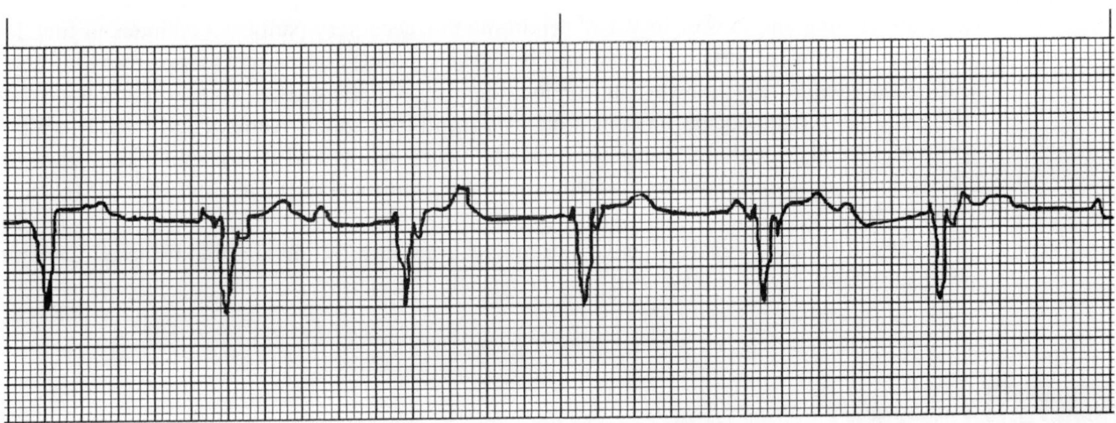

Figure 4-5 Wandering atrial pacemaker.

Box 4-7 Wandering Atrial Pacemaker

Rate: Atrial and ventricular is usually 60 to 100 beats per minute
Rhythm: Atrial and ventricular are both slightly irregular
P waves: The shape, size, and direction change from beat to beat; the P wave may be inverted or absent and may follow the QRS complex; a combination of all of these variations may appear
P-R interval: Is variable; the P-R interval may be normal or shortened
QRS complex: Usually normal configuration and duration, <0.10 second

Wolff-Parkinson-White Syndrome

Wolff-Parkinson-White (WPW) syndrome is one of the most common preexcitation syndromes (Figure 4-6). While developing, a fetus has a special accessory pathway, outside the normal conduction system connecting the atria and ventricles directly. Usually at birth this pathway

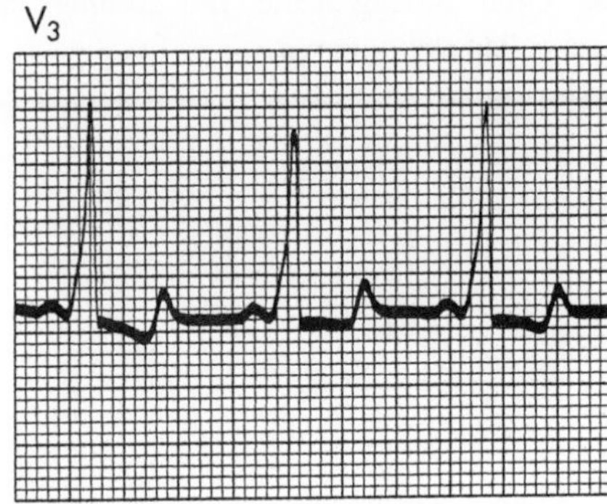

Figure 4-6 Wolff-Parkinson-White (WPW) syndrome.
(From Chou T: *Electrocardiography in clinical practice: adult and pediatric*, ed 4, Philadelphia, 1996, WB Saunders.)

stops functioning and closes. In WPW syndrome this accessory pathway continues to function after birth, keeping the atria connected directly to the ventricles. This accessory pathway is known as the *Kent bundle*. This pathway can conduct impulses to either the atria or the ventricles. When retrograde conduction occurs, a tachycardia may result from circus reentry (Box 4-8). The WPW syndrome usually occurs in young children and young adults and is asymptomatic. When the patient does have symptoms, they include chest pain, shortness of breath, and syncope (because of the rapid tachycardia).

Treatment includes vagal maneuvers or medications such as amiodarone. If these treatments are unsuccessful, then cardioversion may be needed.

Box 4-8 Wolff-Parkinson-White Syndrome

Rate: Usually 60 to 100 beats per minute, sinus in origin

Rhythm: Regular, unless associated with atrial fibrillation

P waves: Normal shape, size, configuration, unless atrial fibrillation is present

P-R interval: If P waves are present, the P-R interval is normal duration, 0.12 to 0.20 second

QRS complex: Usually it will be greater than 0.12 second because of the slurring; upstroke of the QRS complex producing delta waves

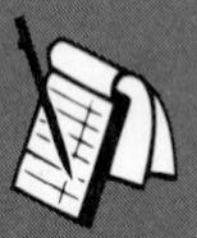

Note

Preexcitation is used to describe rhythms that are associated with the abnormal conduction pathways between the atria and the ventricles that bypass the AV node and the bundle of His and allow electrical impulses to travel via a pathway other than the AV node and bundle of His. This allows for the electrical impulses to excite the ventricles earlier than the usual pattern. Patients with these rhythms are predisposed to tachyarrhythmias because the normal delay at the AV node is not functioning. In addition the accessory pathway allows for reentry. The result is an initial slurring of the QRS complex (in some leads) along with a slow rising onset. These are called *delta waves*.

NARROW COMPLEX TACHYCARDIA

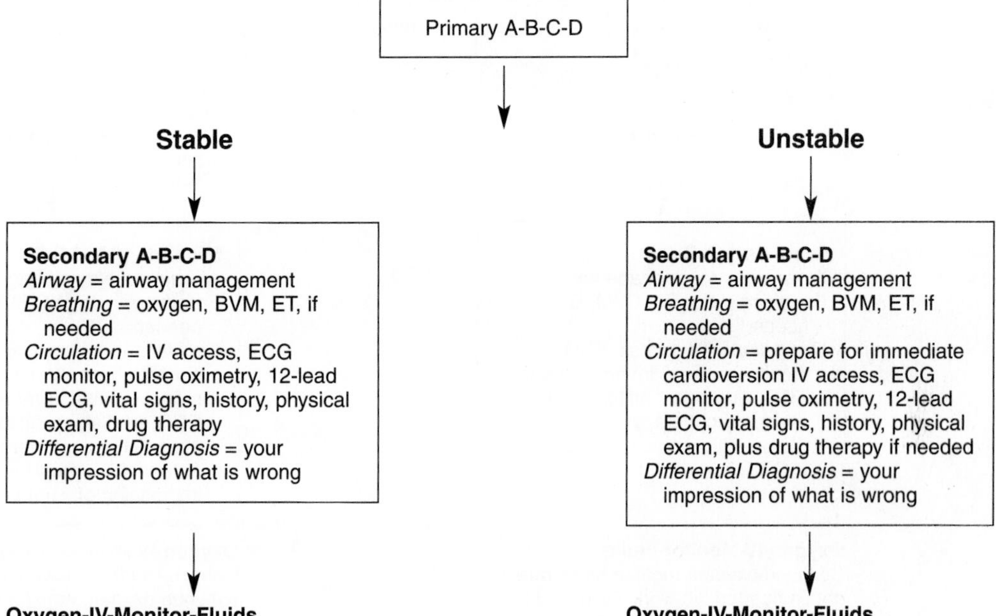

Primary A-B-C-D
Stable
Unstable
Secondary A-B-C-D
Airway = airway management
Breathing = oxygen, BVM, ET, if needed
Circulation = IV access, ECG monitor, pulse oximetry, 12-lead ECG, vital signs, history, physical exam, drug therapy
Differential Diagnosis = your impression of what is wrong
Secondary A-B-C-D
Airway = airway management
Breathing = oxygen, BVM, ET, if needed
Circulation = prepare for immediate cardioversion IV access, ECG monitor, pulse oximetry, 12-lead ECG, vital signs, history, physical exam, plus drug therapy if needed
Differential Diagnosis = your impression of what is wrong

Stable

Oxygen-IV-Monitor-Fluids
Continue oxygen, monitor heart rate, obtain needed lab work. Give fluids if needed. Appropriate drug therapy as needed.

Drug therapy
- Adenosine 6-mg IV bolus rapid IV push. May repeat at 12 mg IV bolus times 2 every 1-2 minutes

NOTE: adenosine is contraindicated in asthmatic patients

OR

- Amiodarone 150 mg IV over 10 minutes and follow with a continuous infusion. May repeat the 150 mg IV bolus

OR

- Beta-blockers such as esmolol, metoprolol, or atenolol
  Esmolol 0.5 mg/kg over 1 minute
  Atenolol 5-mg IV bolus over 5 minutes
  Metoprolol 5-mg IV bolus over 2-5 minutes

OR

- Calcium channel blockers
  Diltiazem – 0.25 mg/kg over 1 minute

OR

- Digoxin 10-15 mcg/kg lean body weight

Unstable

Oxygen-IV-Monitor-Fluids
Continue oxygen, and monitor heart rate. Obtain needed lab work. Continue with cardioversion as needed. Give appropriate drug therapy and fluids as needed

Cardioversion
Begin cardioversion at 100 Joules, may repeat at 200, 300, and 360 J

Algorithm 4-1 Narrow QRS tachycardia. (Modified from Aehlert B: *ACLS quick review study guide,* ed 2, St Louis, 2002, Mosby.)

WIDE COMPLEX TACHYCARDIA

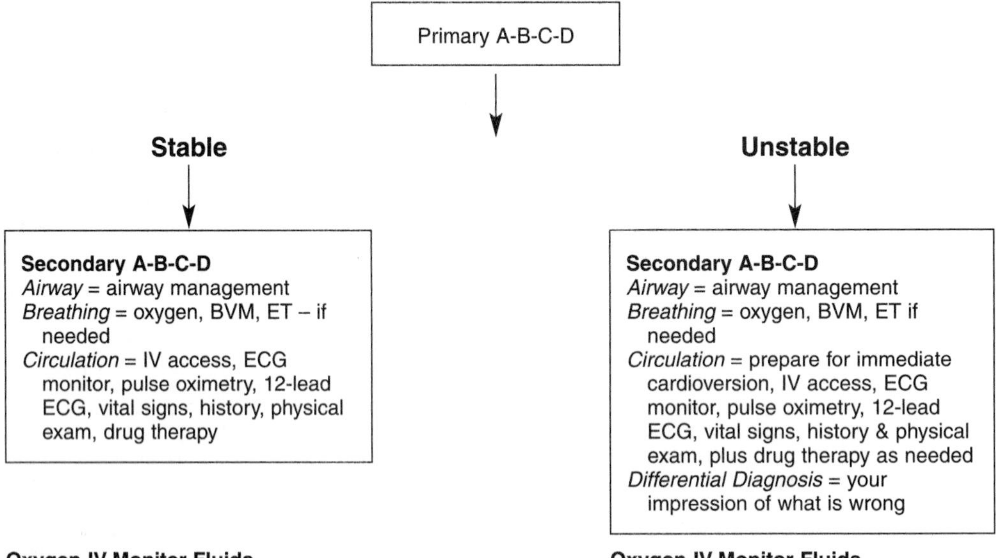
Primary A-B-C-D
Stable
Unstable
Secondary A-B-C-D
Airway = airway management
Breathing = oxygen, BVM, ET – if needed
Circulation = IV access, ECG monitor, pulse oximetry, 12-lead ECG, vital signs, history, physical exam, drug therapy
Secondary A-B-C-D
Airway = airway management
Breathing = oxygen, BVM, ET if needed
Circulation = prepare for immediate cardioversion, IV access, ECG monitor, pulse oximetry, 12-lead ECG, vital signs, history & physical exam, plus drug therapy as needed
Differential Diagnosis = your impression of what is wrong

Oxygen-IV-Monitor-Fluids
Continue oxygen, monitor heart rate, obtain needed lab work. Give fluids if needed. Appropriate drug therapy as needed.

Vital signs
Ongoing vital signs, monitor heart rate, blood pressure, pulse and respirations

Oxygen-IV-Monitor-Fluids
Continue with cardioversion as needed, continue oxygen, monitor heart rate, obtain needed lab work. Give appropriate drug therapy and fluids as needed

Vital signs
Ongoing vital signs, monitor heart rate, blood pressure, pulse and respirations

Note: use the 12-lead ECG and clinical information to help determine the rhythm diagnosis
This rhythm may be defined as one of the following:

SVT
- Junctional tachycardia
- Paroxysmal supraventricular tachycardia
- Atrial tachycardia

Wide Complex Tachycardia
- Wide QRS complex tachycardia of unknown origin

Ventricular Tachycardia
* is the patient stable or unstable? Go to Ventricuar Tachycardia Algorithm 7.1, 7.2

Drug therapy
- Amiodarone
- Procainamide
- Lidocaine

Cardioversion, Defibrillation
Begin cardioversion at 100 Joules, may repeat at 200, 300, 360 J
Begin defibrillation at 200 Joules, Repeat at 300, 360 J

Appropriate drug therapy:
- ☐ Amiodarone 150-mg IV bolus over 10 minutes
- ☐ Procainamide 100-mg IV bolus slowly over 5 minutes; may repeat with a maximum total dose of 17 mg/kg
- ☐ Lidocaine 1- to 1.5-mg/kg IV bolus. May repeat at $^1/_2$ the initial dose or 0.5 to 0.75 mg/kg up to a maximum total dose of 3 mg/kg

Algorithm 4-2 Wide complex tachycardia. (Modified from Aehlert B: *ACLS quick review study guide*, ed 2, St Louis, 2002, Mosby.)

Chapter 4 Self-Test

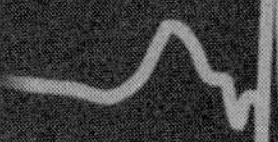

1. Fill in the Blank: Most atrial arrhythmias result from ______________________________ .

2. Multiple Choice: PAC stands for:
   a. Paroxysmal atrial conduction
   b. Premature automaticity
   c. Premature ventricular contraction
   d. Premature atrial contraction

3. Fill in the Blank: List four signs and symptoms of decreased cardiac output.

   ____

   ____

   ____

   ____

4. Multiple Choice: The rate for supraventricular tachycardia or PAT is:
   a. 101 to 150 beats per minute
   b. Less than 200 beats per minute
   c. 150 to 250 beats per minute
   d. None of the above

5. Match the following rhythms with their rates

   ______________________________ Normal sinus rhythm

   ______________________________ Atrial flutter

   ______________________________ Atrial fibrillation

   ______________________________ SVT

   ______________________________ Sinus bradycardia

   ______________________________ Sinus tachycardia

   a. 150 to 250 beats per minute
   b. Atrial rate 250 to 400 beats per minute
   c. 60 to 100 beats per minute
   d. Atrial rate greater than 350, ventricular rate less than 150 beats per minute
   e. 101 to 150 beats per minute
   f. Less than 60 beats per minute

6. True or False: A premature beat is one that occurs early before the next expected beat.

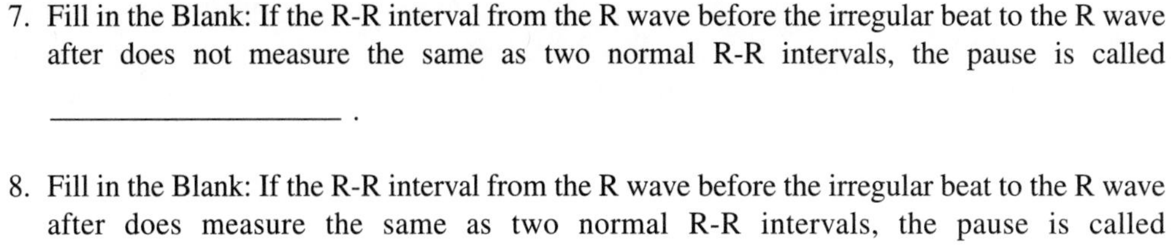

7. Fill in the Blank: If the R-R interval from the R wave before the irregular beat to the R wave after does not measure the same as two normal R-R intervals, the pause is called ____________________.

8. Fill in the Blank: If the R-R interval from the R wave before the irregular beat to the R wave after does measure the same as two normal R-R intervals, the pause is called ____________________.

9. PAT or paroxysmal atrial tachycardia:
   a. Starts and stops suddenly
   b. Is a slow rhythm with a rate less than 60 beats per minute
   c. Has a slow onset and conducts with inverted T waves
   d. None of above

10. True or False: Atrial flutter has the same atrial and ventricular rates, but the P waves form a sawtooth pattern.

11. True or False: The atrial fibrillation rhythm is termed *grossly irregular* or *irregularly irregular*.

12. Multiple Choice: The P-R interval of an atrial fibrillation rhythm:
    a. Is grossly irregular, but the P waves are upright and rounded
    b. Is less than 0.12 but greater than 0.04 second
    c. Is not measurable
    d. Is greater than 0.20 second

13. True or False: WPW syndrome is an accessory pathway of conduction between the atria and the ventricles in the fetus that remains open after birth. Normally this would close after birth.

ECG Practice Strips

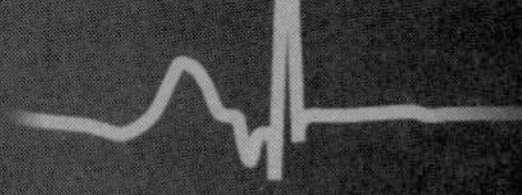

Please calculate the following 15 ECG practice strips:

- Determine the rate.
- Is the rhythm regular or irregular?
- Measure the P-R interval.
- Measure the QRS complex duration.
- Check to see if there is a P wave *before* every QRS complex.
- Check to see if there is a QRS complex *after* every P wave.
- Then give your interpretation of the rhythm.
- All strips are lead II unless otherwise noted.

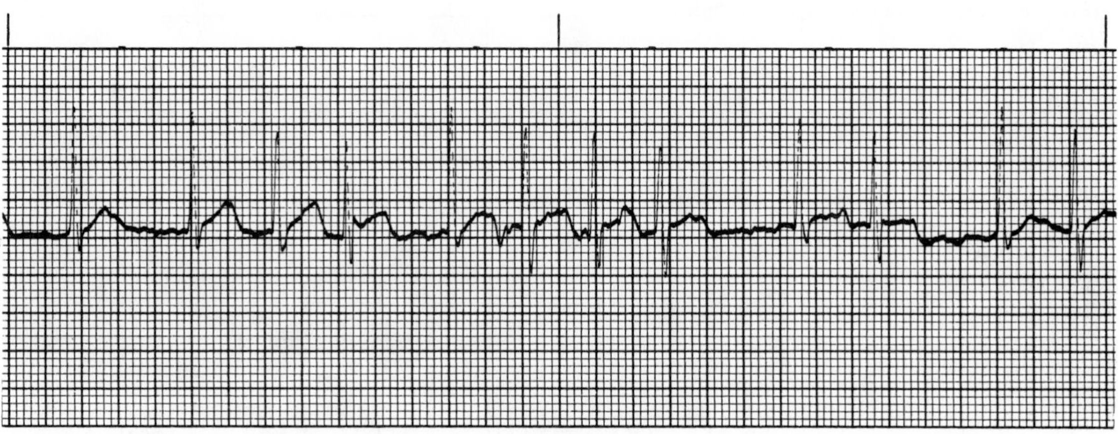

Practice Figure 4-1

Rate: ____________ Rhythm: ____________ P-R interval: ____________ QRS complex: ____________

Is there a P wave before every QRS complex? ____

Is there a QRS complex after every P wave? ____

Interpretation: ____

____

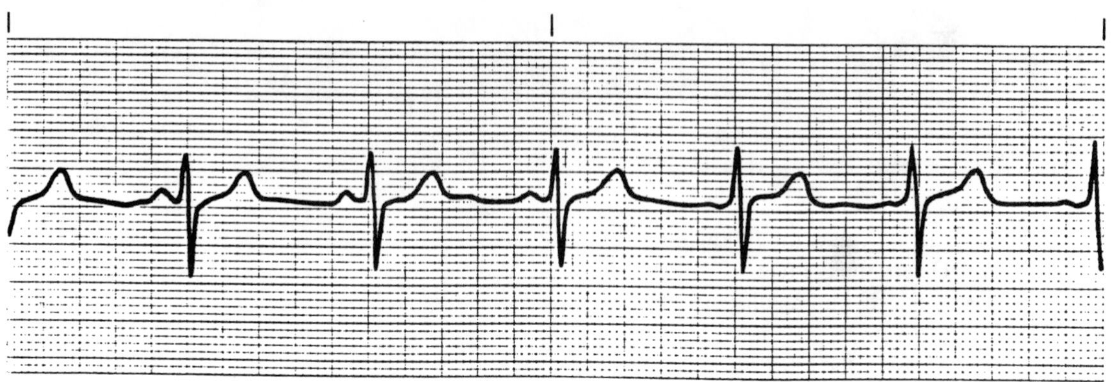

Practice Figure 4-2

Rate: ____________ Rhythm: ____________ P-R interval: ____________ QRS complex: ____________

Is there a P wave before every QRS complex? ____________

Is there a QRS complex after every P wave? ____________

Interpretation: ____________

____

Practice Figure 4-3

Rate: ____________ Rhythm: ____________ P-R interval: ____________ QRS complex: ____________

Is there a P wave before every QRS complex? ____________

Is there a QRS complex after every P wave? ____________

Interpretation: ____________

____

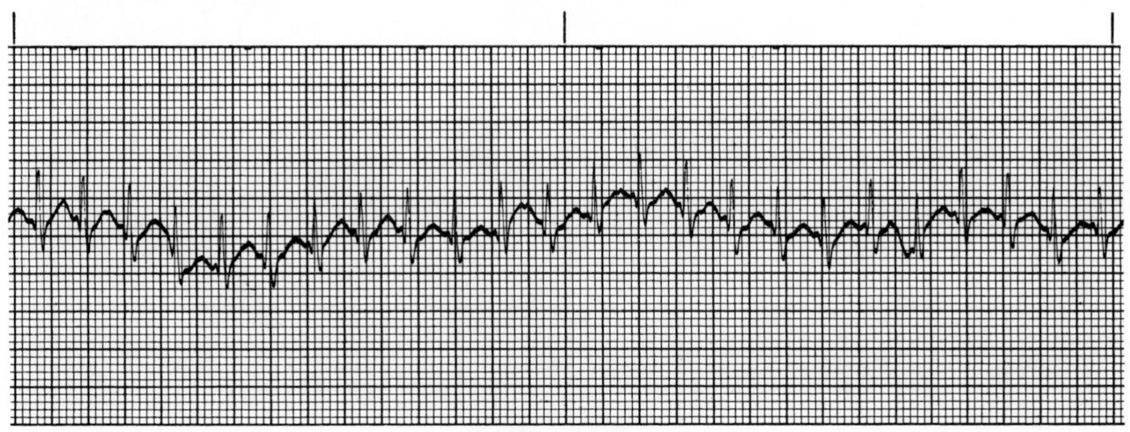

Practice Figure 4-4

Rate: ____________ Rhythm: ____________ P-R interval: ____________ QRS complex: ____________

Is there a P wave before every QRS complex? ________________________________

Is there a QRS complex after every P wave? ________________________________

Interpretation: ________________________________

____

Practice Figure 4-5

Rate: ____________ Rhythm: ____________ P-R interval: ____________ QRS complex: ____________

Is there a P wave before every QRS complex? ________________________________

Is there a QRS complex after every P wave? ________________________________

Interpretation: ________________________________

____

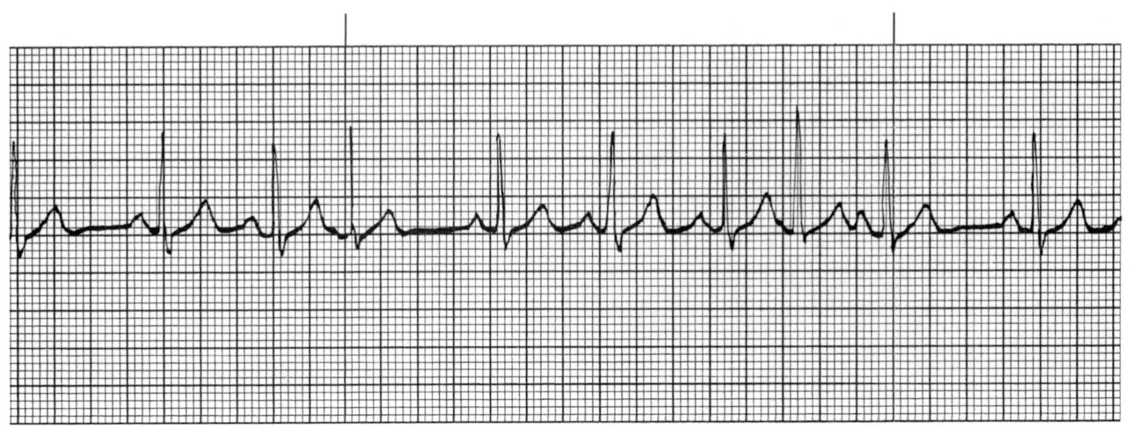

Practice Figure 4-6

Rate: ____________ Rhythm: ____________ P-R interval: ____________ QRS complex: ____________

Is there a P wave before every QRS complex? ____________

Is there a QRS complex after every P wave? ____________

Interpretation: ____________

____

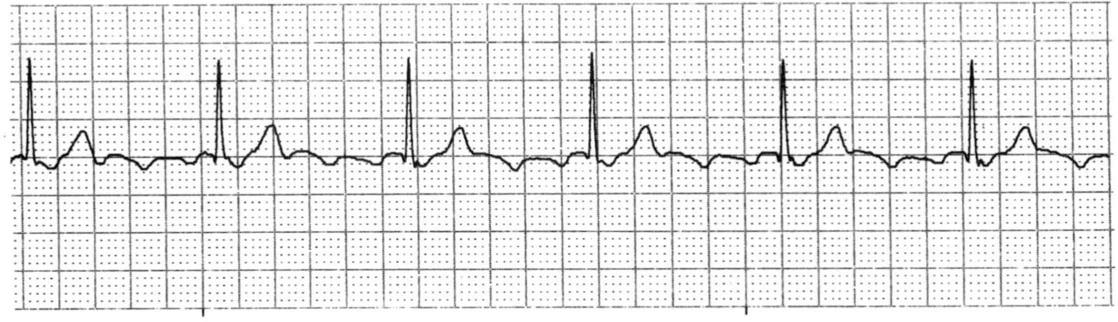

Practice Figure 4-7

Rate: ____________ Rhythm: ____________ P-R interval: ____________ QRS complex: ____________

Is there a P wave before every QRS complex? ____________

Is there a QRS complex after every P wave? ____________

Interpretation: ____________

____

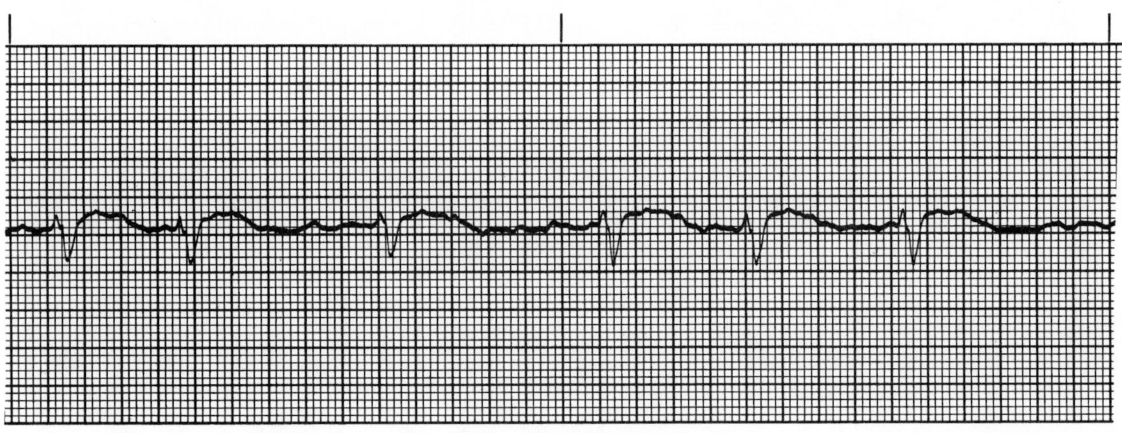

Practice Figure 4-8

Rate: ____________ Rhythm: ____________ P-R interval: ____________ QRS complex: ____________

Is there a P wave before every QRS complex? ____________

Is there a QRS complex after every P wave? ____________

Interpretation: ____________

Practice Figure 4-9

Rate: ____________ Rhythm: ____________ P-R interval: ____________ QRS complex: ____________

Is there a P wave before every QRS complex? ____________

Is there a QRS complex after every P wave? ____________

Interpretation: ____________

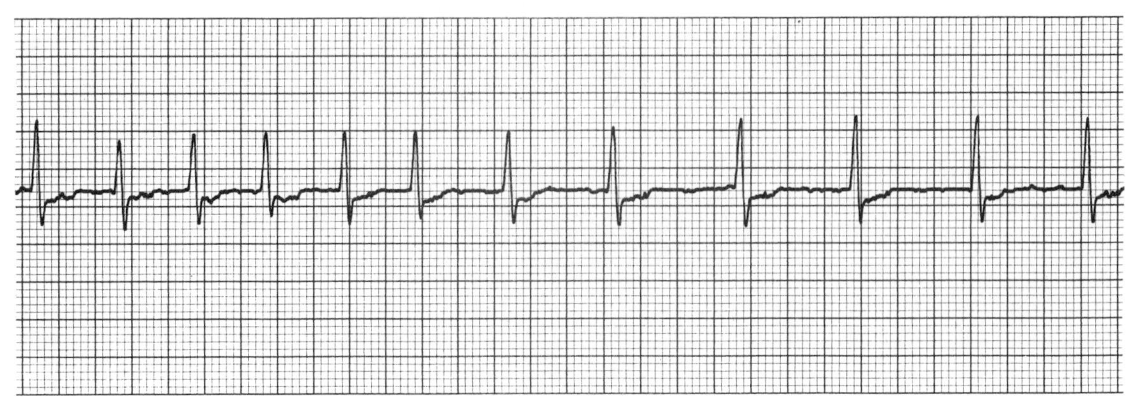

Practice Figure 4-10

Rate: ____________ Rhythm: ____________ P-R interval: ____________ QRS complex: ____________

Is there a P wave before every QRS complex? ____________

Is there a QRS complex after every P wave? ____________

Interpretation: ____________

____

Practice Figure 4-11

Rate: ____________ Rhythm: ____________ P-R interval: ____________ QRS complex: ____________

Is there a P wave before every QRS complex? ____________

Is there a QRS complex after every P wave? ____________

Interpretation: ____________

____

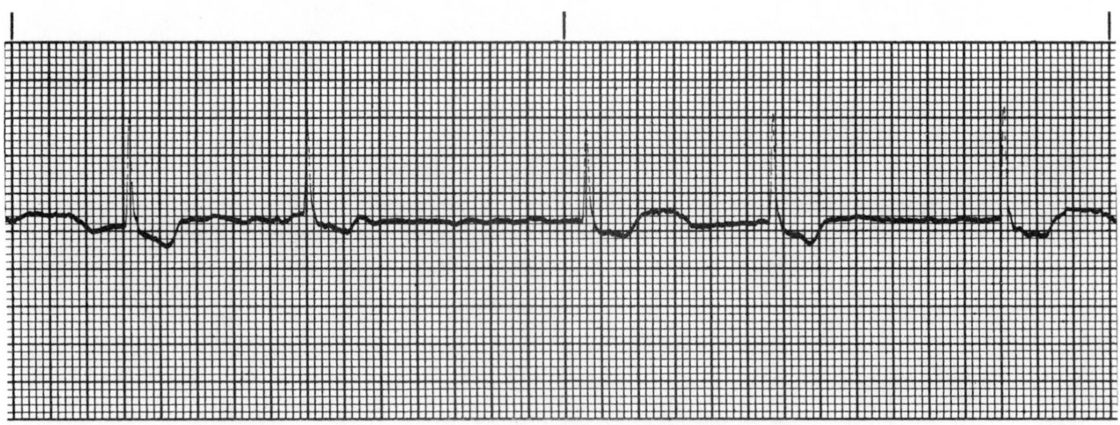

Practice Figure 4-12

Rate: ____________ Rhythm: ____________ P-R interval: ____________ QRS complex: ____________

Is there a P wave before every QRS complex? ____________

Is there a QRS complex after every P wave? ____________

Interpretation: ____________

____

Practice Figure 4-13

Rate: ____________ Rhythm: ____________ P-R interval: ____________ QRS complex: ____________

Is there a P wave before every QRS complex? ____________

Is there a QRS complex after every P wave? ____________

Interpretation: ____________

____

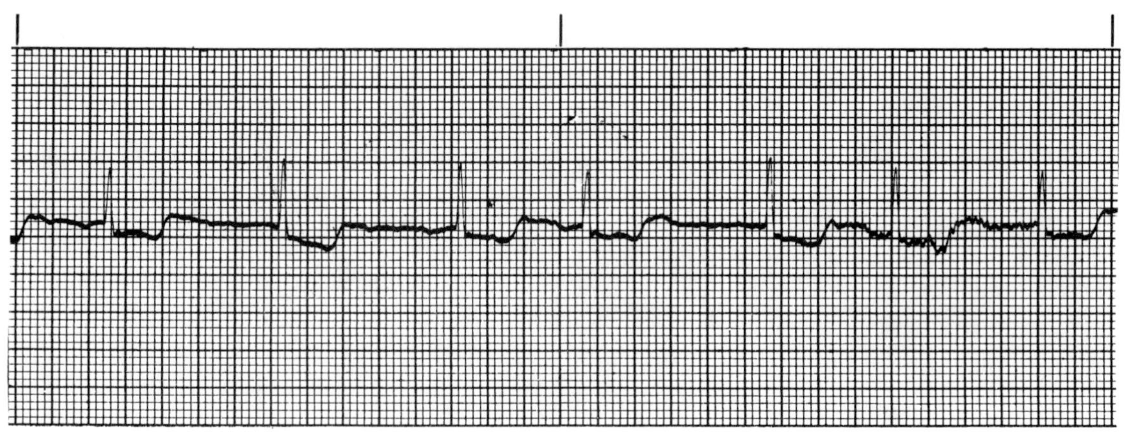

Practice Figure 4-14

Rate: ____________ Rhythm: ____________ P-R interval: ____________ QRS complex: ____________

Is there a P wave before every QRS complex? ____________

Is there a QRS complex after every P wave? ____________

Interpretation: ____________

Practice Figure 4-15

Rate: ____________ Rhythm: ____________ P-R interval: ____________ QRS complex: ____________

Is there a P wave before every QRS complex? ____________

Is there a QRS complex after every P wave? ____________

Interpretation: ____________

Case Scenarios

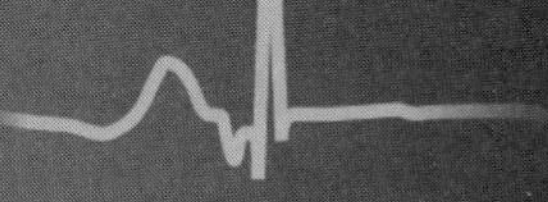

CASE 1

Scenario

Your patient is a 56-year-old man who is complaining of indigestion for the past 3 hours. He states he had lunch, then began not feeling well and became nauseated. His medical history includes non–insulin-dependent diabetes mellitus (NIDDM), arthritis, and angina. Medications include Micronase, ibuprofen, and nitroglycerin SL, as needed. He says this is not the type of angina pain he usually has, and he feels very light-headed. Vital signs are BP, 150/98; P, 158; R, 24, and Sao_2 = 98%. His ECG rhythm is the following:

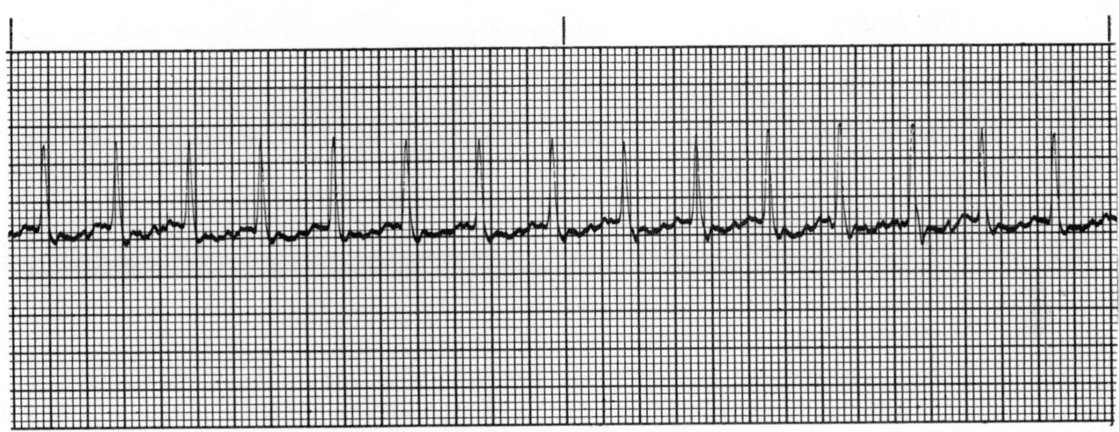

Identify the Rhythm

What is the rate? ____________ What is the rhythm (regular or irregular)? ____________

Is there a P wave before every QRS complex? ____________ Is there a QRS complex after every P wave? ____________

What is the P-R interval? ______________ QRS complex duration? ______________

Interpretation:

____

____

Case 1 Self-Test

In the spaces below give your treatment for the Primary Survey and Secondary Survey, plus the continued care under Oxygen-IV-Monitor-Fluids and Vital Signs. How would you care for this patient and what orders would you expect from the physician? At the bottom list your potential diagnosis or impression of the patient's problem.

Primary Survey	***Secondary Survey***
A.	A.
B.	B.
C.	C.
D.	D.

Oxygen-IV-Monitor-Fluids: ______________________________

____

Vital Signs: ______________________________

____

Your Impression: ______________________________

____

CASE 2

Scenario

You see an 81-year-old woman who is complaining of shortness of breath for the past 2 days, and it is becoming worse today. She has a medical history of CHF, angina, arthritis, and mild COPD. Her medications include nitroglycerin SL, as needed, Lasix, 40 mg/day, potassium, one aspirin per day, and a Proventil inhaler to use as needed. Her vital signs are stable. Lung sounds are decreased breath sounds with wheezes throughout and crackles at the bases. Her ECG strip is the following:

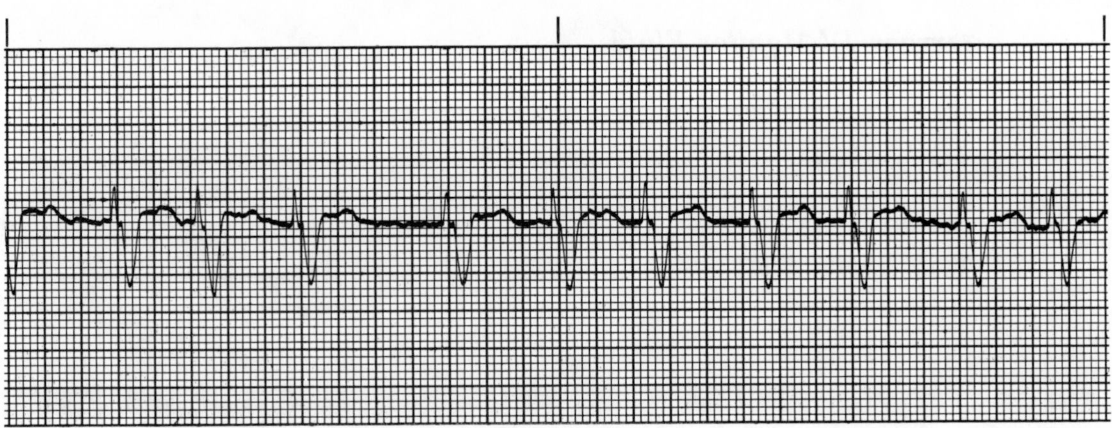

Identify the Rhythm

What is the rate? ____________ What is the rhythm (regular or irregular)? ____________

Is there a P wave before every QRS complex? ____________ Is there a QRS complex after every P wave? ____________

What is the P-R interval? ____________ QRS complex duration? ____________

Interpretation:

____

____

Case 2 Self-Test

In the spaces below give your treatment for the Primary Survey and Secondary Survey, plus the continued care under Oxygen-IV-Monitor-Fluids and Vital Signs. How would you care for this patient and what orders would you expect from the physician? At the bottom list your potential diagnosis or impression of the patient's problem.

Primary Survey

A.

B.

C.

D.

Secondary Survey

A.

B.

C.

D.

Oxygen-IV-Monitor-Fluids: ______________________________

____

Vital Signs: ______________________________

____

Your Impression: ______________________________

____

CASE 3

Scenario

You are called for a 32-year-old woman who had an episode of syncope while shopping. At present she is alert and oriented to person, place, and time only. Her skin is pink, warm, and dry. Lung sounds are clear, and the Sao_2 = 99%. Vital signs are stable. A finger stick reveals a blood sugar level of 104. At present she has no complaints. She is concerned about why she passed out. She tells you she has been working 16-hour days for the past several weeks and has been under a considerable amount of stress. You see the following ECG rhythm on the monitor:

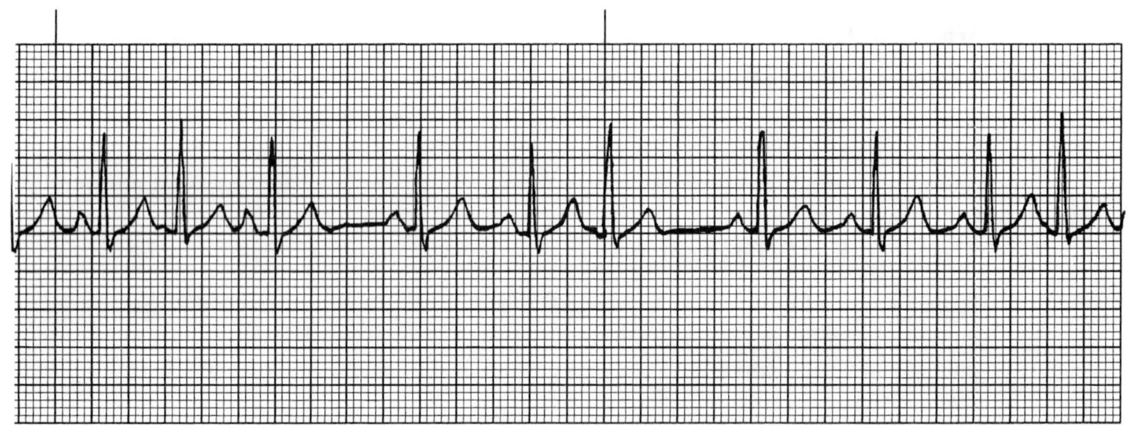

Identify the Rhythm

What is the rate? ____________ What is the rhythm (regular or irregular)? ____________

Is there a P wave before every QRS complex? ____________ Is there a QRS complex after every P wave? ____________

What is the P-R interval? ______________ QRS complex duration? ______________

Interpretation:

____

____

Case 3 Self-Test

In the spaces below give your treatment for the Primary Survey and Secondary Survey, plus the continued care under Oxygen-IV-Monitor-Fluids and Vital Signs. How would you care for this patient and what orders would you expect from the physician? At the bottom list your potential diagnosis or impression of the patient's problem.

Primary Survey

A.

B.

C.

D.

Secondary Survey

A.

B.

C.

D.

Oxygen-IV-Monitor-Fluids: ______________________________

____

Vital Signs: ______________________________

____

Your Impression: ______________________________

____

CASE 4

Scenario

A man comes into the emergency department carrying his 49-year-old wife. They were out walking, when she began to race him up a hill. Shortly after, she collapsed. At present she is awake but not alert. There is nothing in her medical history, and she does not take any medications. Her husband tells you she did eat her regular meals today. Her vital signs are BP, 96/50; P, rapid and weak; R, 22; and Sao_2 = 96%. Her lung sounds are clear. Her husband tells you that his wife has been under a lot of stress at work in addition to putting in long hours at her church for the past few weeks. This is why they decided to walk today, just to relax. You see the following on the monitor:

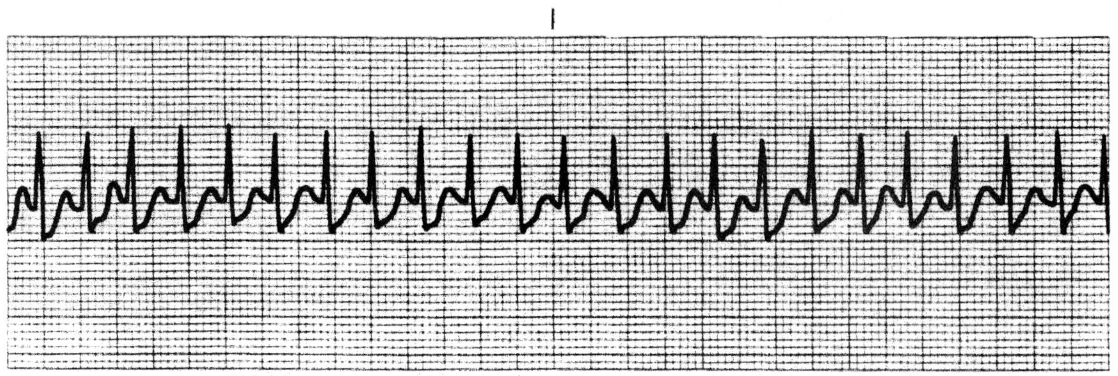

Identify the Rhythm

What is the rate? ____________ What is the rhythm (regular or irregular)? ____________

Is there a P wave before every QRS complex? ____________ Is there a QRS complex after every P wave? ____________

What is the P-R interval? ______________ QRS complex duration? ______________

Interpretation:

____

____

Case 4 Self-Test

In the spaces below give your treatment for the Primary Survey and Secondary Survey, plus the continued care under Oxygen-IV-Monitor-Fluids and Vital Signs. How would you care for this patient and what orders would you expect from the physician? At the bottom list your potential diagnosis or impression of the patient's problem.

Primary Survey

A.

B.

C.

D.

Secondary Survey

A.

B.

C.

D.

Oxygen-IV-Monitor-Fluids: ______________________________

____

Vital Signs: ______________________________

____

Your Impression: ______________________________

____

CASE 5

Scenario

Mary, a 22-year-old woman, was on her way to work at the local hospital when she suddenly could not catch her breath. She pulled over and then slumped over the wheel of the car. When you arrive, you find her conscious but definitely not alert. She appears very groggy but tells you she has not been drinking and does not take any drugs, plus there is nothing in her medical history. Her vital signs are BP, 94/60; P, very weak and rapid; R, 26; and Sao_2 = 97%. You see the following ECG rhythm:

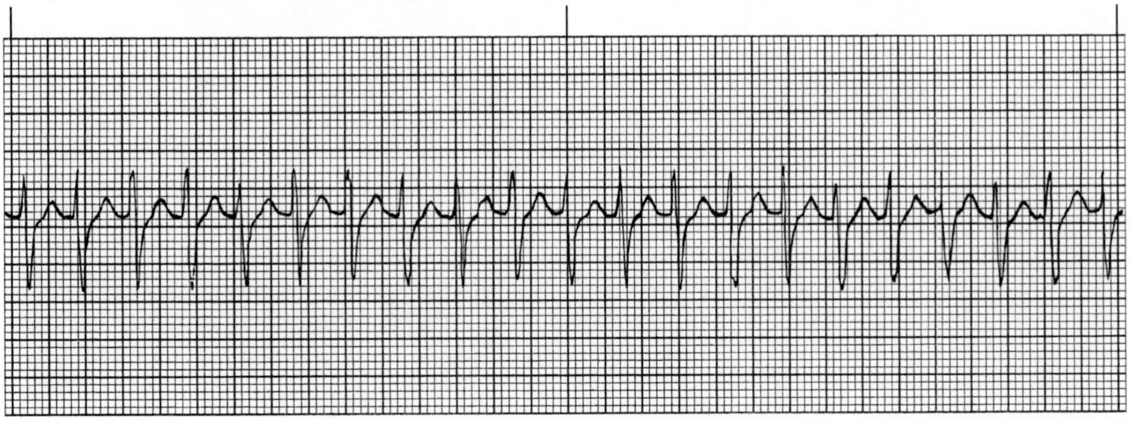

Identify the Rhythm

What is the rate? ____________ What is the rhythm (regular or irregular)? ____________

Is there a P wave before every QRS complex? ____________ Is there a QRS complex after every P wave? ____________

What is the P-R interval? ____________ QRS complex duration? ____________

Interpretation:

____

____

Case 5 Self-Test

In the spaces below give your treatment for the Primary Survey and Secondary Survey, plus the continued care under Oxygen-IV-Monitor-Fluids and Vital Signs. How would you care for this patient and what orders would you expect from the physician? At the bottom list your potential diagnosis or impression of the patient's problem.

Primary Survey

A.

B.

C.

D.

Secondary Survey

A.

B.

C.

D.

Oxygen-IV-Monitor-Fluids: ____________________

____

Vital Signs: ____________________

____

Your Impression: ____________________

____

5

Junctional Rhythms

OBJECTIVES

By the end of this chapter, the student will be able to do the following:

- **Explain the ECG characteristics of the following junctional rhythms:**
  - **Junctional rhythm**
  - **Accelerated junctional rhythm**
  - **Premature junctional complex**
  - **Junctional tachycardia**
- **Describe the signs, symptoms, and treatment of the following:**
  - **Junctional rhythm**
  - **Accelerated junctional rhythm**
  - **Premature junctional complex**
  - **Junctional tachycardia**

OUTLINE

Junctional rhythms originate at the AV node, the bundle of His, and the area around the AV node. The AV node is located in the lower portion of the right atrium. The bundle of His is located in the upper part of the interventricular septum. The bundle of His connects the AV with the bundle branches. The AV junction basically contains the AV node and the top (nonbranching part) of the bundle of His. When the SA node fails to fire, the AV junction or the bundle of His may become the dominant pacemaker site; this is called a *junctional escape beat*. When they take over, the impulses fire at a rate of only 40 to 60 beats per minute. Also note that when the AV junction and bundle of His acquire control, the impulses travel up to the atria and down to the ventricles. If they travel backward to the atria, this is known as *retrograde conduction*. When the impulses travel forward to the ventricles, it is known as *antegrade conduction*. With junctional rhythms the P waves are usually negative deflection, and they may be before, during, or after the QRS complex. The P waves may be completely absent. Where the P wave occurs depends on several factors:

- *Retrograde conduction*. The impulse travels up to the atria first; thus the P wave occurs before the QRS complex.
- *Antegrade conduction*. The impulse travels down to the ventricles first; then the P wave follows the QRS complex.
- If both atrial and ventricular conduction occur at the same time, the P wave is hidden in the QRS complex.
- If the atria are not stimulated at all, the P wave is absent.

The ability of the AV junction to initiate impulses, thus producing a junctional rhythm, acts as a safety mechanism to prevent cardiac standstill. The AV junction takes over if the SA node fails to send an electrical impulse or if the impulse is blocked.

Junctional rhythms may be caused by the following:

- Disease of the SA node, such as sick sinus syndrome
- Acute myocardial infarction
- Valvular disease
- Rheumatic fever
- Digitalis toxicity
- Increased vagal tone in patients

Patients who have undergone surgical procedures for heart disease may also experience junctional rhythms.

The patient may be symptom free or may show the signs and symptoms of reduced cardiac output (e.g., chest pain, shortness of breath, hypotension, syncope, and altered level of consciousness). Again, assessing your patient is the most important factor, not just interpreting the ECG rhythm on the monitor.

JUNCTIONAL RHYTHM

This is a rhythm originating in the AV junction and is known as a *safety mechanism* or an *escape rhythm* (Figure 5-1). The pacemaker rate is 40 to 60 beats per minute. If the junctional rhythm has a rate greater than 60 beats per minute, it is an accelerated junctional rhythm. P waves may or may not be present and are usually negative deflection or inverted if present (Box 5-1).

Treatment depends on the patient and any signs and symptoms of reduced cardiac output. Usually with a junctional rhythm, treatment is not needed. If, however, treatment is needed, it includes a 0.5- to 1.0-mg atropine IV push and possibly a transcutaneous pacer along with dopamine and epinephrine IV, to increase the heart rate, or possibly a permanent pacemaker, to ensure adequate cardiac output.

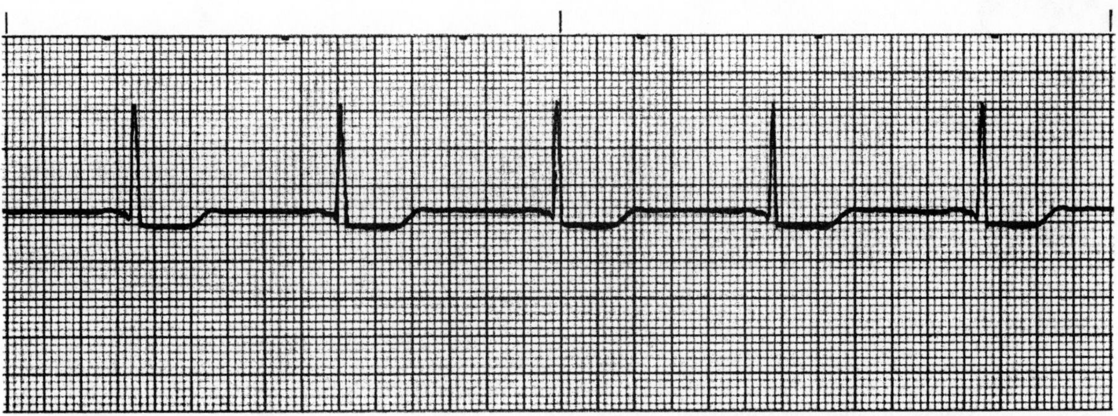

Figure 5-1 Junctional rhythm.

Box 5-1 Junctional Rhythm

Rate: 40-60 beats per minute
Rhythm: Atrial and ventricular are regular
P waves: Usually inverted; may be before, during, or after the QRS complex
P-R interval: If P waves occur before the QRS complex, the PR interval is shortened; if the P wave occurs during or after the QRS complex the P-R interval cannot be measured
QRS complex: Configuration and duration are within normal limits, but a P wave is not always present before every QRS complex; the duration of the QRS complex is less than 0.10 second

Accelerated Junctional Rhythm

An accelerated junctional rhythm originates in the bundle of His or in the junctional tissue and fires impulses at a rate of 60 to 100 beats per minute (Figure 5-2, Box 5-2).

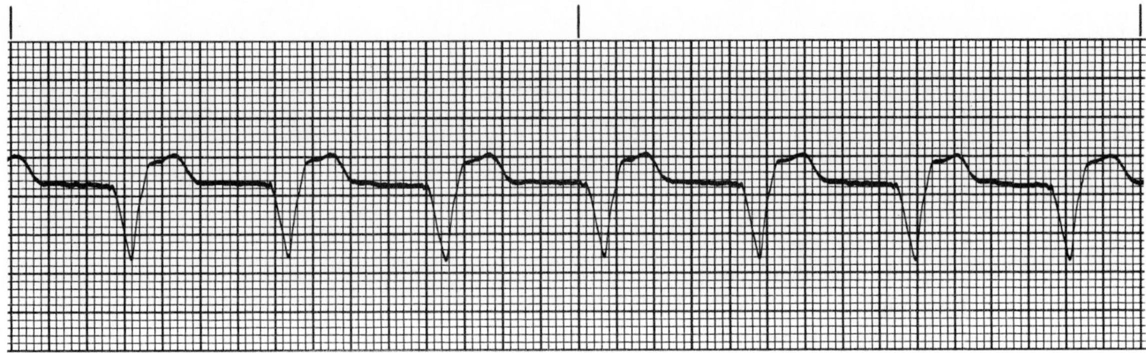

Figure 5-2 Accelerated junctional rhythm.

Box 5-2 Accelerated Junctional Rhythm

Rate: 60-100 beats per minute
Rhythm: Atrial and ventricular are regular
P waves: May be before, during, or after the QRS complex and are usually inverted; P waves may also be absent
P-R interval: If the P wave falls before the QRS complex, the P-R interval is shortened less than 0.12 second; if the P wave occurs during or after the QRS complex, the P-R interval is not measurable
QRS complex: Usually normal configuration and duration, less than 0.10 second

Causes

Causes include the following:

- Hypoxia
- Increased parasympathetic tone (increased vagal tone)
- SA node disease
- Medications such as beta blockers and calcium channel blockers
- Digitalis toxicity

An accelerated junctional rhythm can sometimes be found in patients immediately after a cardiac operation.

Treatment

Treatment is needed if the patient shows signs of a reduced heart rate and reduced cardiac output. Such signs include hypotension, syncope, weakness, chest pain or pressure, shortness of breath, and an altered level of consciousness.

Treatment includes a 0.5- to 1.0-mg atropine IV push up to a maximum dose of 0.04 mg/kg. Treatment may also include transcutaneous pacing, a dopamine IV and an epinephrine IV, or a permanent pacemaker.

Premature Junctional Contraction

A premature junctional contraction (PJC) is an early beat that occurs before the next expected sinus beat (Figure 5-3). The focus or origin is at the AV junction or the bundle of His. When the impulse begins in the bundle of His and travels down to the ventricles first, the P wave is seen after the QRS complex. If the impulse travels up to the atria at the same time it travels to the ventricles, then the P wave falls in the QRS complex and is not visible (Box 5-3).

Causes

A PJC is a single beat, not an extra rhythm, so you will need to identify the underlying rhythm. PJCs are not common, but when they are present, it is usually due to any of the following:

- Digitalis toxicity
- Increased vagal tone
- Myocardial infarction
- Excessive caffeine
- Amphetamine ingestion
- Ischemia
- Congestive heart failure
- Valvular disease
- Rheumatic heart disease

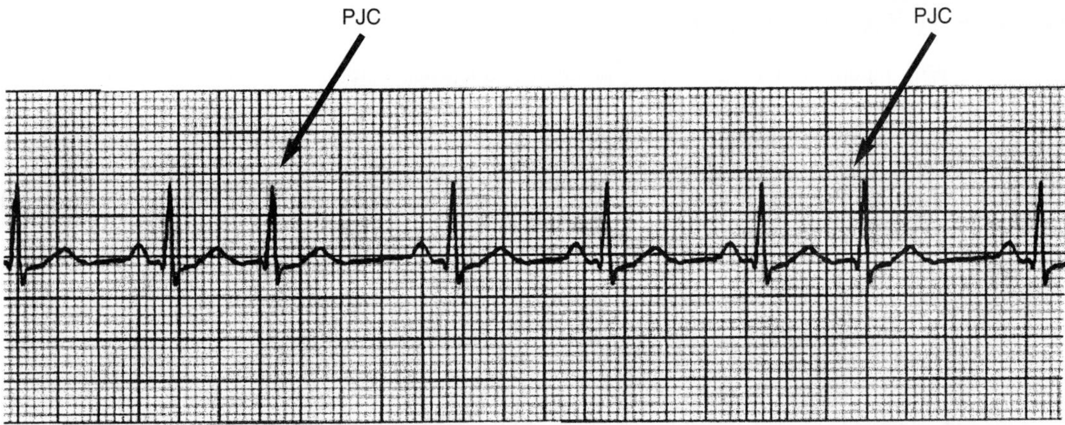

Figure 5-3 Premature junctional contractions (PJCs).

Box 5-3 Premature Junctional Contraction

Rate: Depends on the underlying rhythm, but usually normal
Rhythm: Underlying rhythm may be regular, but an irregular rhythm is noted during the PJCs
P waves: May occur before, during, or after the QRS complex and are usually inverted
P-R interval: If there is a P wave before the QRS complex, the P-R interval is shortened; if the P wave is during or after the QRS complex it cannot be measured
QRS complex: Configuration and duration are usually normal, less than 0.10 second; a P wave does not always occur before every QRS complex

PJC, Premature junctional contraction.

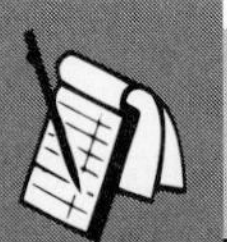

Note

A PJC is a single beat, not an entire rhythm, so you still need to identify the underlying rhythm.

Treatment

The significance of PJCs depends on the patients and their underlying medical problems. Typically, PJCs are unusual in young, healthy patients and if seen are considered harmless, unless more than six occur per minute. Usually PJCs do not require treatment. If the patient is showing signs and symptoms of decreased cardiac output or palpitations, then atropine or cardiac pacing may be needed. Management depends on the underlying rhythm and the cause of the PJCs.

Junctional Tachycardia

With junctional tachycardia the preceding junctional parameters remain the same as seen in a junctional rhythm, but the ventricular rate is greater than 100 beats per minute (Figure 5-4). The usual range is 101 to 180 beats per minute (Box 5-4). The rhythm originates in the bundle of His and is usually due to enhanced automaticity. Junctional tachycardia is described as three or more premature beats in a row. The rhythm may also be a paroxysmal junctional tachycardia, which means it *suddenly starts* and *suddenly stops*.

Causes

Causes of junctional tachycardia include the following:

- Ischemia
- MI
- Hypoxia
- Acute rheumatic fever
- Hypotension
- CHF
- Cardiogenic shock
- Cardiomyopathy
- Myocarditis
- Vagal stimulation
- Valve replacement

Treatment

Treatment is not usually necessary, unless the rate is more than 150 beats per minute or the patient has symptoms of decreased cardiac output. Treatment would be aimed at managing the underlying cause. Drug therapy may include digitalis, verapamil or propranolol, and adenosine. Other measures used are cardioversion and vagal maneuvers, such as carotid sinus massage (Algorithm 4-1, Narrow Complex Tachycardia).

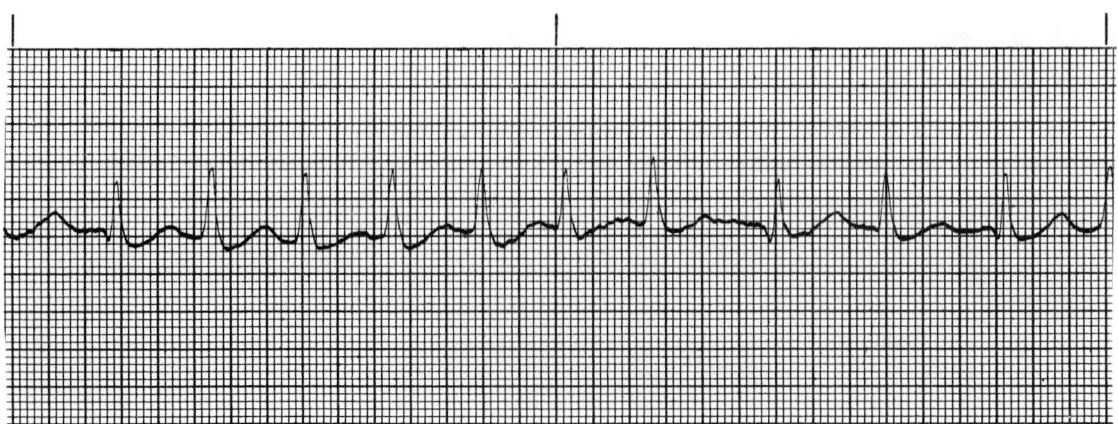

Figure 5-4 Junctional tachycardia.

Box 5-4 Junctional Tachycardia

Rate: 101-180 beats per minute
Rhythm: Usually regular, both atrial and ventricular
P waves: May occur before, during, or after the QRS complex and are usually inverted
P-R interval: If there is a P wave before the QRS complex, the P-R interval is shortened and the duration is less than 0.10 second; if the P wave is during or after the QRS complex, the P-R interval cannot be measured
QRS complex: Usually of normal configuration and duration, less than 0.10 second; there is not always a P wave before every QRS complex

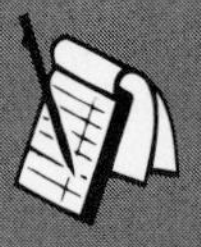

Note

If you are going to perform carotid massage, first check for carotid bruits. You do not want to dislodge plaque and cause an MI or a stroke.

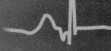

Chapter 5 Self-Test

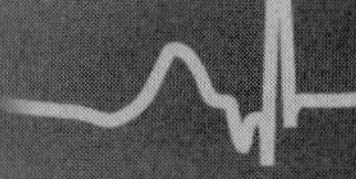

1. Fill in the Blank: A junctional rhythm has a rate of __________________ to __________________ .

2. Circle the Correct Word: A junctional rhythm is usually *regular/irregular*.

3. True or False: A rhythm with a premature junctional contraction usually has no R-R interval that is regular except for the premature beat.

4. Fill in the Blank: In junctional rhythms, the pacemaker site is in the __________________ __________________.

5. Fill in the blank: The P-R interval of a junctional rhythm, if present, is less than __________________ seconds.

6. List four common causes for PJCs and junctional rhythms:

   ____

   ____

   ____

   ____

7. Circle the Correct Word: A rhythm with PJCs *seldom/often* produces clinical symptoms.

8. Fill in the Blank: A sinus rhythm with PJCs usually has a rate of __________________ to __________________ beats per minute.

9. Fill in the Blank: __________________ conduction through the atria causes an inverted P wave in a junctional rhythm.

10. Fill in the Blank: A rate of 60 to 100 beats per minute is found in a/an __________________ junctional rhythm.

11. Fill in the Blank: A rate of 101 to 180 beats per minute is found in a junctional __________________ .

12. Fill in the Blank: In a junctional __________________ complex, the SA node fails to fire intermittently and the AV junction takes over as a protective mechanism.

13. Fill in the Blank: A junctional escape rhythm usually has an R-to-R rate of ________________ to ________________ beats per minute.

14. Fill in the Blank: Ventricular fibrillation or ventricular tachycardia may result from this junctional rhythm: ____

15. List the three possible places to find a P wave in a junctional rhythm:

    ____

    ____

    ____

ECG Practice Strips

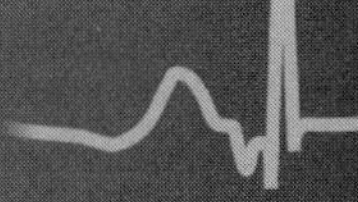

Please calculate the following 15 ECG practice strips:

- Determine the rate.
- Is the rhythm regular or irregular?
- Measure the P-R interval.
- Measure the QRS complex duration.
- Check to see if there is a P wave *before* every QRS complex.
- Check to see if there a QRS complex *after* every P wave.
- Then give your interpretation of the rhythm.
- All strips are lead II unless otherwise noted.

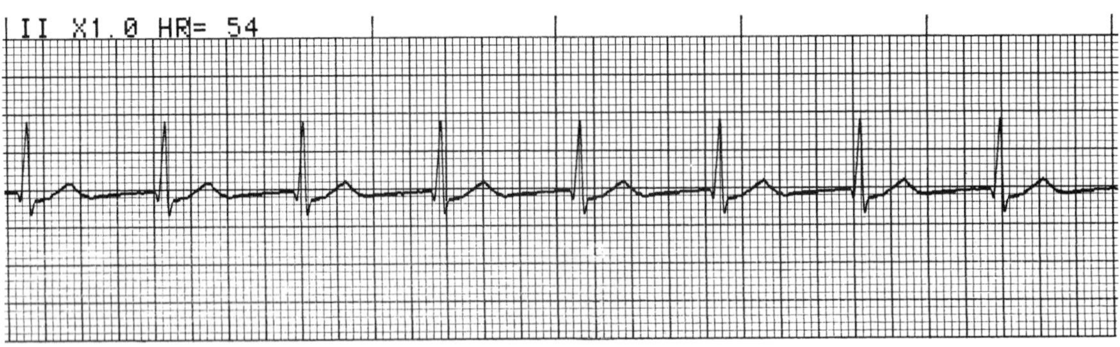

Practice Figure 5-1

Rate: ____________ Rhythm: ____________ P-R interval: ____________ QRS complex: ____________

Is there a P wave before every QRS complex? ______________________________

Is there a QRS complex after every P wave? ______________________________

Interpretation: ______________________________

____

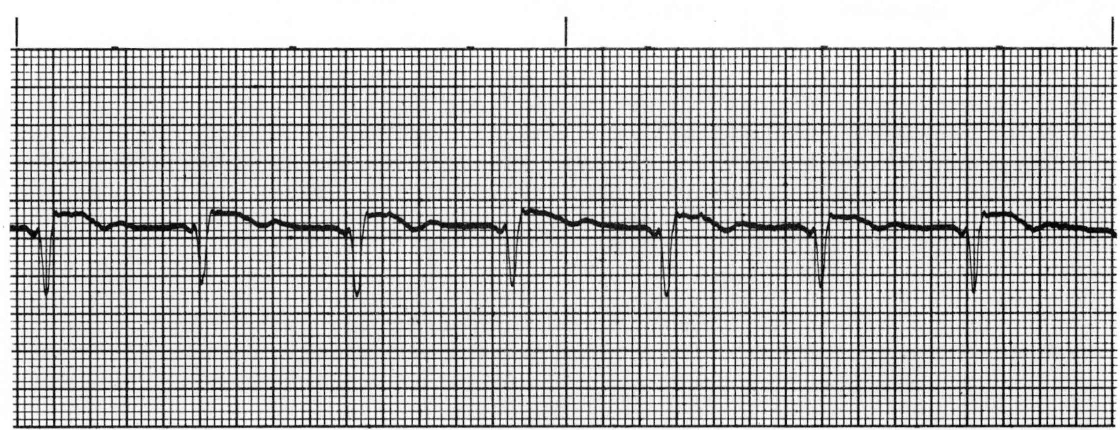

Practice Figure 5-2

Rate: ____________ Rhythm: ____________ P-R interval: ____________ QRS complex: ____________

Is there a P wave before every QRS complex? ______________________________

Is there a QRS complex after every P wave? ______________________________

Interpretation: ______________________________

____

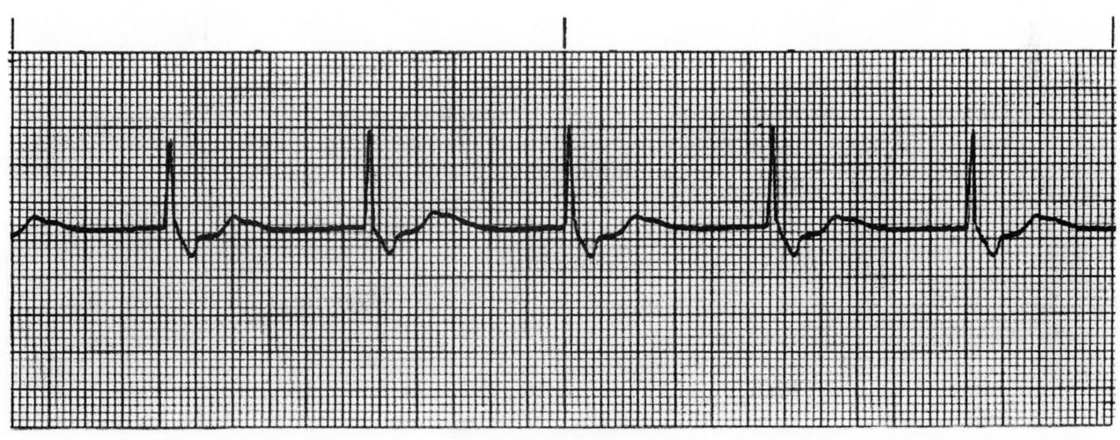

Practice Figure 5-3

Rate: ____________ Rhythm: ____________ P-R interval: ____________ QRS complex: ____________

Is there a P wave before every QRS complex? ______________________________

Is there a QRS complex after every P wave? ______________________________

Interpretation: ______________________________

____

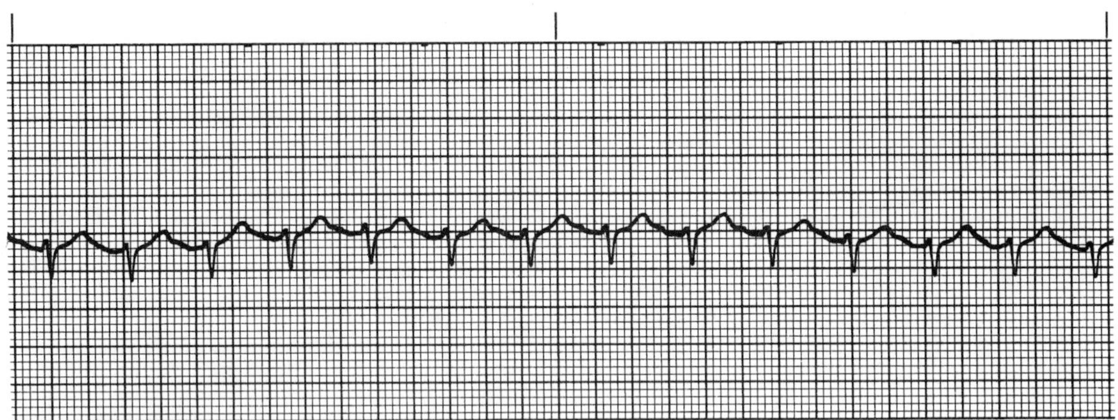

Practice Figure 5-4

Rate: __________ Rhythm: __________ P-R interval: __________ QRS complex: __________

Is there a P wave before every QRS complex? __________

Is there a QRS complex after every P wave? __________

Interpretation: __________

Practice Figure 5-5

Rate: __________ Rhythm: __________ P-R interval: __________ QRS complex: __________

Is there a P wave before every QRS complex? __________

Is there a QRS complex after every P wave? __________

Interpretation: __________

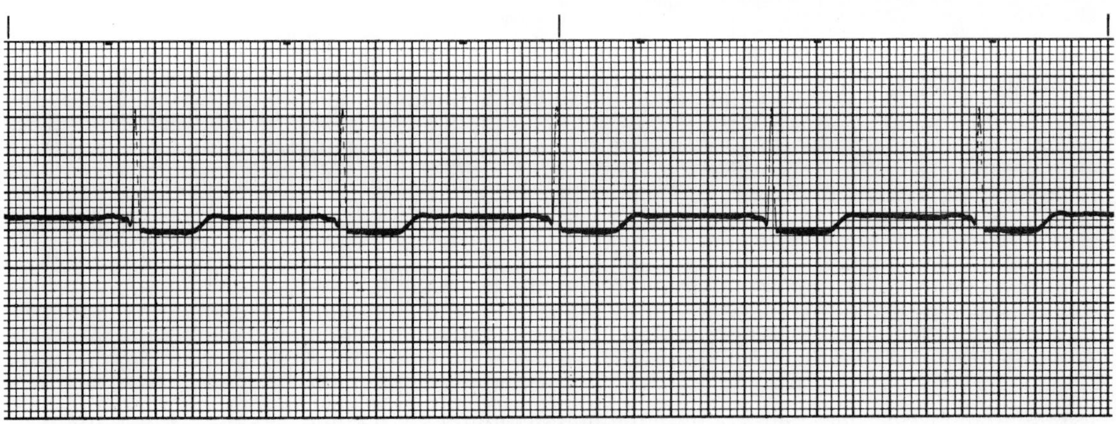

Practice Figure 5-6

Rate: ____________ Rhythm: ____________ P-R interval: ____________ QRS complex: ____________

Is there a P wave before every QRS complex? ____________

Is there a QRS complex after every P wave? ____________

Interpretation: ____________

____

Practice Figure 5-7

Rate: ____________ Rhythm: ____________ P-R interval: ____________ QRS complex: ____________

Is there a P wave before every QRS complex? ____________

Is there a QRS complex after every P wave? ____________

Interpretation: ____________

____

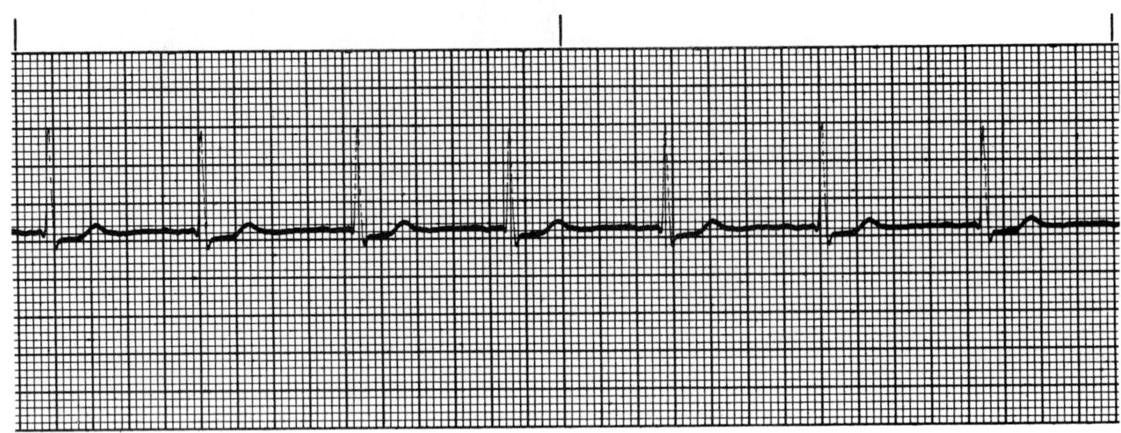

Practice Figure 5-8

Rate: ____________ Rhythm: ____________ P-R interval: ____________ QRS complex: ____________

Is there a P wave before every QRS complex? ____________

Is there a QRS complex after every P wave? ____________

Interpretation: ____________

____

Practice Figure 5-9

Rate: ____________ Rhythm: ____________ P-R interval: ____________ QRS complex: ____________

Is there a P wave before every QRS complex? ____________

Is there a QRS complex after every P wave? ____________

Interpretation: ____________

____

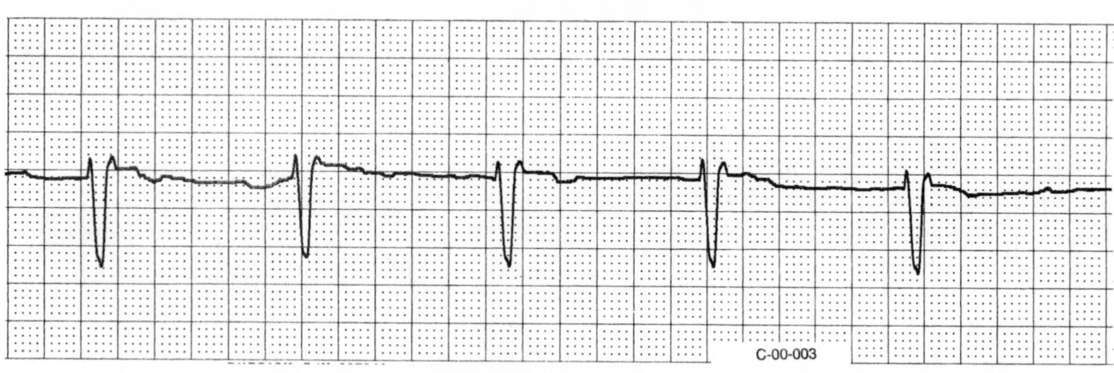

Practice Figure 5-10

Rate: ____________ Rhythm: ____________ P-R interval: ____________ QRS complex: ____________

Is there a P wave before every QRS complex? ____________

Is there a QRS complex after every P wave? ____________

Interpretation: ____________

____

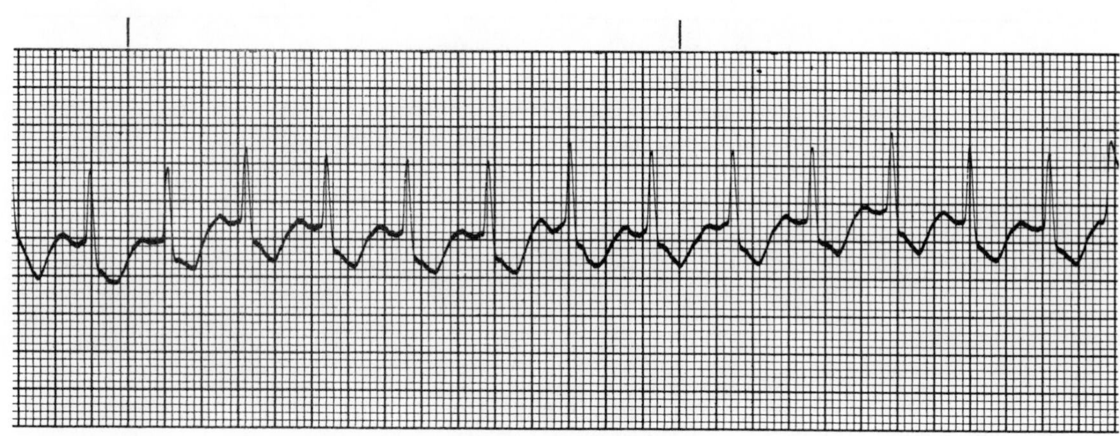

Practice Figure 5-11

Rate: ____________ Rhythm: ____________ P-R interval: ____________ QRS complex: ____________

Is there a P wave before every QRS complex? ____________

Is there a QRS complex after every P wave? ____________

Interpretation: ____________

____

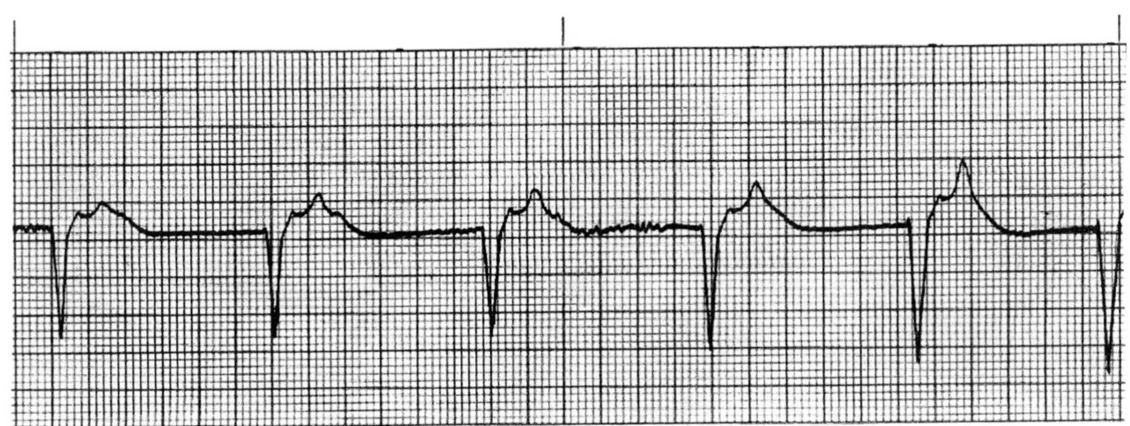

Practice Figure 5-12

Rate: ______ Rhythm: ______ P-R interval: ______ QRS complex: ______

Is there a P wave before every QRS complex? ______

Is there a QRS complex after every P wave? ______

Interpretation: ______

______

Practice Figure 5-13

Rate: ______ Rhythm: ______ P-R interval: ______ QRS complex: ______

Is there a P wave before every QRS complex? ______

Is there a QRS complex after every P wave? ______

Interpretation: ______

______

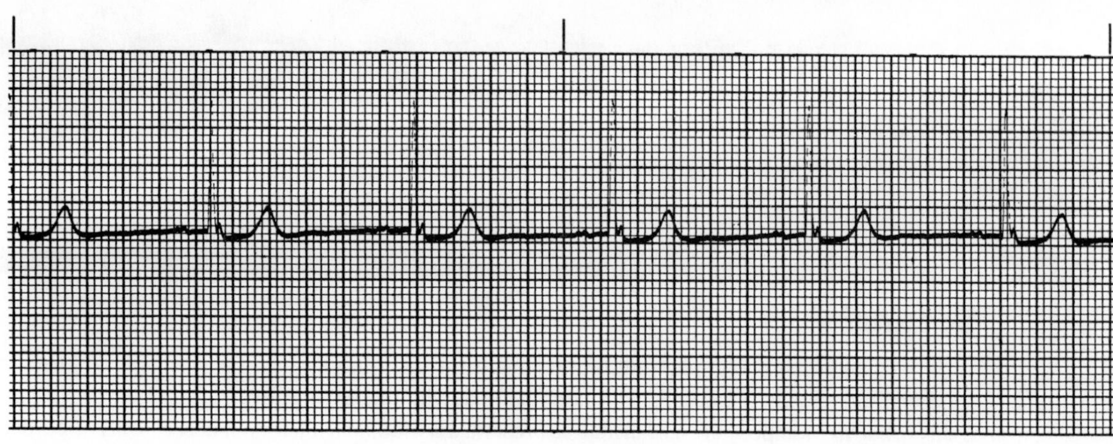

Practice Figure 5-14

Rate: ____________ Rhythm: ____________ P-R interval: ____________ QRS complex: ____________

Is there a P wave before every QRS complex? ____________

Is there a QRS complex after every P wave? ____________

Interpretation: ____________

Practice Figure 5-15

Rate: ____________ Rhythm: ____________ P-R interval: ____________ QRS complex: ____________

Is there a P wave before every QRS complex? ____________

Is there a QRS complex after every P wave? ____________

Interpretation: ____________

Case Scenarios

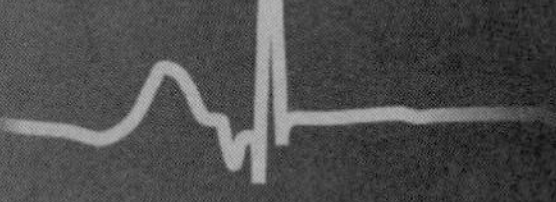

CASE 1

Scenario

A 41-year-old man is complaining that he has been vomiting all day. He is unable to keep any food or fluids down. He denies any pain and states he did have a fever off and on for the past 2 days, but his temperature is normal at present. His medical history includes only rheumatic fever as a child. He is taking no medications. Vital signs are BP, 112/60; P, 52; and R, 20. You see the following on the monitor:

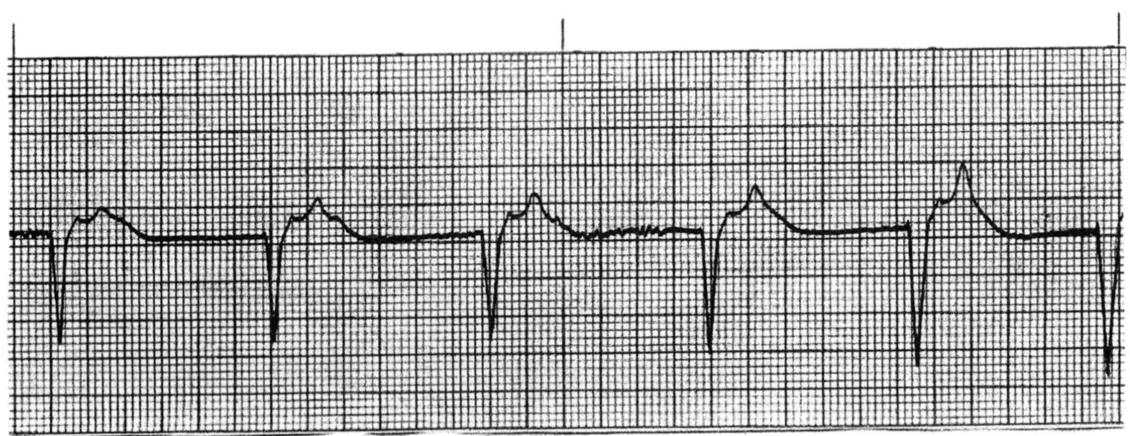

Identify the Rhythm

What is the rate? ____________ What is the rhythm (regular or irregular)? ____________

Is there a P wave before every QRS complex? ____________ Is there a QRS complex after every P wave? ____________

What is the P-R interval? ____________ QRS complex duration? ____________

Interpretation:

____

____

Case 1 Self-Test

In the spaces below give your treatment for the Primary Survey and the Secondary Survey, plus the continued care under Oxygen-IV-Monitor-Fluids and Vital Signs. How would you care for this patient, and what orders would you expect from the physician? At the bottom, list your potential diagnosis or impression of what the patient's problem is.

Primary Survey

A.

B.

C.

D.

Secondary Survey

A.

B.

C.

D.

Oxygen-IV-Monitor-Fluids: ______________________________

____

Vital Signs: ______________________________

____

Your Impression: ______________________________

____

CASE 2

Scenario

A 47-year-old woman comes into the emergency department complaining of epigastric discomfort accompanied with slight chest discomfort. She says she has been working extra hours at the office lately, she has had a recent divorce, and her mother died 3 months ago. She has nothing in her medical history and no known allergies. Vital signs are BP, 104/62; P, 72; R, 20; and Sao_2 = 99%. You see the following on the monitor:

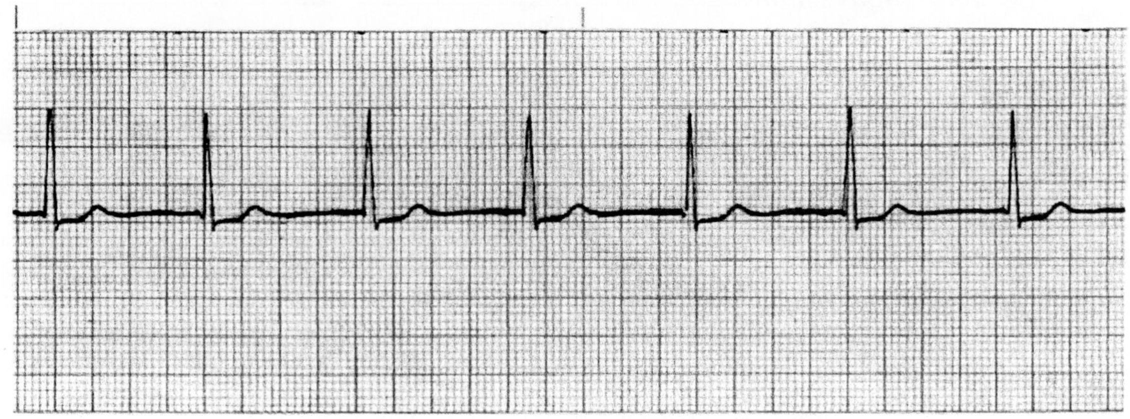

Identify the Rhythm

What is the rate? ______________ What is the rhythm (regular or irregular)? ______________

Is there a P wave before every QRS complex? ______________ Is there a QRS complex after every P wave? ______________

What is the P-R interval? ______________ QRS complex duration? ______________

Interpretation:

____

____

Case 2 Self-Test

In the spaces below give your treatment for the Primary Survey and the Secondary Survey, plus the continued care under Oxygen-IV-Monitor-Fluids and Vital Signs. How would you care for this patient, and what orders would you expect from the physician? At the bottom, list your potential diagnosis or impression of what the patient's problem is.

Primary Survey	***Secondary Survey***
A.	A.
B.	B.
C.	C.
D.	D.

Oxygen-IV-Monitor-Fluids: ____

____

Vital Signs: ____

____

Your Impression: ____

____

CASE 3

Scenario

A 67-year-old woman comes in by EMS after being in a one-car motor vehicle crash. She was driving at 40 mph with a seat belt on when her car skidded on a patch of ice. She tells you she felt faint just before skidding on the ice. She has bruising across her chest from the seat belt and is complaining of pain in the right forearm. She did not lose consciousness and is fully immobilized. She has nothing in her medical history, but says she has had chest pressure for the past several days. She has no known allergies. Vital signs are BP, 122/74; P, 93; R, 18; and Sao_2 = 100%. You see the following on the monitor:

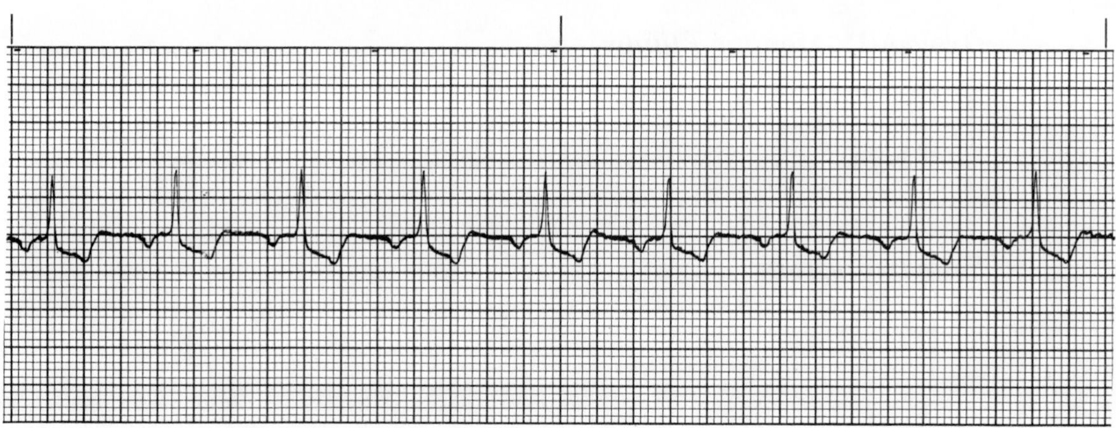

Identify the Rhythm

What is the rate? ____________ What is the rhythm (regular or irregular)? ____________

Is there a P wave before every QRS complex? ____________ Is there a QRS complex after every P wave? ____________

What is the P-R interval? ______________ QRS complex duration? ______________

Interpretation:

____

____

Case 3 Self-Test

In the spaces below give your treatment for the Primary Survey and the Secondary Survey, plus the continued care under Oxygen-IV-Monitor-Fluids and Vital Signs. How would you care for this patient, and what orders would you expect from the physician? At the bottom, list your potential diagnosis or impression of what the patient's problem is.

Primary Survey

A.

B.

C.

D.

Secondary Survey

A.

B.

C.

D.

Oxygen-IV-Monitor-Fluids: ______________________________

____

Vital Signs: ______________________________

____

Your Impression: ______________________________

____

CASE 4

Scenario

An 89-year-old woman is brought in by ambulance. She has been disoriented for the past 2 days, and her blood glucose level is elevated. She has a history of CHF, polio as a child, and arthritis. Her medications include Lanoxin, Lasix, potassium, Diflucan, and one baby aspirin per day, but she cannot remember if she has taken them. She has no known allergies and is somewhat nauseated at this moment. Vital signs are BP, 192/106; P, 142; R, 24; and Sao_2 = 94%. You see the following on the monitor:

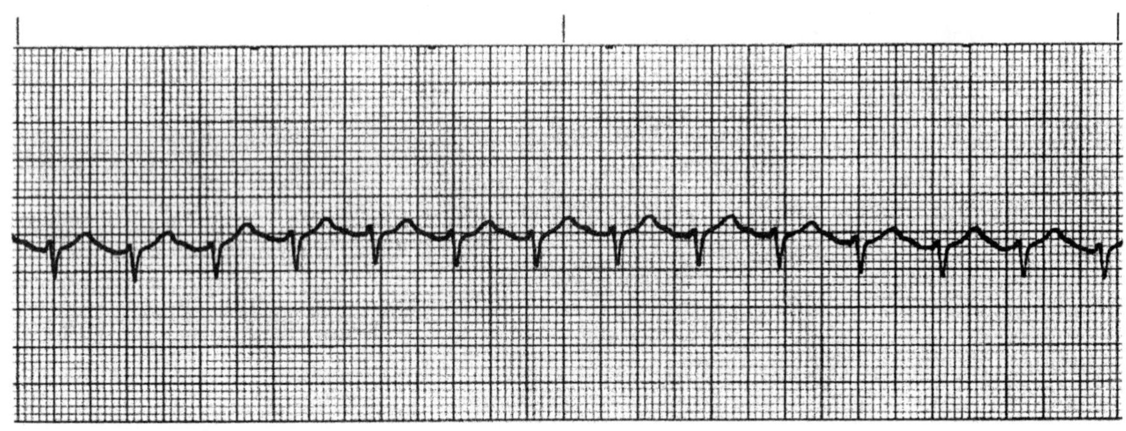

Identify the Rhythm

What is the rate? ______________ What is the rhythm (regular or irregular)? ______________

Is there a P wave before every QRS complex? ______________ Is there a QRS complex after every P wave? ______________

What is the P-R interval? ______________ QRS complex duration? ______________

Interpretation:

____

____

Case 4 Self-Test

In the spaces below give your treatment for the Primary Survey and the Secondary Survey, plus the continued care under Oxygen-IV-Monitor-Fluids and Vital Signs. How would you care for this patient, and what orders would you expect from the physician? At the bottom, list your potential diagnosis or impression of what the patient's problem is.

Primary Survey	***Secondary Survey***
A.	A.
B.	B.
C.	C.
D.	D.

Oxygen-IV-Monitor-Fluids: ______________________________

____

Vital Signs: ______________________________

____

Your Impression: ______________________________

____

CASE 5

Scenario

The patient comes to your emergency department with chest pain for the past 2 days, accompanied with shortness of breath and nausea. He says he has never had a pain like this and rates it as 9 on a scale of 1 to 10. There is nothing in his medical history, even though he is 61-years-old. He not taking any medications except for over-the-counter vitamins, and he is allergic to Ceclor. Vital signs are BP, 160/72; P, 75; R 16, and Sao_2 = 97%. You see the following on the monitor:

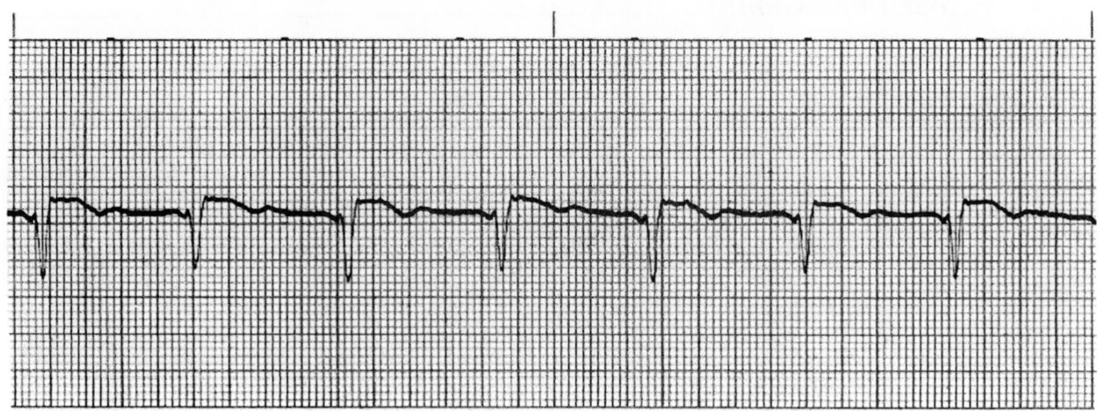

Identify the Rhythm

What is the rate? ____________ What is the rhythm (regular or irregular)? ____________

Is there a P wave before every QRS complex? ____________ Is there a QRS complex after every P wave? ____________

What is the P-R interval? ______________ QRS complex duration? ______________

Interpretation:

____

____

Case 5 Self-Test

In the spaces below give your treatment for the Primary Survey and the Secondary Survey, plus the continued care under Oxygen-IV-Monitor-Fluids and Vital Signs. How would you care for this patient, and what orders would you expect from the physician? At the bottom, list your potential diagnosis or impression of what the patient's problem is.

Primary Survey	***Secondary Survey***
A.	A.
B.	B.
C.	C.
D.	D.

Oxygen-IV-Monitor-Fluids: ____

____

Vital Signs: ____

____

Your Impression: ____

____

6

Atrioventricular Heart Block Rhythms

OBJECTIVES

By the end of this chapter, the student will be able to do the following:

- **Specify the characteristics for the following atrioventricular (AV) heart blocks:**
  - **First-degree AV heart block**
  - **Mobitz type I (Wenckebach) second-degree AV heart block**
  - **Mobitz type II (classical) second-degree AV heart block**
  - **Complete or third-degree heart block**
- **Recognize the signs, symptoms, causes, and treatment of each of the following rhythms:**
  - **First-degree AV heart block**
  - **Second-degree AV heart block (Mobitz I, type I, or Wenckebach)**
  - **Second-degree AV heart block (Mobitz II, type II)**
  - **Third-degree AV heart block (complete heart block)**
- **Define and understand the following terms:**
  - **Mobitz type I block**
  - **Mobitz type II block**
  - **Incomplete heart block**
  - **Complete heart block**

OUTLINE

Atrioventricular Heart Blocks

First-Degree Atrioventricular Block

Second-Degree Atrioventricular Block, Type I: Mobitz I (Wenckebach)

OUTLINE—cont'd

An atrioventricular (AV) heart block may be caused by partial or complete blockage involving the conduction system or may be due to a delay in conduction. The block may occur at the AV node, in the atrium, in the bundle of His, or in the His-Purkinje system. The interruption in impulse conduction may result in a partial or complete blockage. Signs and symptoms manifested by the patient depend on the degree of the blockage.

Frequently, these AV blocks occur during an MI and are caused by ischemia or a lack of blood flow to the AV node/AV junction. This restricted blood flow may be temporary or permanent. AV blocks are most commonly associated with anterior and inferior infarctions.

AV blocks are classified by severity, not by their location.

First and second heart blocks are incomplete blocks; there is a delay or an interruption in the electrical impulse being conducted. The AV junction is the area containing specialized tissue and provides a pathway for the electrical impulses traveling from the atria to the ventricles. When a delay or interruption occurs at the AV node, AV junction, or bundle of His, it is known as an *AV block*. The P waves and the P-R interval are the key to identifying an AV block. The P waves tell you an impulse was initiated, and the P-R interval reflects depolarization across the atria.

A first-degree AV block indicates the impulses from the SA node are delayed but not blocked (longer than normal P-R interval). With a second-degree AV block you find an incomplete blockage. There is an intermittent disturbance in the electrical impulses being conducted from the atria to the ventricles. A second-degree AV block is indicated because either there are more P waves than QRS complexes or the P-R intervals become longer and longer until the QRS complex is completely dropped.

Third-degree AV blocks are *complete* heart blocks between the atria and the ventricles; the electrical conduction to the ventricles is completely interrupted, with severe consequences. The severity of the consequences of a heart block is determined by the patient's signs and symptoms, the ventricular rate, and the heart's ability to perfuse the peripheral system with oxygen.

ATRIOVENTRICULAR HEART BLOCKS

First-Degree Atrioventricular Block

In a first-degree AV block, pacing is usually initiated by the SA node (Figure 6-1). The impulse travels through the atria but is delayed at the AV node/AV junction or bundle of His. Because of this delay, the P-R interval is longer than normal (0.12 to 0.20 second is normal), but there is a P wave before every QRS complex and a QRS complex after every P wave (Box 6-1).

Causes

Causes of first-degree AV block include the following:

- Increased vagal tone
- MI
- Hypokalemia
- Hyperkalemia

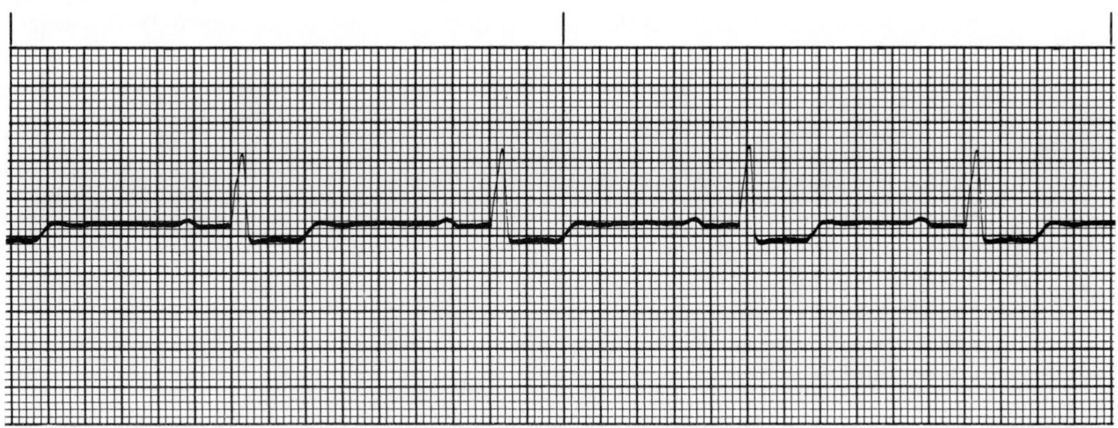

Figure 6-1 First-degree atrioventricular (AV) block.

Box 6-1 First-Degree Atrioventricular Block

Rate: Atrial and ventricular are both the same and within normal limits of 60-100 beats per minute
Rhythm: Regular
P wave: Normal size and configuration; there is a P wave before every QRS complex
P-R interval: Prolonged, greater than 0.20 second but is constant; a P-R interval of 0.20-0.24 second is minor, 0.25 -0.29 second is a moderate first-degree AV block, and >0.30 second is a severe first-degree AV block
QRS complex: Duration is usually normal if the conduction delay is at the AV node

- Hypothyroidism
- Degenerative disease of the conduction system *(common cause)*
- Rheumatic fever
- Drugs such as digoxin, quinidine, procainamide, calcium channel blockers, and beta blockers

AV block may also normally be seen in an athlete.

Treatment

If the pulse rate is normal, the patient is usually symptom free. Therefore no treatment is needed. However, if the patient is showing signs of decreased cardiac output (e.g., syncope, hypotension, or altered mental status), then treatment is mandatory. Treatment may include transcutaneous pacing and/or atropine and possibly dopamine and epinephrine (*Emergency Cardiovascular Care 2000 Guidelines*). If there is no improvement, a temporary pacemaker may be considered.

Second-Degree Atrioventricular Block, Type I: Mobitz I (Wenckebach)

Second-degree AV block, type I is known by all of the following names:
- Second-degree type I
- Wenckebach
- Mobitz I AV block

The conduction delay in a second-degree type I block usually occurs at the AV node/AV junction (Figure 6-2). With this type of block, you will see the P-R interval become progressively longer with each consecutive cardiac cycle, until a QRS complex is dropped (Box 6-2). This suggests that the atria are being polarized normally but some of the impulses are being blocked from reaching the ventricles. The significance is usually benign, and the patient is without symptoms.

Causes

Causes of second-degree AV block include the following:
- Cardiac glycoside toxicity
- Parasympathetic stimulation
- Inferior-wall MI
- Cardiac surgery
- Ischemic heart disease
- Rheumatic fever

Treatment

Treatment is only indicated if the patient has symptoms. Symptoms may include shortness of breath, chest pain, hypotension, weakness, or dizziness. When any of these signs and symptoms occur in conjunction with a Wenckebach rhythm, producing a bradycardia, prepare to give atropine 0.5- to 1.0-mg IV push or do transcutaneous pacing. The atropine may be repeated every 3 to 5 minutes up to a total dose of 0.03 to 0.04 mg/kg depending on the severity of the bradycardia, signs, and symptoms.

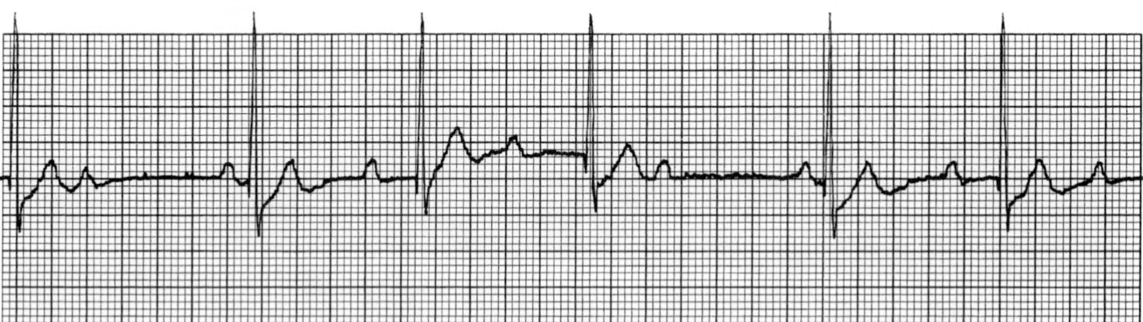

Figure 6-2 Second-degree type I (Mobitz I) atrioventricular (AV) block.

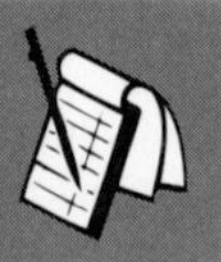

Note

The Mobitz I or Wenckebach is the least serious of the second-degree AV blocks.

Box 6-2 Second-Degree Atrioventricular Block: Mobitz I (Wenckebach)

Rate: Atrial rate is greater than the ventricular rate; however, the ventricular rate is usually within normal limits
Rhythm: Atrial is regular; ventricular is irregular; the R-R interval shortens progressively until a QRS complex is dropped
P wave: Normal in size and configuration, but not every P wave is followed by a QRS complex
P-R interval: The P-R interval becomes progressively longer until a QRS complex is dropped; then the procedure begins all over again, with a short P-R interval, which becomes progressively longer until a QRS complex is dropped; this occurs usually every third or fourth beat
QRS complex: Duration is within normal limits, less than 0.10 second, but with the dropped complexes; there is not a QRS complex after every P wave

Second-Degree Atrioventricular Block, Type II: Mobitz II

A second-degree AV block type II is also known as a Mobitz II (Figure 6-3). It is imperative that you are familiar with both of the associated names, because these AV blocks may be called by either of the names in a question, in the emergency department, in the critical care unit (CCU), in the intensive care unit (ICU), or in the back of an ambulance. In a type II AV block, the conduction is delayed below the AV node, usually at the bundle of His or further down in the bundle branches. The P waves appear on the ECG, but not every P wave is followed by a QRS complex (Box 6-3).

There are usually multiple P waves for each QRS complex, resulting in a 2:1, 3:1, or 4:1 conduction. A type II AV block is much more serious than a type I because cardiac output is usually reduced. A Mobitz II AV block may rapidly progress to a third-degree AV block.

Recognizing a high-degree AV block (Mobitz II) is important, because it may cause severe complications, such as a reduced heart rate and decreased cardiac output. This in turn may precipitate Stokes-Adams syncopal attacks. In addition, a high-degree AV block may rapidly become a third-degree heart block. When two or more successive atrial impulses are blocked, it creates a major conduction disturbance. Usually this is expressed in terms of an atrial to ventricular ratio, with the block being at least 3:1 (three atrial beats for every ventricular beat). This is why it is called a *high-degree AV block*.

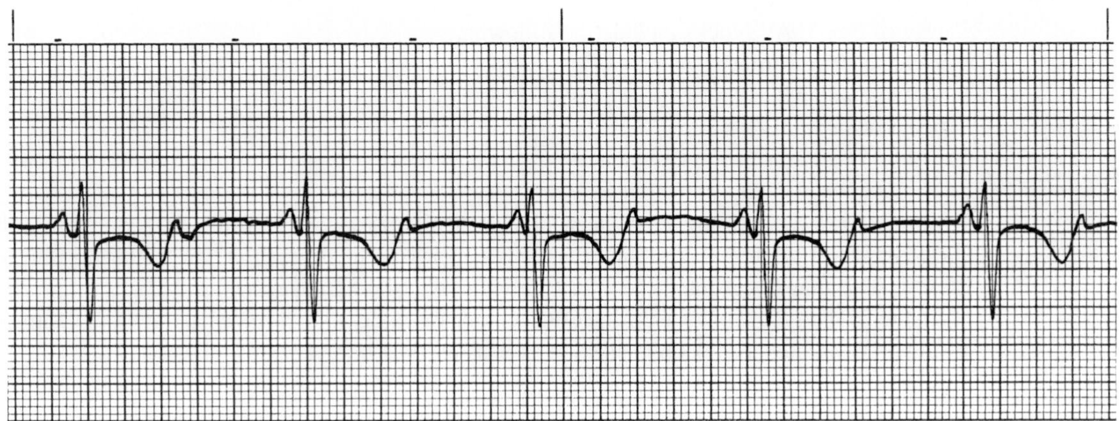

Figure 6-3 Second-degree type II (Mobitz II) atrioventricular (AV) block.

Box 6-3 Second-Degree Atrioventricular Block, Type II: Mobitz II

Rate: Atrial is regular, but greater than the ventricular. Depending on the conduction—2:1, 3:1, 4:1—the atrial rate will be twice as fast, or three times as fast as the ventricular rate.

Rhythm: Atrial is regular; ventricular may be regular or irregular. If the AV block is intermittent, the rhythm is irregular, and pauses correspond to any dropped beats.

P wave: All impulses for the P wave originate at the SA node. It is of normal size, shape, and configuration. Not all P waves are followed by QRS complexes. The atrial rate varies according to the underlying rhythm, but the P-P interval is the same.

P-R interval: The P-R interval may be within normal limits or may be prolonged, if there is a QRS complex after the P wave.

QRS complex: The QRS complex may be normal or wide, depending on where the block occurs. If the block is at the bundle of His, the QRS complex duration is of normal duration, <0.10 second. When the block occurs below the bundle of His, the QRS complex duration is wide. The R-R interval may be regular or irregular depending on if the block ratio is constant or variable. Also, QRS complexes are periodically absent.

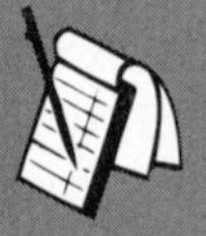

Note

In a Mobitz I AV block the QRS complexes are usually of normal duration. With a Mobitz II AV block, the QRS complexes usually have a duration that is wider than normal or greater than 0.10 second because of a bundle branch block.

Causes

Causes of type II AV blocks include the following:

- Severe coronary artery disease
- Anterior wall MI
- Acute myocarditis

Treatment

Treatment for a second-degree AV heart block (Mobitz II) depends on the QRS complex. If the QRS complex is of normal duration or is narrow, then your treatment is a 0.5- to 1.0-mg atropine IV push. This may be repeated every 3 to 5 minutes and should not exceed a total maximum dose of 0.03 to 0.04 mg/kg. However, if the QRS complex is wider than the normal duration, treatment should be transcutaneous pacing, as soon as possible Just remember:

Narrow QRS complex = Atropine
Wide QRS complex = Transcutaneous pacing
(Emergency Cardiovascular Care 2000 Guidelines)

Third-Degree Atrioventricular Block

With a third-degree AV block, the atria and the ventricles are functioning electrically, independently of each other (Figure 6-4). The impulses generated from the SA node are completely blocked before reaching the ventricles. When all of these supraventricular impulses are prevented from traveling the normal conduction pathway and prevented from reaching the ventricles, it is recognized as a third-degree AV heart block. Depending on the location of the block, a junctional or ventricular escape rhythm may be generated, which controls the ventricles. A third-degree block may be associated with a supraventricular rhythm, but you will not see any relationship between the P waves and the QRS complexes (Box 6-4).

Causes

Causes of a complete third-degree block include the following:

- Anterior or inferior wall MI
- Congenital heart disease
- Damage to the AV node
- Drugs such as digitalis, propranolol, and verapamil
- Rheumatic fever
- Mitral valve replacement complications
- Cardiac catheterization or angioplasty

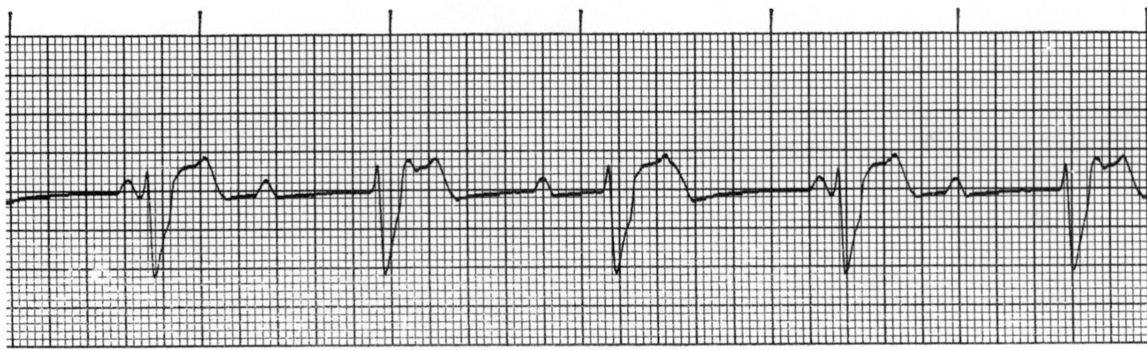

Figure 6-4 Third-degree atrioventricular (AV) block.

Box 6-4 Third-Degree Atrioventricular Block

Rate: Atrial rate is faster than ventricular. Atrial rate is faster than ventricular because the ventricular rate is determined by the origin of the escape rhythm. The ventricular rate is usually 20 to 40 beats per minute.

Rhythm: Both atrial and ventricular are regular, but there is no relationship between the two.

P wave: The P wave is usually of normal size and configuration, but there is not necessarily a P wave before every QRS complex.

P-R interval: The P-R interval is not measurable because there is no relationship between the P waves and the QRS complexes.

QRS complex: The QRS complex may be a narrow complex or a wide complex depending on where the ventricular rhythm originates. If the QRS complex is narrow, then the pacemaker site is at the AV junction. A wide QRS complex indicates a ventricular pacemaker site.

A complete AV block with narrow QRS complexes usually results from a blockage above the bundle of His and has a ventricular rate greater than 40 beats per minute. A complete AV block with wide QRS complexes is usually due to a blockage in either the right or left bundle branch and has a ventricular rate of less than 40 beats per minute.

If the block is due to congenital heart disease, it usually occurs at the AV node and the resulting QRS complex is normal, with a heart rate of approximately 60 beats per minute. However, if the block involves the bundle of His and the bundle branches, the resulting heart rate is 20 to 30 beats per minute. A third-degree heart block can rapidly progress to asystole.

Treatment

Treatment includes immediate transcutaneous pacing, atropine IV push, dopamine, and epinephrine. A permanent pacemaker may be needed.

Treatment really depends on the degree of AV block. If the blockage is occurring in the AV node or AV junction and the QRS complex is normal or narrow, give a 0.5- to 1.0-mg atropine IV push to increase the ventricular rate. However, if the AV block is lower in the bundle of His–Purkinje system with a wide QRS complex, then you should go immediately to transcutaneous pacing to increase the ventricular rate.

Chapter 6 Self-Test

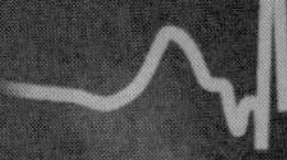

1. Multiple Choice: One characteristic of a first-degree AV block is:
   a. The P-R interval is greater than 0.20 second
   b. The P-R interval is not measurable
   c. The P-R interval is greater than 0.12 second
   d. The P wave is dropped every second beat

2. List the three other names for a type I AV block

   ____

   ____

   ____

3. True or False: With a type I second-degree AV block the P-R interval becomes longer until a QRS complex is dropped.

4. Match the following heart blocks with the statement that describes them best

   ______________________________ First-degree AV block

   ______________________________ Mobitz I

   ______________________________ Mobitz II

   ______________________________ Third-degree AV block

   a. The P-R interval becomes progressively longer until the QRS complex is dropped
   b. The atria and ventricles are functioning independently of each other. There is no relationship between the P waves and the QRS complexes.
   c. The P-R interval is longer than normal or greater than 0.20 second
   d. Atrial rate is greater than the ventricular rate depending on the conduction, which may be 2:1, 3:1, or 4:1

5. True of False: When you have a type I AV block, the ventricular rhythm is usually regular.

6. Fill in the Blank: Another name for a type II AV block is ______________ ,

7. Multiple Choice: With a second-degree type II AV block, you will find:
   a. Atrial and ventricular rates are the same
   b. The blockage is above the AV node
   c. The atrial rate will be faster than the ventricular rate, resulting in a 2:1, 3:1, or 4:1 conduction
   d. The atrial rate is irregular because it is faster than the ventricular rate

8. True or False: A Mobitz type II AV block is more serious than a Mobitz type I AV block because cardiac output is most likely reduced at times.

9. True or False: The P waves of a third-degree AV block are usually of normal size and configuration.

10. Circle the Correct Answer: The atrial rate of a third-degree AV block is *faster/slower* than the ventricular rate.

11. True or False: First- and second-degree AV blocks are partial or incomplete blocks, because all or at least some of the P waves are conducted to the ventricles.

12. Fill in the Blank: Third-degree heart blocks can be complete blockage of the ____________ ______________________ and the conduction is completely interrupted to the ventricles.

ECG Practice Strips

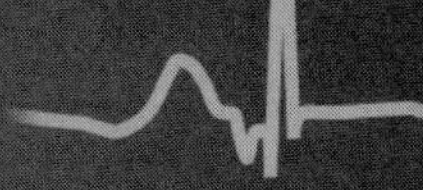

Please calculate the following 15 ECG practice strips

- Determine the rate.
- Is the rhythm regular or irregular?
- Measure the P-R interval.
- Measure the QRS complex duration.
- Check to see if there is a P wave *before* every QRS complex.
- Check to see if there is a QRS complex *after* every P wave.
- Then give your interpretation of the rhythm.
- All strips are lead II unless otherwise noted.

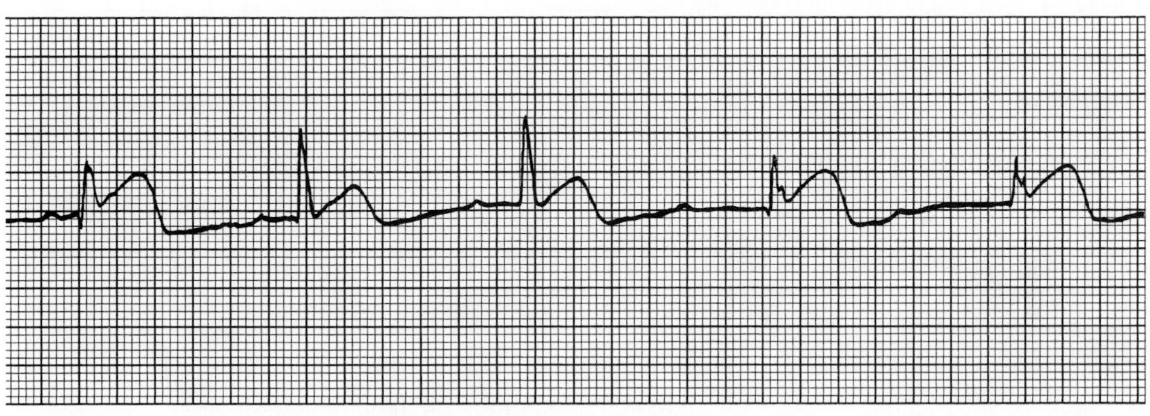

Practice Figure 6-1

Rate: ____________ Rhythm: ____________ P-R interval: ____________ QRS complex: ____________

Is there a P wave before every QRS complex? ____

Is there a QRS complex after every P wave? ____

Interpretation: ____

____

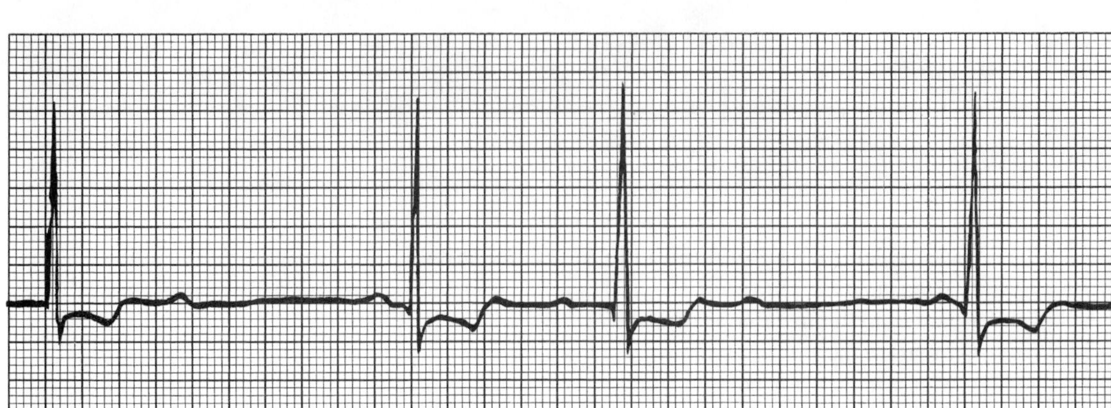

Practice Figure 6-2

Rate: ____________ Rhythm: ____________ P-R interval: ____________ QRS complex: ____________

Is there a P wave before every QRS complex? ____________

Is there a QRS complex after every P wave? ____________

Interpretation: ____________

____

Practice Figure 6-3

Rate: ____________ Rhythm: ____________ P-R interval: ____________ QRS complex: ____________

Is there a P wave before every QRS complex? ____________

Is there a QRS complex after every P wave? ____________

Interpretation: ____________

____

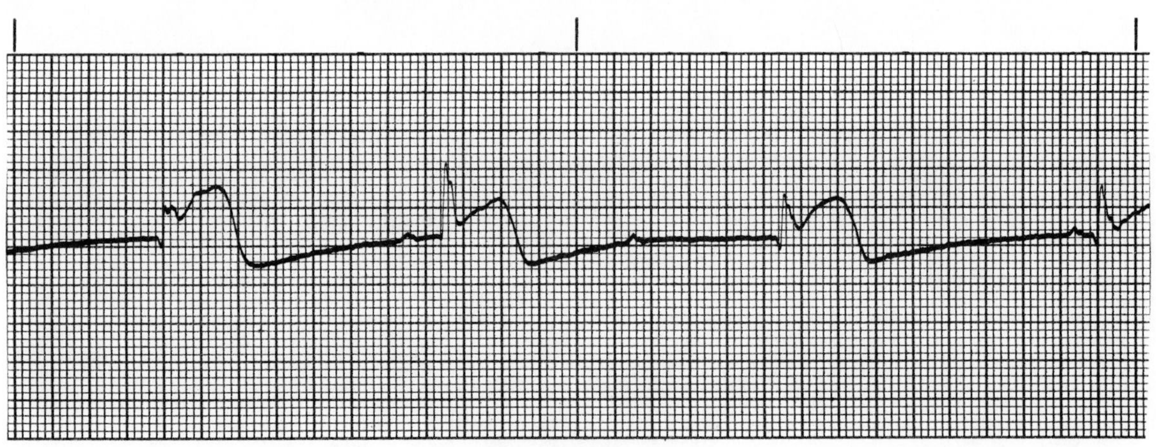

Practice Figure 6-4

Rate: ____________ Rhythm: ____________ P-R interval: ____________ QRS complex: ____________

Is there a P wave before every QRS complex? ________________________________

Is there a QRS complex after every P wave? ________________________________

Interpretation: ________________________________

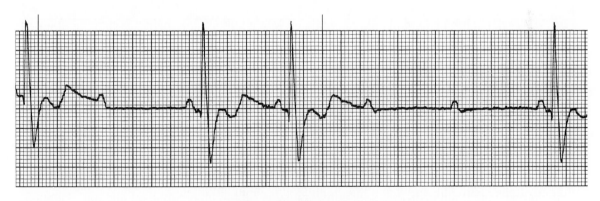

____

Practice Figure 6-5

Rate: ____________ Rhythm: ____________ P-R interval: ____________ QRS complex: ____________

Is there a P wave before every QRS complex? ________________________________

Is there a QRS complex after every P wave? ________________________________

Interpretation: ________________________________

____

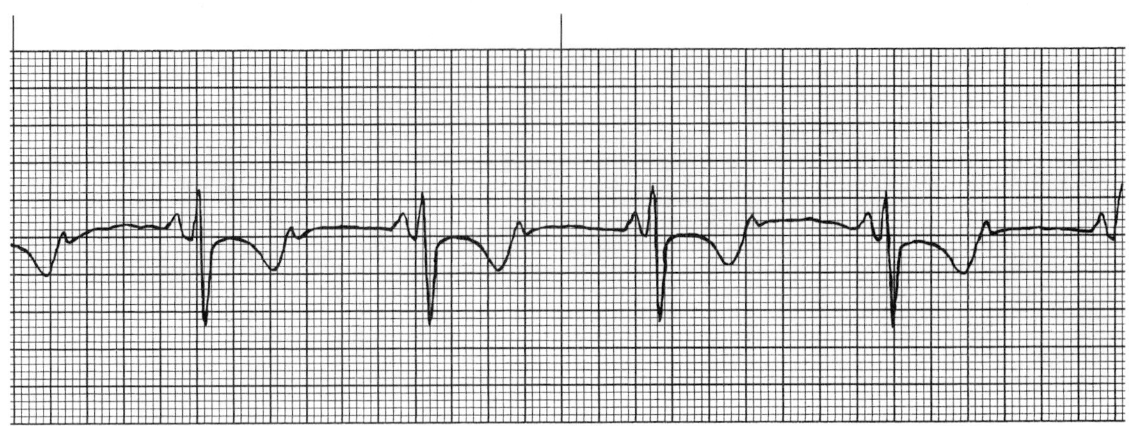

Practice Figure 6-6

Rate: ____________ Rhythm: ____________ P-R interval: ____________ QRS complex: ____________

Is there a P wave before every QRS complex? ____________

Is there a QRS complex after every P wave? ____________

Interpretation: ____________

____

Practice Figure 6-7

Rate: ____________ Rhythm: ____________ P-R interval: ____________ QRS complex: ____________

Is there a P wave before every QRS complex? ____________

Is there a QRS complex after every P wave? ____________

Interpretation: ____________

____

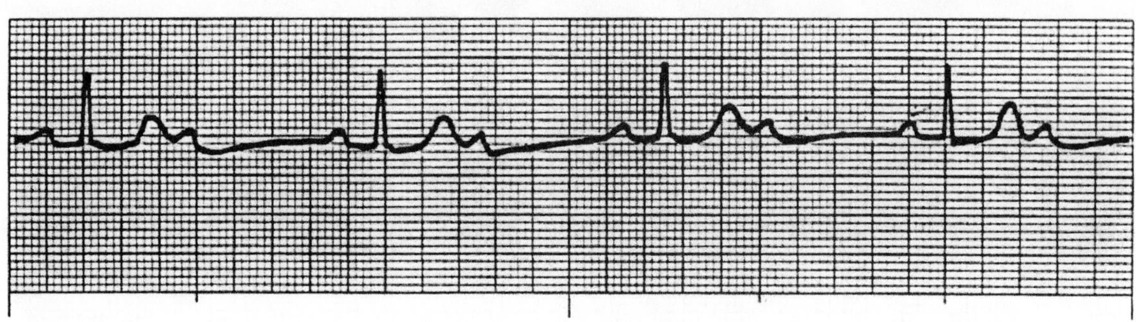

Practice Figure 6-8

Rate: ____________ Rhythm: ____________ P-R interval: ____________ QRS complex: ____________

Is there a P wave before every QRS complex? ____

Is there a QRS complex after every P wave? ____

Interpretation: ____

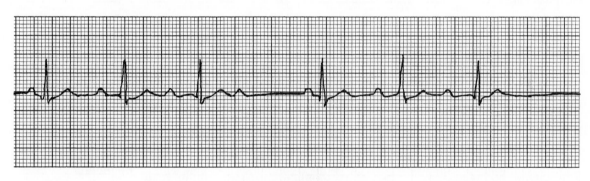

____

Practice Figure 6-9

Rate: ____________ Rhythm: ____________ P-R interval: ____________ QRS complex: ____________

Is there a P wave before every QRS complex? ____

Is there a QRS complex after every P wave? ____

Interpretation: ____

____

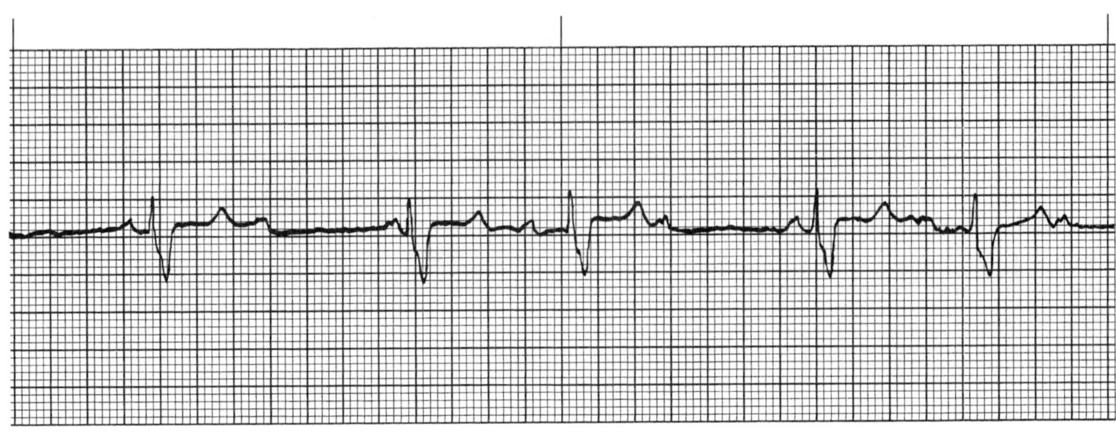

Practice Figure 6-10

Rate: ____________ Rhythm: ____________ P-R interval: ____________ QRS complex: ____________

Is there a P wave before every QRS complex? ____________

Is there a QRS complex after every P wave? ____________

Interpretation: ____________

Practice Figure 6-11

Rate: ____________ Rhythm: ____________ P-R interval: ____________ QRS complex: ____________

Is there a P wave before every QRS complex? ____________

Is there a QRS complex after every P wave? ____________

Interpretation: ____________

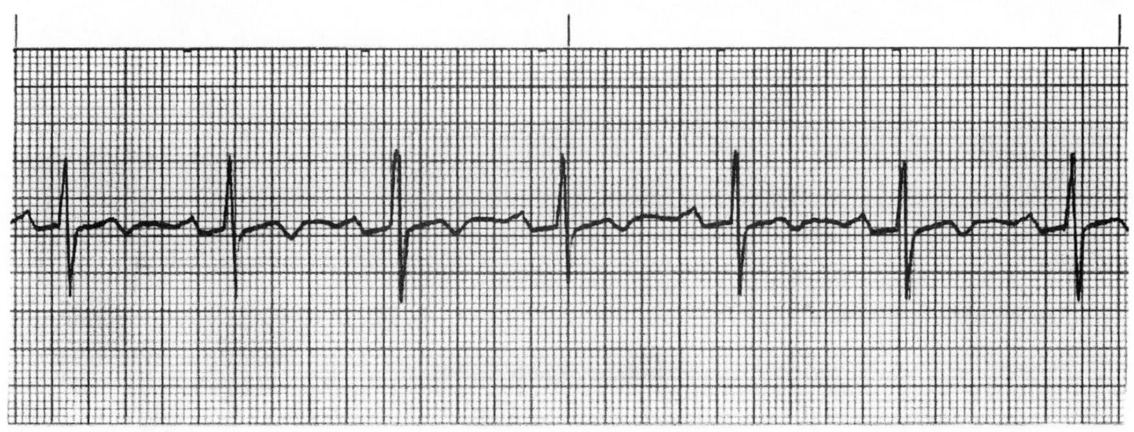

Practice Figure 6-12

Rate: ____________ Rhythm: ____________ P-R interval: ____________ QRS complex: ____________

Is there a P wave before every QRS complex? ____________

Is there a QRS complex after every P wave? ____________

Interpretation: ____________

____

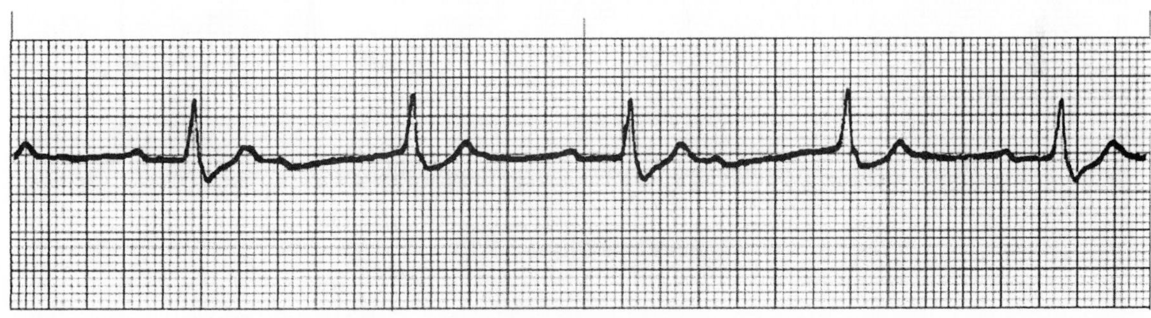

Practice Figure 6-13

Rate: ____________ Rhythm: ____________ P-R interval: ____________ QRS complex: ____________

Is there a P wave before every QRS complex? ____________

Is there a QRS complex after every P wave? ____________

Interpretation: ____________

____

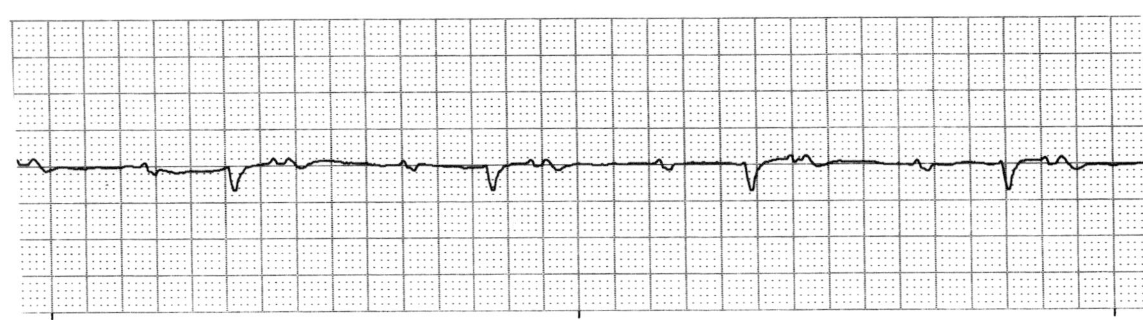

Practice Figure 6-14

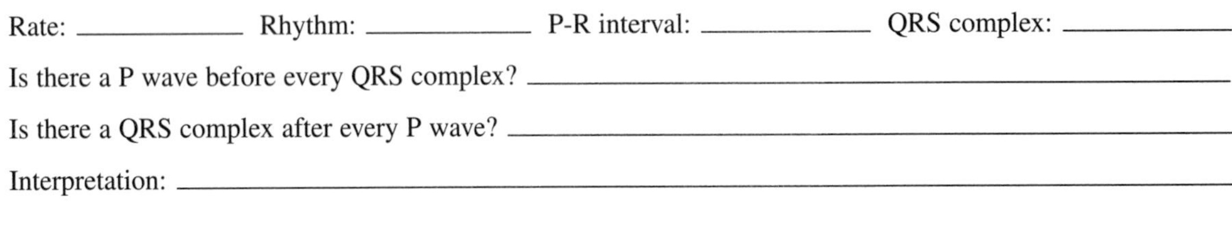

Rate: ____________ Rhythm: ____________ P-R interval: ____________ QRS complex: ____________

Is there a P wave before every QRS complex? ____________

Is there a QRS complex after every P wave? ____________

Interpretation: ____________

____

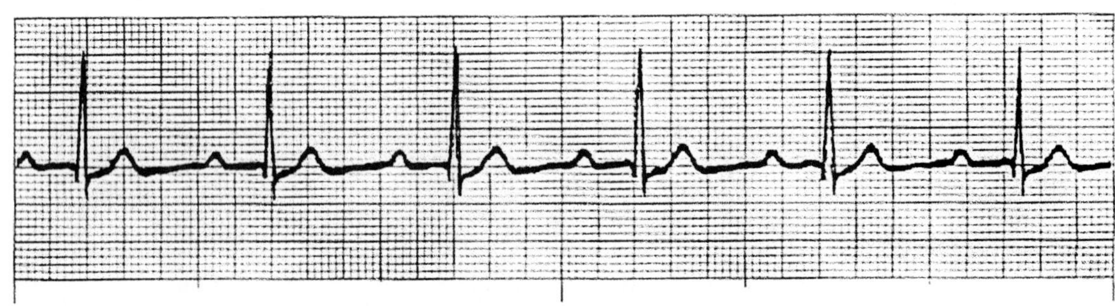

Practice Figure 6-15

Rate: ____________ Rhythm: ____________ P-R interval: ____________ QRS complex: ____________

Is there a P wave before every QRS complex? ____________

Is there a QRS complex after every P wave? ____________

Interpretation: ____________

____

Case Scenarios

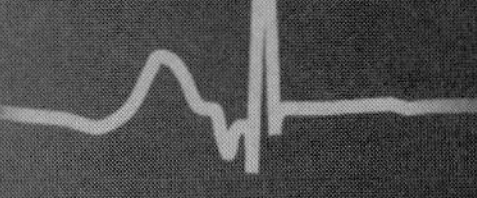

CASE 1

Scenario

A 71-year-old man brought in by his family is complaining of chest pain. He states the pain is nonradiating and is located on the left side of his chest. He is also complaining of nausea and has diaphoresis. When asked, he rates his pain as 5 on the 1 to 10 scale and says it began about 2 hours ago. His medical history includes coronary artery disease, angina, hypertension, and arthritis. Medications include digoxin; nitroglycerin SL, as needed; Vasotec; and Naprosyn. His vital signs are BP, 114/76; P, 62; R, 20, and Sao_2 = 96%. You see the following on the monitor:

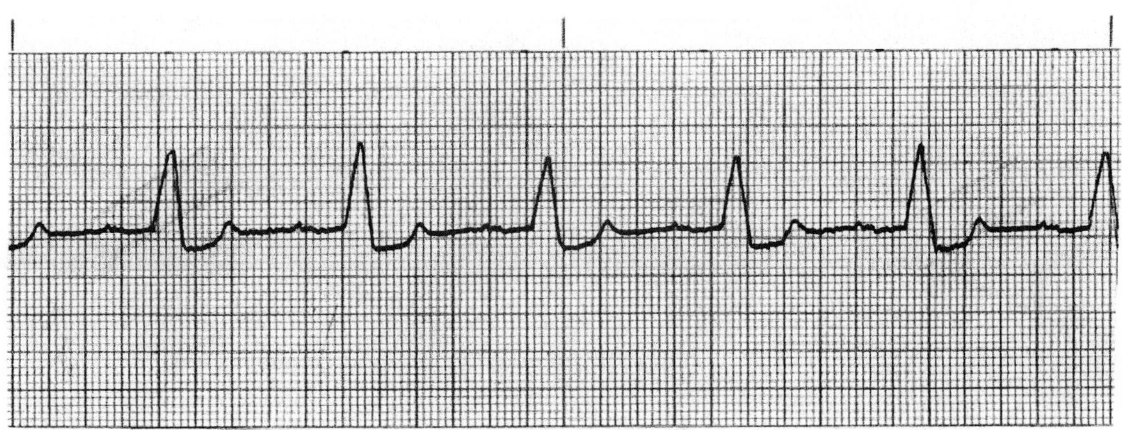

Identify the Rhythm

What is the rate? ______________ What is the rhythm (regular or irregular)? ______________

Is there a P wave before every QRS complex? ______________ Is there a QRS complex after every P wave? ______________

What is the P-R interval? __________________ QRS complex duration? __________________

Interpretation:

____

____

Case 1 Self-Test

In the spaces below give your treatment for the Primary Survey and the Secondary Survey, plus the continued care under Oxygen-IV-Monitor-Fluids and Vital Signs. How would you care for this patient, and what orders would you expect from the physician? At the bottom, list your potential diagnosis or impression of what the patient's problem is.

Primary Survey	***Secondary Survey***
A.	A.
B.	B.
C.	C.
D.	D.

Oxygen-IV-Monitor-Fluids: ______________________________

____

Vital Signs: ______________________________

____

Your Impression: ______________________________

____

CASE 2

Scenario

A 48-year-old woman complains of fatigue for the past several weeks and shortness of breath with chest discomfort for the past 2 days. She has also been complaining of intermittent fever for the past 2 weeks. Today she feels dizzy, weak, and sweaty. She appears pale. She has nothing significant in her medical history, and she takes no medications. She does tell you that she works in an x-ray department, but does not know if that would make any difference. After much questioning, she tells you that 6 months ago her doctor diagnosed myocarditis, but she never really followed up for the treatment. However, she says she has never experienced symptoms like those she is having today. Vital signs are BP, 98/66; P, 52; R, 26, and Sao_2 = 96%. You see the following on the monitor:

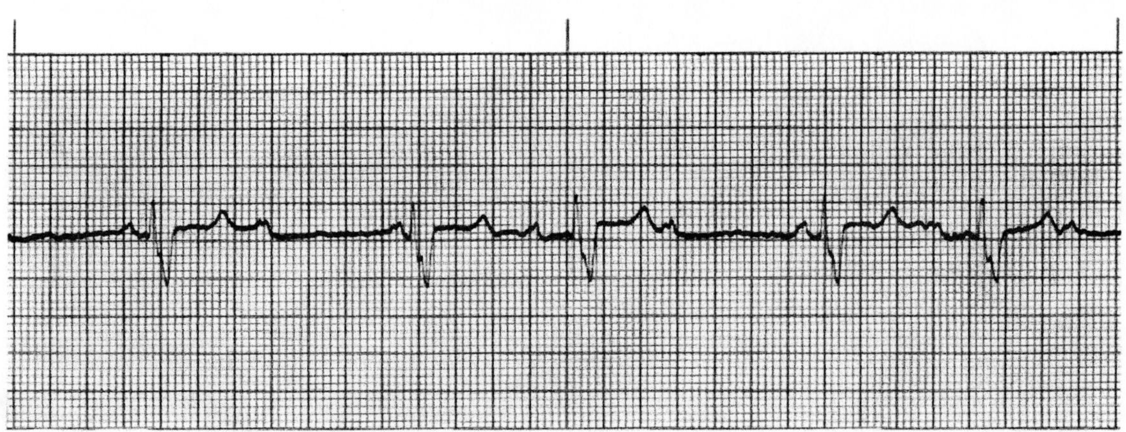

Identify the Rhythm

What is the rate? ____________ What is the rhythm (regular or irregular)? ____________

Is there a P wave before every QRS complex? ____________ Is there a QRS complex after every P wave? ____________

What is the P-R interval? ____________ QRS complex duration? ____________

Interpretation:

____

____

Case 2 Self-Test

In the spaces below give your treatment for the Primary Survey and Secondary Survey, plus the continued care under Oxygen-IV-Monitor-Fluids and Vital Signs. How would you care for this patient, and what orders would you expect from the physician? At the bottom, list your potential diagnosis or impression of what the patient's problem is.

Primary Survey

A.

B.

C.

D.

Secondary Survey

A.

B.

C.

D.

Oxygen-IV-Monitor-Fluids: ______________________________

____

Vital Signs: ______________________________

____

Your Impression: ______________________________

____

CASE 3

Scenario

You have a 59-year-old man with a sudden episode of syncope. He has no associated symptoms. His medical history includes an MI 3 months ago and a valve replacement 3 weeks ago. He has been recovering nicely until 30 minutes ago. His medications are aspirin, once a day; nitroglycerin SL, as needed; and digoxin, 0.25 mg once a day. At present his vital signs are BP, 110/66; P, 72; R, 18, and Sao_2 = 98%. His skin is pink, warm, and dry, and he has no difficulty breathing. You see the following on the monitor:

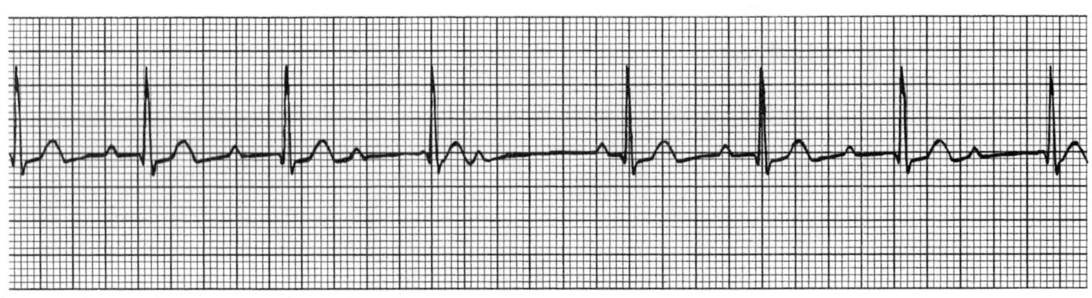

Identify the Rhythm

What is the rate? ____________ What is the rhythm (regular or irregular)? ____________

Is there a P wave before every QRS complex? ____________ Is there a QRS complex after every P wave? ____________

What is the P-R interval? ____________ QRS complex duration? ____________

Interpretation:

____

____

Case 3 Self-Test

In the spaces below give your treatment for the Primary Survey and Secondary Survey, plus the continued care under Oxygen-IV-Monitor-Fluids and Vital Signs. How would you care for this patient, and what orders would you expect from the physician? At the bottom, list your potential diagnosis or impression of what the patient's problem is.

Primary Survey

A.

B.

C.

D.

Secondary Survey

A.

B.

C.

D.

Oxygen-IV-Monitor-Fluids: ______________________________

____

Vital Signs: ______________________________

____

Your Impression: ______________________________

____

CASE 4

Scenario

A man arrives in the ER with chest pain and says it feels like his angina pain, but this time he also feels light-headed, which he says is different. He had a mitral valve replacement 6 weeks ago with no complications. He has a history of angina and diverticulitis. His medications include nitroglycerin (as needed) and one aspirin a day. Vital signs are BP, 100/52; P, 55; and R, 20 and nonlabored. Lungs are clear. He is oriented ×3, and his skin is pale, but warm and dry. You see the following on the monitor:

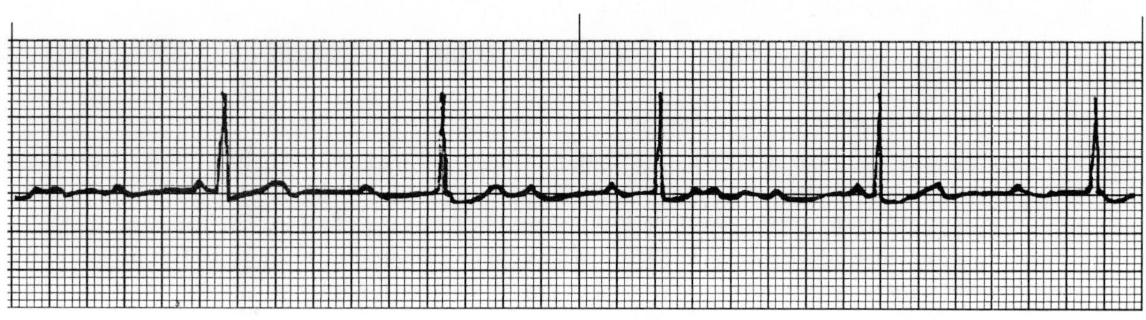

Identify the Rhythm

What is the rate? ____________ What is the rhythm (regular or irregular)? ____________

Is there a P wave before every QRS complex? ____________ Is there a QRS complex after every P wave? ____________

What is the P-R interval? ______________ QRS complex duration? ______________

Interpretation:

____

____

Case 4 Self-Test

In the spaces below give your treatment for the Primary Survey and Secondary Survey, plus the continued care under Oxygen-IV-Monitor-Fluids and Vital Signs. How would you care for this patient, and what orders would you expect from the physician? At the bottom, list your potential diagnosis or impression of what the patient's problem is.

Primary Survey	***Secondary Survey***
A.	A.
B.	B.
C.	C.
D.	D.

Oxygen-IV-Monitor-Fluids: ____

____

Vital Signs: ____

____

Your Impression: ____

____

CASE 5

Scenario

An 89-year-old female with nausea, vomiting, and fever for the last 4 days is brought in by EMS. Her family says they just cannot take care of her any longer. She has urinary incontinence, is extremely weak, and is even combative at times. At present she is awake but not alert. Her history includes high blood pressure, CHF, and COPD. She smoked an average of $1^1/_2$ packs per day (PPD) for more than 45 years. Vital signs are BP, 196/70; P, 47; R, 24; and Sao_2 = 93% on room air. On the monitor you see the following:

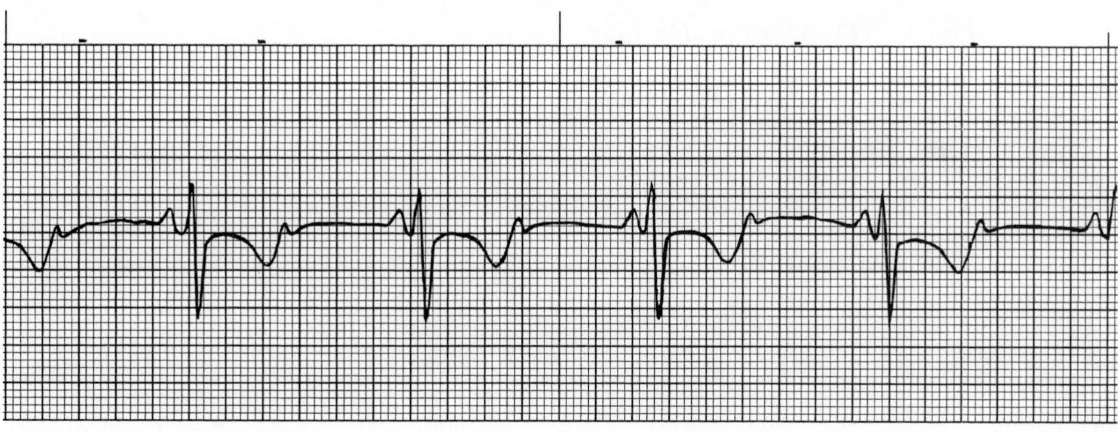

Identify the Rhythm

What is the rate? __________ What is the rhythm (regular or irregular)? __________

Is there a P wave before every QRS complex? __________ Is there a QRS complex after every P wave? __________

What is the P-R interval? __________ QRS complex duration? __________

Interpretation:

____

____

Case 5 Self-Test

In the spaces below give your treatment for the Primary Survey and Secondary Survey, plus the continued care under Oxygen-IV-Monitor-Fluids and Vital Signs. How would you care for this patient, and what orders would you expect from the physician? At the bottom, list your potential diagnosis or impression of what the patient's problem is.

Primary Survey

A.

B.

C.

D.

Secondary Survey

A.

B.

C.

D.

Oxygen-IV-Monitor-Fluids: ______________________________

____

Vital Signs: ______________________________

____

Your Impression: ______________________________

____

7

Ventricular Rhythms

OBJECTIVES

By the end of this chapter, the student will be able to do the following:

- **Specify characteristics of the following dysrhythmias:**
  - **Premature ventricular complex**
  - **Idioventricular rhythm (ventricular escape)**
  - **Accelerated ventricular rhythm**
  - **Torsades de pointes**
  - **Ventricular tachycardia (V-tach)**
  - **Ventricular fibrillation (V-fib)**
  - **Asystole**
  - **Pulseless electrical activity (PEA)**
- **Know and understand the signs, symptoms, causes, and treatment of the following dysrhythmias:**
  - **Premature ventricular complexes**
  - **Idioventricular rhythms**
  - **Ventricular escape beats**
  - **Accelerated ventricular rhythm**
  - **Torsades de pointes**
  - **V-tach**
  - **V-fib**
  - **Asystole**
  - **PEA**
- **Describe the indications for defibrillation**
- **Describe the indications for cardioversion**
- **Explain the terms *bigeminy, trigeminy,* and *quadrigeminy* in relation to premature ventricular contractions**
- **Know and understand "A-B-C-D"–primary and secondary survey**

OUTLINE

Some of the most common, but also the most deadly of rhythms, are ventricular rhythms. As you can imagine their origin is in the ventricles, below the bifurcation of the bundle of His, often in the Purkinje fibers. Because they arise from the ventricles, the rate is less than 40 beats per minute. There is no atrial activity or depolarization; therefore, the P wave is absent and the QRS complex is wide and bizarre.

These abnormal rhythms may result from any of the following:

- Circus reentry
- R on T phenomenon
- Enhanced automaticity

VENTRICULAR RHYTHMS

Characteristics of ventricular rhythms include the following:

1. QRS complex is wider than 0.12 second.
2. QRS complex has a bizarre appearance.
3. A T wave that deflects in the opposite direction from the QRS complex.
4. The rate is less than 40 beats per minute, unless it is a tachycardia or an accelerated rhythm.
5. The patient may or may not have a *pulse* and *blood pressure*.

Premature Ventricular Contractions

Premature ventricular contractions (PVCs) are among the most common ventricular dysrhythmias. PVCs may be found in young healthy persons or in diseased hearts. They may be caused by enhanced automaticity or reentry and usually arise from an irritable site that is called "ectopic focus." A PVC is a premature beat that occurs earlier than the next expected sinus beat, and the pause is compensatory (Box 7-1). The underlying rhythm may be sinus, atrial, junctional, or ventricular, but is usually sinus or atrial.

The PVCs may or may not look alike. If they do look alike, then all originate from the same ectopic focus and are called *uniform* or *unifocal PVCs* (Figure 7-1). When they do not all look alike, then the impulses are arising from two or more ventricular sites and are called *multifocal PVCs*. Research has shown that warning dysrhythmias such as PVCs are evident before ventricular fibrillation. Some of the characteristics of worrisome PVCs are the following:

1. More than six PVCs per minute
2. PVCs that fall on the downslope of a T wave of the preceding beat; the R wave of the next beat falls on the downslope of the preceding T wave
3. PVCs that occur in bigeminy, trigeminy, and quadrigeminy
4. Two PVCs in a row, which by definition are *couplets or paired PVCs*
5. A run of three PVCs or more in a row, which by definition is *ventricular tachycardia*
6. Multifocal PVCs arising from different ventricular sites

Multifocal PVCs usually indicate severe heart disease. In many cases it is difficult to tell if it is a PVC, so use with your calipers as discussed in Chapter 2 to see if there is a compensatory pause or a noncompensatory pause.

Box 7-1 Premature Ventricular Contractions

Rate: Atrial and ventricular rate is usually normal, depending on underlying rhythm
Rhythm: Atrial and ventricular rhythm is irregular during PVCs, underlying rhythm usually regular, again depending on the rhythm
P wave: Absent with PVCs, but usually present in underlying rhythm
P-R interval: Not measurable during PVCs
QRS complex: Appears as wide and bizarre; occurs earlier than expected and the duration is >0.12 second

PVC, Premature ventricular contraction.

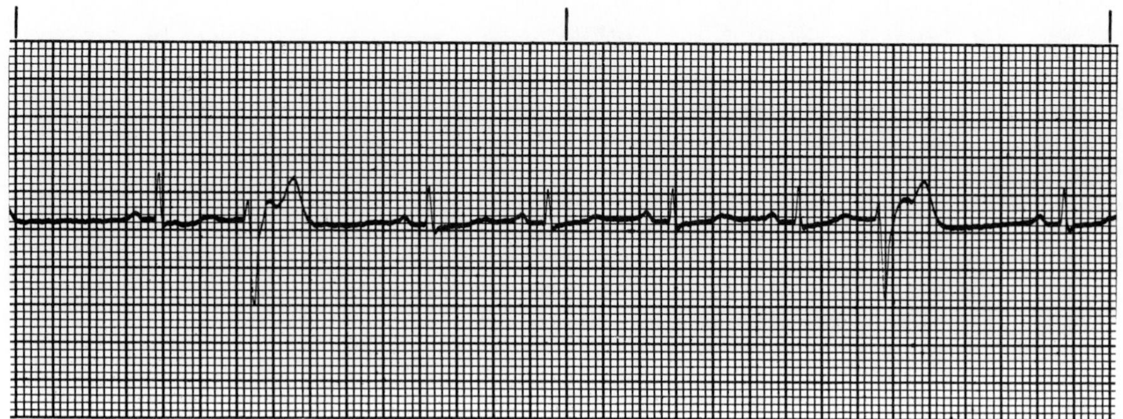

Figure 7-1 Premature ventricular contractions (PVCs).

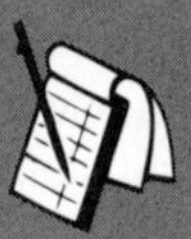

Note

A *compensatory pause* is when the R-R interval with the pause or irregular beat (from the R wave before the irregular beat to the R wave after the irregular beat) *is equal to* the sum of two normal R-R intervals of the underlying rhythm. A *noncompensatory pause* is when the R-R interval with the pause or irregular beat (from the R wave before the irregular beat to the R wave after the irregular beat) *is not equal to* the sum of two normal R-R intervals of the underlying rhythm.

Interpolated PVCs are ones that occur between two normal QRS complexes. They do not interrupt the underlying rhythm.

Causes

PVCs may occur in healthy persons who have normal hearts and in whom there is no apparent cause for the PVCs. These PVCs are benign, and the patients have no symptoms. Asymptomatic and symptomatic causes are shown in Box 7-2.

Signs and Symptoms

Usually the heart rate is between 60 and 100 beats per minute, but often the heart rate on the monitor does not match the patient's pulse rate. The pulse will be less if the PVCs are not producing a mechanical contraction of the heart. The patient may complain of palpitations or skipped beats. When the patient's circulatory system is unable to compensate for the PVCs, there are signs/symptoms of decreased cardiac output, syncope, low blood pressure, diaphoresis, angina, or chest pain.

Box 7-2 Causes of Premature Ventricular Contractions

Exercise
Stress
Caffeine
Hypoxia
Anxiety
Alcohol
Tobacco
Acid-base imbalance
Electrolyte imbalance
Digitalis toxicity
Myocardial ischemia
Drugs such as epinephrine, dopamine, sympathomimetics, tricyclic antidepressants, phenothiazines
Increased sympathetic tone
AMI
CHF

AMI, Acute myocardial infarction; *CHF*, congestive heart failure.

Treatment

Treatment is usually aimed at correcting the underlying problem. However, if the patient is showing signs/symptoms of decreased cardiac output, then an antiarrhythmic or a beta blocker drug may be considered because it aids in suppressing PVCs. Oxygen is always the first choice in the treatment line. Oxygen may help to improve cardiac output and may begin to provide relief of any pain especially if the PVCs are in the setting of an MI.

If bradycardia is present along with the PVCs, then atropine or transcutaneous pacing should be administered to increase the heart rate. By eliminating the bradycardia you may eliminate the PVCs. Drug therapy may include antiarrhythmic agents such as amiodarone, procainamide, lidocaine, or a beta-blocking agent such as esmolol, atenolol, or metoprolol. Usually the beta blockers are used if the PVCs are being caused by an acute coronary event.

Idioventricular Rhythm

An idioventricular rhythm originates in the ventricles with a rate of 20 to 40 beats per minute (Figure 7-2). This occurs when the SA node or the AV junction fails to initiate an electrical impulse. The idioventricular rhythm is a protective mechanism because the pacemaker site is in the ventricles or Purkinje system. As with most ventricular rhythms, the QRS complex is wide and bizarre, lasting more than 0.12 second (Box 7-3).

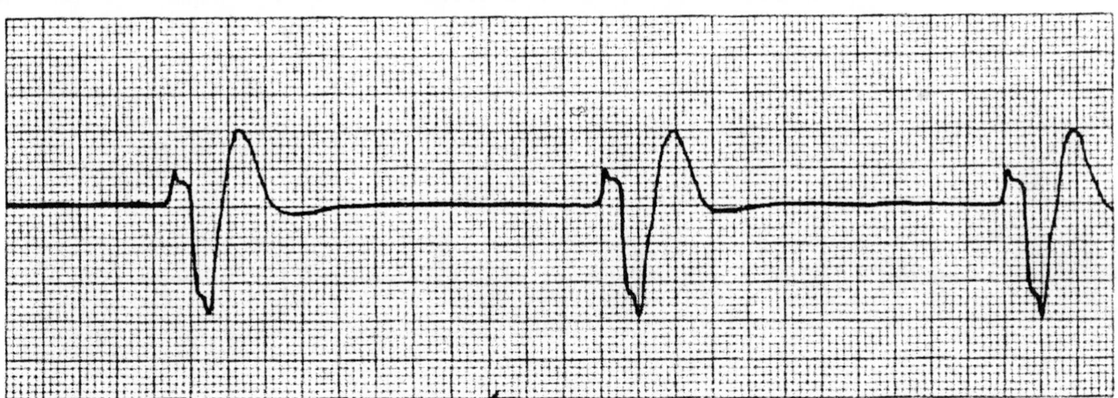

Figure 7-2 Idioventricular rhythm.

Box 7-3 Idioventricular Rhythm

Rate: Ventricular rate of 20-40 beats per minute
Rhythm: Usually regular
P waves: Absent
P-R interval: Not measurable
QRS complex: Wide, bizarre with T wave deflection in opposite direction, >0.12 second

Causes

Causes of idioventricular rhythms include MI, digitalis toxicity, metabolic imbalances, and hyperkalemia.

Treatment

The use of lidocaine is avoided for an idioventricular rhythm because this may cease all ventricular activity. Atropine is the drug of choice if the patient has a pulse and has symptoms. Other forms of treatment include transcutaneous pacing and a dopamine infusion if the patient has hypotension. If there is no pulse, then cardiopulmonary resuscitation (CPR) should be administered in conjunction with all advanced life support measures.

Accelerated Idioventricular Rhythm

An accelerated idioventricular rhythm (accelerated ventricular rhythm) is an idioventricular rhythm but with a rate of 41 to 100 beats per minute (Figure 7-3). This arrhythmia occurs because of enhanced automaticity of an irritable ventricular focus. An accelerated ventricular rhythm may occur in young healthy adults and may be without symptoms, or it may occur in the presence of an acute inferior wall MI or digitalis toxicity (Box 7-4).

This rhythm may be mistaken for ventricular tachycardia.

Treatment is only indicated if the patient is showing signs of decreased cardiac output and hypotension. Treatment is the same as for an idioventricular rhythm: an atropine sulfate 0.5- to 1.0-mg IV push if the rate is below 60 beats per minute, administered every 5 minutes to a maximum total of 0.04 mg/kg. A temporary or transcutaneous pacemaker should be considered.

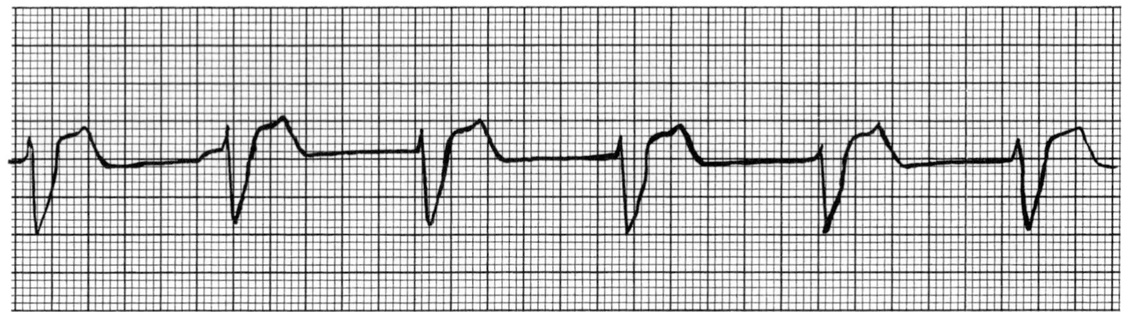

Figure 7-3 Accelerated idioventricular rhythm.

Box 7-4 Accelerated Ventricular (Idioventricular) Rhythm

Rate: No atrial rate; ventricular rate is 41-100 beats per minute
Rhythm: Ventricular usually regular
P waves: Absent
P-R interval: Not measurable
QRS complex: Wide and bizarre with a duration >0.12 second; the T wave deflection is in the opposite direction of the QRS complex

Ventricular Tachycardia

Ventricular tachycardia (V-tach) is a rhythm originating from the ventricles, but with a rate greater than 100 beats per minute (Figure 7-4). In fact, the perimeters for V-tach are 101 to 250 beats per minute. V-tach occurs when there is a run of three or more PVCs in a row and a rate of more than 101 beats per minute (Box 7-5).

V-tach may be a short run, lasting less than 30 seconds. It may be sustained, lasting longer than 30 seconds up to several hours.

V-tach is strange because it may or may not occur with pulse, and the patient may or may not be conscious. Thus the patient may be stable with normal vital signs or unstable with hypotension or no vital signs. Young healthy people may tolerate this rhythm for several hours, yet in other patients, the rhythm may deteriorate into ventricular fibrillation within a matter of minutes.

Causes

V-tach is usually caused by myocardial irritability. The rhythm originates in the ventricles, the same as PVCs through reentry or enhanced automaticity. It may be triggered by the R on T phenomenon before the cells have fully repolarized. When a PVC lands on a T wave of the preceding beat during this vulnerable period, a reentrant impulse may be initiated. V-tach may also be caused by the ischemia associated with an AMI.

Other causes include CHF, electrolyte imbalance, coronary artery disease, ventricular aneurysms, acid-base imbalances, mitral valve prolapse, rheumatic heart disease and toxicity from cardiac drugs such as digitalis, procainamide, and quinidine. Some noncardiac conditions that may lead to V-tach include pulmonary embolism and hypokalemia.

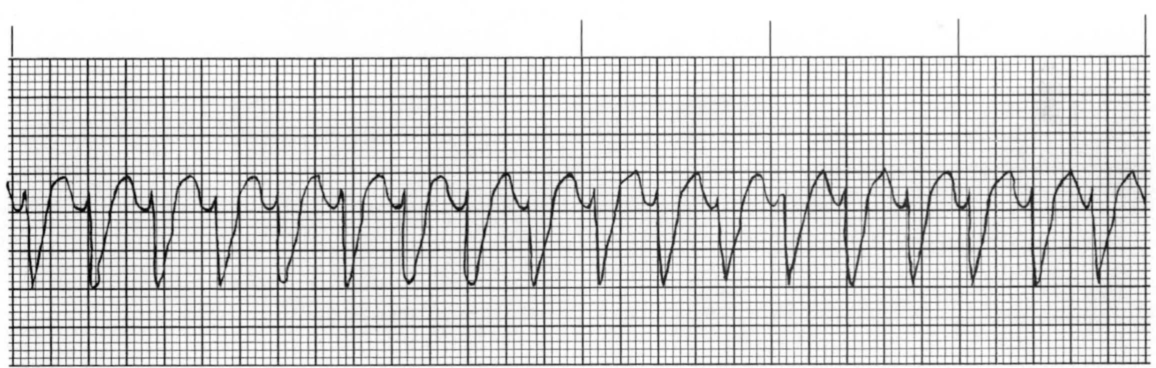

Figure 7-4 Ventricular tachycardia (V-tach).

Box 7-5 Ventricular Tachycardia

Rate: No atrial rate, ventricular rate 101-250 beats per minute
Rhythm: Essentially regular
P waves: Absent
P-R interval: Not measurable
QRS complex: Wide, bizarre appearance, duration >0.12 second

Treatment

Treatment of V-tach depends solely on the patient's symptoms. If the rhythm is sustained and the patient is stable with no signs and symptoms of cardiac compromise, then give oxygen and establish IV access. Amiodarone, lidoaine, or other antiarrhythmics should also be initiated.

If the patient is unstable, with signs and symptoms of cardiac compromise, cardioversion may be considered. If the patient is unconscious or without pulses, defibrillation should be initiated.

Defibrillation is the delivery of electrical current through the chest wall for the purpose of terminating nonperfusing rhythms such as ventricular fibrillation, unstable V-tach with a pulse, pulseless V-tach, and sustained torsades de pointes into a sinus rhythm. Defibrillation may be performed with a manual or automatic defibrillator. Defibrillation is initiated at 200 joules (J), the second shock at 200 to 300 J, and the third and consecutive shocks at 360 J (Box 7-6; Algorithms 7-1 and 7-2).

Electrical cardioversion is a synchronized countershock used to deliver an electrical shock through the chest wall for the purpose of terminating nonperfusing rhythms. An example is a V-tach in a patient with a pulse and who is conscious. Diazepam, midazolam (Versed), or fentanyl are some of the medications that might be used to sedate the patient before cardioversion. Unlike defibrillation, where the shock is delivered randomly, in synchronized cardioversion the shock is delivered approximately right after the peak of the R wave of the cardiac cycle. This is done to avoid the vulnerable period of the relative refractory period. Start with 100 J, then 200 J, 300 J, and 360 J for synchronized cardioversion (see Box 7-6). See Algorithms 7-1 and 7-2.

When you are unsure if the rhythm is V-tach or an SVT due to a regular wide QRS complex and the patient cardiac output is compromised, then treat the rhythm as V-tach until proven otherwise (see Algorithm 4-2).

Box 7-6 Procedure for Any Unstable Arrhythmia That Requires Electrical Intervention

Electrical Therapy

Defibrillation

1. Apply conductive gel to paddles (remove nitroglycerin patches, paste from chest wall).
2. Turn on defibrillator power.
3. Select correct energy level.
4. Position paddles on the chest wall using firm pressure (25 #).
5. Charge paddles and recheck the rhythm.
6. *Look* to make sure all personnel are clear. Visually check patient area from head to toe and call **"Clear."**
7. Depress both paddle discharge buttons simultaneously to deliver the shock.
8. Check the rhythm on the monitor and check the pulse.

Cardioversion

1. Turn on defibrillator and select the synchronous mode.
2. Observe the monitor to make sure the R wave coincides with the marker.
3. Put gel on the paddles and place on the patient's chest.
4. Select the energy level per protocol.
5. Ensure the patient area is clear and call **"Clear."**
6. Depress the discharge buttons simultaneously and *hold* them until the defibrillator fires on the next R wave.

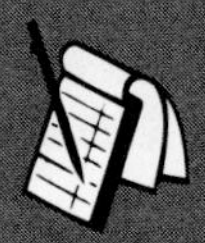

Note

Always treat the patient, not the monitor. Identify the rhythm on the monitor, but then look at the patient. Is he or she having problems breathing? Chest pain? Does he or she have normal vital signs? Are there any compromising situations going on? Everything is compiled, and then you may reach a decision about the method of treatment.

Torsades de Pointes

Torsades de pointes is a form of ventricular tachycardia in which there is a twisting of the points. The QRS complex changes in width and shape and appears to "twist" around the isoelectric line. The ventricular rate is 150 to 250 beats per minute (Figure 7-5). The QRS complexes may deflect downward for several beats and then upward for several beats. This dysrhythmia may have a sudden onset AND MAY SUDDENLY STOP (Box 7-7).

Causes

Any condition that causes a prolonged Q-T interval may precipitate torsades de pointes. Causes of long Q-T intervals include the following:

- Electrolyte imbalances
- Hypomagnesemia
- Hypocalcemia
- Hypokalemia
- Organophosphate poisonings
- Eating disorders
- Drug induced
- Phenothiazines
- Cyclic antidepressants
- Type IA antidysrhythmics
- Quinidine, procainamide

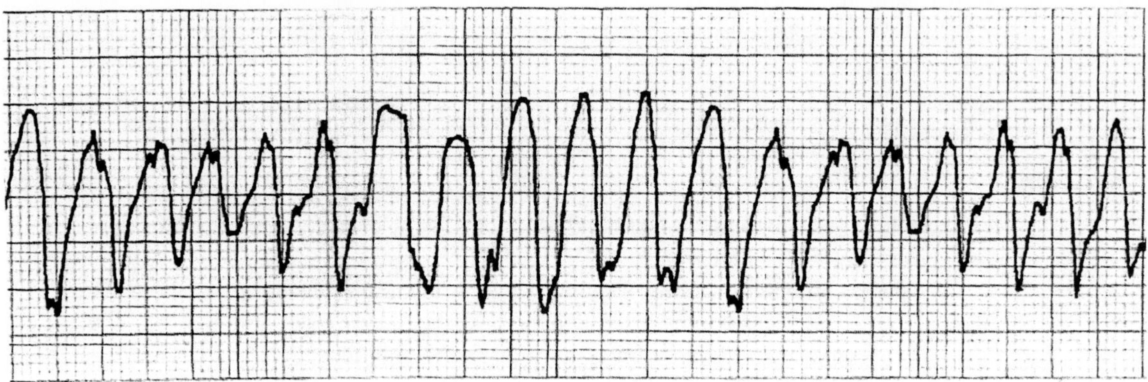

Figure 7-5 Torsades de pointes.

Box 7-7 Torsades de Pointes

Rate: Ventricular rate 150-250 beats per minute
Rhythm: Regular or irregular
P waves: Absent
P-R interval: Not measurable
QRS complex: Wide, bizarre with some complexes deflecting downward and some deflecting upward for several beats

Treatment

The treatment for torsades de pointes is different compared with V-tach, even though the signs and symptoms are similar. Treatment includes magnesium sulfate and over-drive pacing. It is extremely important to discontinue using any drugs such as lidocaine and quinidine because these may actually make the dysrhythmia worse because they prolong the Q-T interval.

Ventricular Fibrillation

Ventricular fibrillation (V-fib) is by far the most important rhythm for the health care provider to recognize. V-fib originates in the ventricles, most usually as a result of a reentry impulse and is a chaotic, rapid rhythm. With V-fib the heart is actually quivering instead of contracting; therefore there is no cardiac output and no systemic perfusion. V-fib results in cardiac arrest and is usually caused by MI or ischemia (Box 7-8).

There are two kinds of V-fib: coarse and fine. Coarse V-fib indicates that there is a recent onset of V-fib, whereas fine V-fib indicates that there has been a delay since the patient collapsed. Coarse V-fib indicates there is a considerable amount of electrical activity left in the heart; it may be easily converted with prompt defibrillation action (Figure 7-6). Fine V-fib shows little electrical activity in the heart, and it will be more difficult to resuscitate the patient. Fine V-fib may result in asystole (Figure 7-7).

Causes

V-fib is caused by any of the following:

- AMI
- Untreated V-tach
- Electrolyte imbalance such as hypokalemia, hyperkalemia, and hypercalcemia
- Acid-base imbalance
- Electrical shock, hypothermia
- R on T PVCs
- Drug overdose
- Trauma

Treatment

First, look at your patient for signs and symptoms. Is he or she conscious or unconscious? Is there any pulse or blood pressure?

If the patient is conscious, check the electrode leads to make sure they are not loose. Also check to see if the patient is shivering. Shivering may cause the rhythm monitor to look like V-fib. If the patient is unconscious with no pulse or respirations, then initiate CPR and defibrillation. Next intubate and establish IV access, and follow with drug therapy in conjunction with continued defibrillation.

Box 7-8 Ventricular Fibrillation

Rate: Cannot be determined
Rhythm: No pattern, fibrillatory waves
P waves: Absent
P-R interval: Not measurable
QRS complex: Cannot be determined

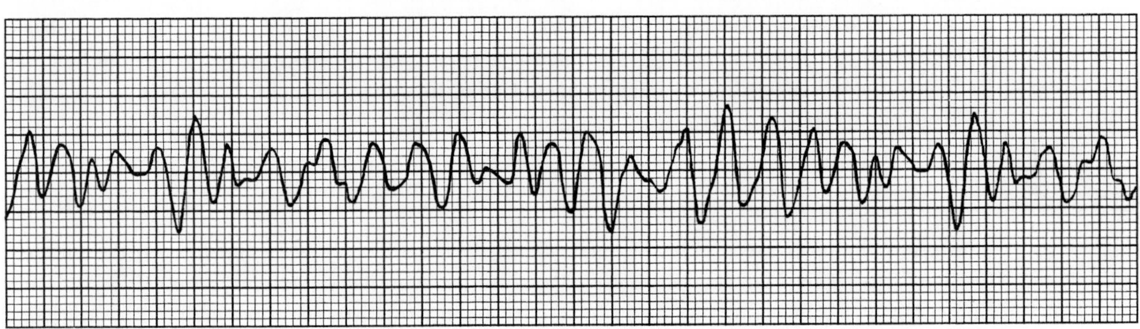

Figure 7-6 Coarse ventricular fibrillation (V-fib).

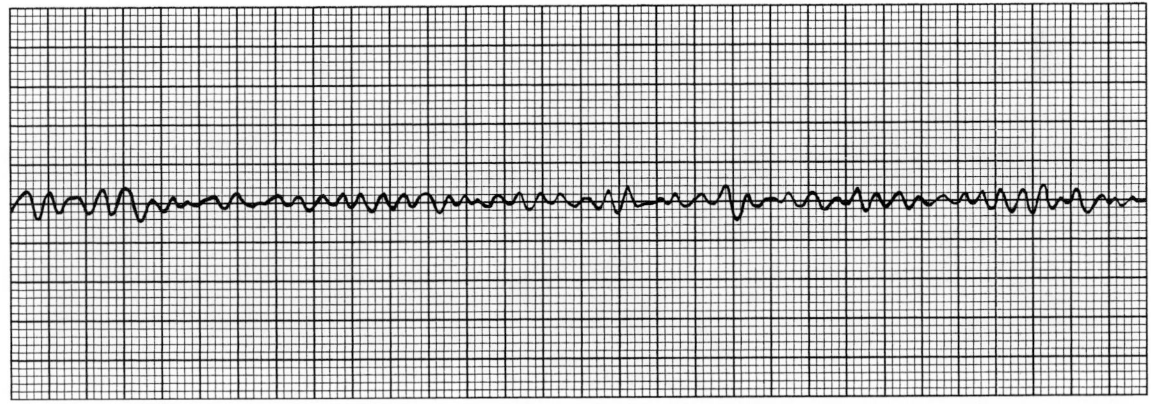

Figure 7-7 Fine ventricular fibrillation (V-fib).

Defibrillation is the delivery of an electrical charge through the chest wall. Hopefully, this charge of electricity will convert nonperfusing rhythms into perfusing sinus rhythms. Defibrillation is performed with the use of two paddles applied with approximately 25 lb of pressure on the chest wall. Treatment is aimed at early defibrillation, either with automatic or manual defibrillators. With a manual defibrillator, start at 200 J, then 200 to 300 J, then 360 J. See Algorithm 7-3 and Box 7-6.

Automatic Defibrillators

The resuscitation of a patient undergoing cardiac arrest depends solely on the "chain of survival" according to *Emergency Cardiovascular Care 2000 Guidelines*. Early access, early recognition, early CPR, and early defibrillation followed by ACLS provide the patient with the best chance of survival. Automatic defibrillators or AEDs provide this chance. There are two types available: automatic and semiautomatic. The automatic external defibrillator (AED) requires you to hook up the patient with two defibrillatory patches, connect the leads, and turn on the machine and press *analyze*. The machine does the rest, advising you, for example, when it is going to shock and when to stand clear. The semiautomatic is connected in the same fashion; however, you must press the analyze button to analyze the rhythm. Then the machine, in a computer-generated voice, tells you what steps to take. You manually deliver the shocks by pressing another button on the advice of the machine. The AED is available for First-Responder units and basic emergency medical technicians (EMTs), and it is becoming commonplace in many public areas such as golf courses, stadiums, and airplanes. Use of the AED is rapidly becoming part of every CPR course across the nation.

Asystole

Asystole is the term used for ventricular standstill; the ECG shows a flat line on the monitor (Figure 7-8). There is no electrical activity because the heart has completely stopped functioning. Sometimes you may see some fine atrial activity, but no impulses are conducted to the ventricles.

This is definitely a life-threatening situation. The patient has no blood pressure, has no pulse, and is not breathing. Airway and circulatory status are the major concern. The patient is in need of CPR (Box 7-9)!

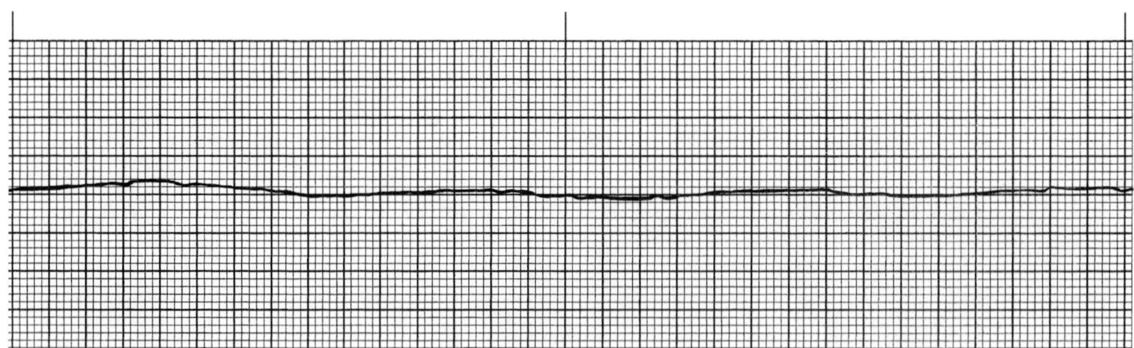

Figure 7-8 Asystole.

Box 7-9 Asystole

Rate: Atrial—usually indiscernible; ventricular—none
Rhythm: Atrial—usually indiscernible; ventricular—none
P waves: May be present, but not usually
P-R interval: Not measurable
QRS complex: Absent

Causes

Asystole can be caused by any of the following:

- Prolonged V-fib
- AMI
- Cardiac tamponade
- Metabolic acidosis
- Any condition that may cause inadequate blood flow, resulting in hypoxia
- Hypokalemia, hyperkalemia
- Pulmonary embolism
- Air embolism
- Electric shock
- Heart failure
- AV block
- Cocaine overdose

Treatment

Treatment is instituted as follows: CPR; monitor—always check this rhythm and confirm in two different leads on the cardiac monitor; intubate and establish IV access; and provide drug therapy as indicated by *Emergency Cardiovascular Care 2000 Guidelines*. Consider immediate transcutaneous pacing. Pacing needs to be applied during the first 10 minutes of asystole. Drug therapy should include epinephrine 1-mg IV push every 3 to 5 minutes of arrest and atropine 1-mg IV push every 3 to 5 minutes of arrest up to a total of 0.04 mg/kg. When you have run the complete code and tried everything in the algorithm, consider terminating the code. Today more and more asystole arrest situations are being terminated in the home. Asystole is more the confirmation of death rather than a treatable rhythm (Algorithm 7-4).

Pulseless Electrical Activity

Pulseless electrical activity is a condition that arises when there is dissociation of the electrical and mechanical activities of the heart. This can quickly lead to asystole. On the ECG you will see complexes and organized electrical activity, but the patient has no palpable pulse or blood pressure (Figure 7-9). Mechanical contraction of the myocardial fibers does not take place, and

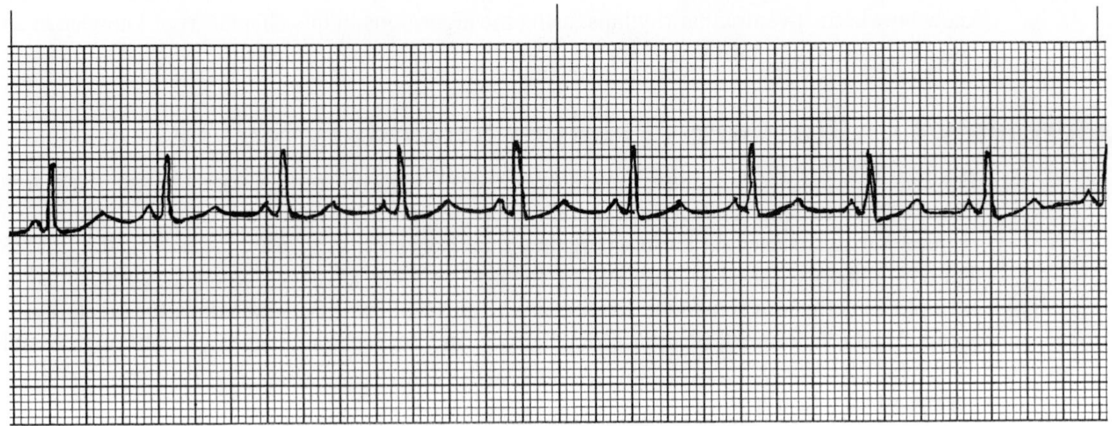

Figure 7-9 Pulseless electrical activity (PEA).

as a result the patient has no cardiac output or perfusion. Pulseless electrical activity is also known as *PEA* or *electromechanical dissociation* (EMD).

Causes

The causes of PEA are shown in Box 7-10.

Box 7-10 Causes of Pulseless Electrical Activity

- Left ventricular failure
- MI
- Hypovolemia
- Hypoxia
- Hyperkalemia
- Hypothermia
- Tension pneumothorax
- Pulmonary embolism
- Cardiac tamponade
- Acidosis
- Drug overdose

MI, Myocardial infarction.

Treatment

Management of PEA is the same as for any cardiac arrest situation: quickly evaluate electrical activity on the monitor, recheck that you do not feel a pulse, begin CPR, and intubate and establish IV access. Drug therapy includes epinephrine, in addition to atropine if the rate you are seeing on the monitor is less than 60 beats per minute. Refer to Algorithm 7-5.

VENTRICULAR SURVEYS

Now is the time for quick action! Ventricular rhythms are dangerous, life-threatening rhythms. To care for your patient you must have a good knowledge base of the rhythms and algorithms. Because you are eager to learn how to identify and interpret ECG strips, it is imperative you know how to treat ventricular rhythms, using the algorithms in this chapter. Your knowledge and quick actions may in turn save someone's life.

Emergency Cardiac Care—Primary-Secondary Survey

The *Emergency Cardiovascular Care 2000 Guidelines* recommend a series of specific actions that are easy to learn and definitely help keep you focused in an emergency situation. The primary survey focuses on basic emergency measures such as airway, rescue breathing, CPR, and defibrillation. The secondary survey focuses on more advanced emergency measures, for example, endotracheal intubation for the airway, positive-pressure ventilations for breathing, IV access, fluid replacement, pharmacology therapy, and hopefully a diagnosis identifying possible causes for the critical situation you have encountered.

- **Preliminary first actions**
- **Primary survey**
- **Secondary survey**

Preliminary first actions are performed immediately when you arrive on the scene or discover a patient in distress, if the setting is an in-hospital situation. First actions include three components:

- **A = Assess responsiveness**
- **C = Call for help**
- **P = Position yourself and the patient**

Primary survey includes four steps: **A-B-C-D**.

- **A = Airway**
- **B = Breathing**
- **C = Circulation**
- **D = Defibrillation**

Secondary survey includes four steps: **A-B-C-D**.

- **A = Airway**
- **B = Breathing**
- **C = Circulation**
- **D = Differential diagnosis**

Primary Survey

In the primary survey your focus is aimed at two components: CPR and defibrillation. The secondary survey also focuses on advanced procedures and a possible diagnosis. Both surveys are composed of one simple concept (Box 7-11).

Box 7-11 Primary A-B-C-D

A—Is the airway open? If not open the airway; may use oropharyngeal airway to keep it open.

B—Is the patient breathing? Assess respiratory status; is it adequate? If not initiate rescue breathing, using head tilt-chin lift method and provide positive-pressure ventilations. Stabilize the head if there is any question of trauma involvement.

C—Does the patient have a pulse? If not begin chest compressions!

D—Is defibrillation (electricity) needed? Shock is given in V-fib and pulseless V-tach; cardioversion is delivered in an unstable SVT.

SVT, Supraventricular tachycardia; *V-fib*, ventricular fibrillation; *V-tach*, ventricular tachycardia.

Secondary Survey

The secondary survey encompasses the same A, B, C, D, but this time, each letter stands for more advanced and in-depth interventions (Box 7-12).

Potential underlying or precipitating causes of cardiac arrest include the following:

- Hypoxia
- Tension pneumothorax
- Hypovolemia
- Cardiac tamponade
- AMI
- Severe acidosis
- Electrolyte disturbances
- Shock

Box 7-12 Secondary A-B-C-D

A—Establish an advanced airway with endotracheal or nasotracheal intubation
B—Now assess the adequacy of ventilations through the ET; provide positive-pressure ventilations through ET
C—Obtain IV access to administer fluids and medications; continue CPR; provide drug therapy appropriate for the ECG rhythm
D—Differential diagnosis; identify any possible causes for the arrest or critical situation; you need a differential diagnosis to be able to find and treat reversible causes of the arrest

CPR, Cardiopulmonary resuscitation; *ECG*, electrocardiogram; *ET*, endrotracheal tube; *IV*, intravenous.

- Drug overdose
- Fluid imbalance
- Trauma
- Pulmonary embolism
- Hypothermia, hyperthermia

SUMMARY

Preliminary first actions
- Assess responsiveness
- Call for help
- Position patient/rescuer

First A-B-C-D (primary survey)
- **A**irway:Open the airway
- **B**reathing: Provide positive-pressure ventilation
- **C**irculation: Chest compressions
- **D**efibrillation: Shock–V-fib/V-tach

Second A-B-C-D (secondary survey)
- **A**irway: Perform ET intubation; maintain advanced airway control
- **B**reathing: Assess ventilations through endotracheal tube (ET); continue positive pressure ventilations
- **C**irculation: Obtain IV access for fluids and drug administration; continue CPR; apply medications appropriate to rhythm
- **D**ifferential diagnosis: Identify possible reasons for cardiac arrest; differential diagnosis to identify reversible causes that have a specific therapy

VENTRICULAR TACHYCARDIA

MONOMORPHIC: QRS complexes that are basically the same shape, size, and duration

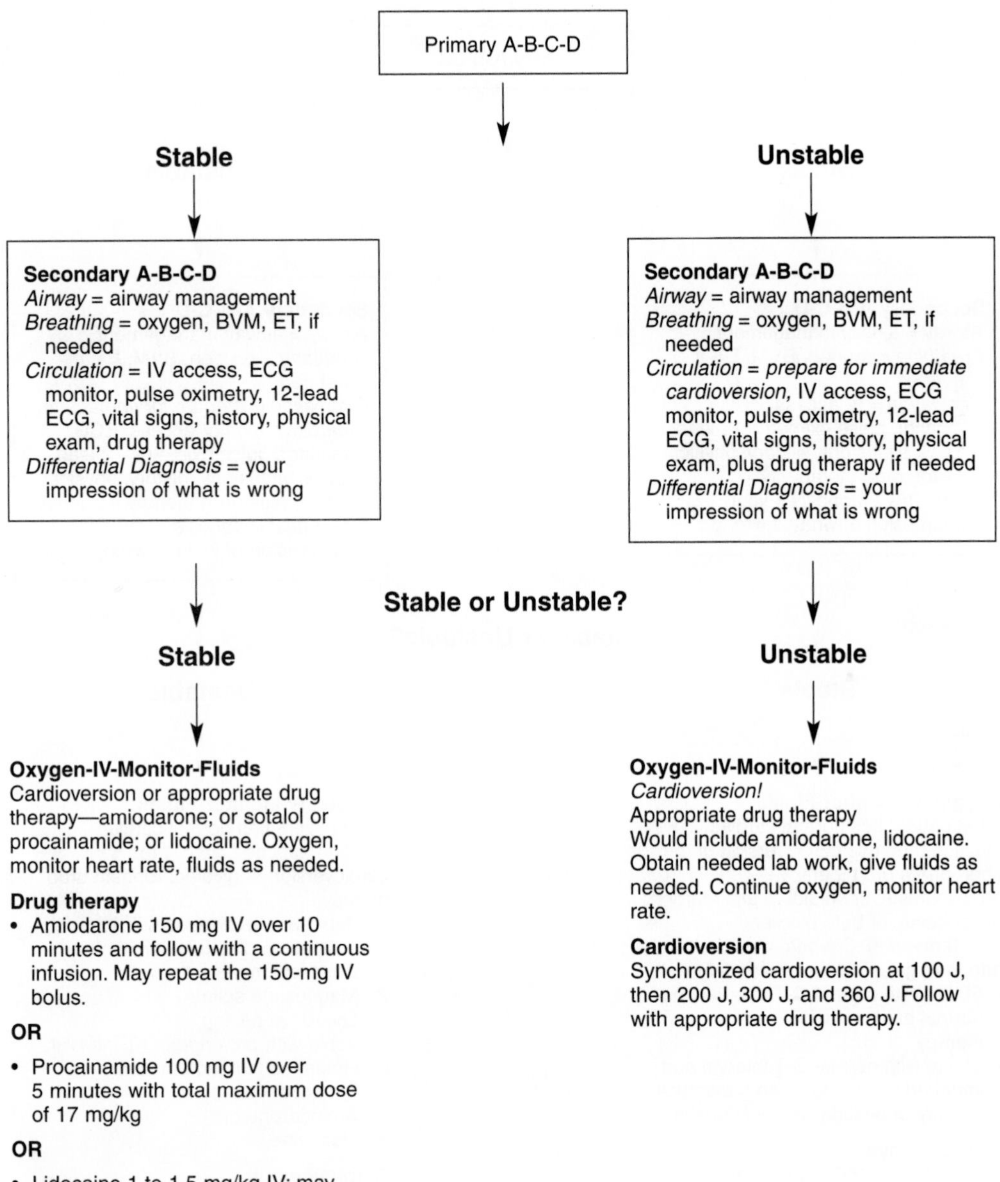
Primary A-B-C-D
Stable
Unstable
Secondary A-B-C-D
Airway = airway management
Breathing = oxygen, BVM, ET, if needed
Circulation = IV access, ECG monitor, pulse oximetry, 12-lead ECG, vital signs, history, physical exam, drug therapy
Differential Diagnosis = your impression of what is wrong
Secondary A-B-C-D
Airway = airway management
Breathing = oxygen, BVM, ET, if needed
Circulation = prepare for immediate cardioversion, IV access, ECG monitor, pulse oximetry, 12-lead ECG, vital signs, history, physical exam, plus drug therapy if needed
Differential Diagnosis = your impression of what is wrong
Stable or Unstable?
Stable
Unstable
Oxygen-IV-Monitor-Fluids
Cardioversion or appropriate drug therapy—amiodarone; or sotalol or procainamide; or lidocaine. Oxygen, monitor heart rate, fluids as needed.
Drug therapy
• Amiodarone 150 mg IV over 10 minutes and follow with a continuous infusion. May repeat the 150-mg IV bolus.
OR
• Procainamide 100 mg IV over 5 minutes with total maximum dose of 17 mg/kg
OR
• Lidocaine 1 to 1.5 mg/kg IV; may repeat at 0.5 to 0.75 mg/kg (half-dose) up to a total of 3 mg/kg
Oxygen-IV-Monitor-Fluids
Cardioversion!
Appropriate drug therapy
Would include amiodarone, lidocaine. Obtain needed lab work, give fluids as needed. Continue oxygen, monitor heart rate.
Cardioversion
Synchronized cardioversion at 100 J, then 200 J, 300 J, and 360 J. Follow with appropriate drug therapy.

Algorithm 7-1 Ventricular tachycardia (V-tach), monomorphic. (Modified from Aelhert B: *ACLS quick review study guide*, ed 2, St Louis, 2002, Mosby.)

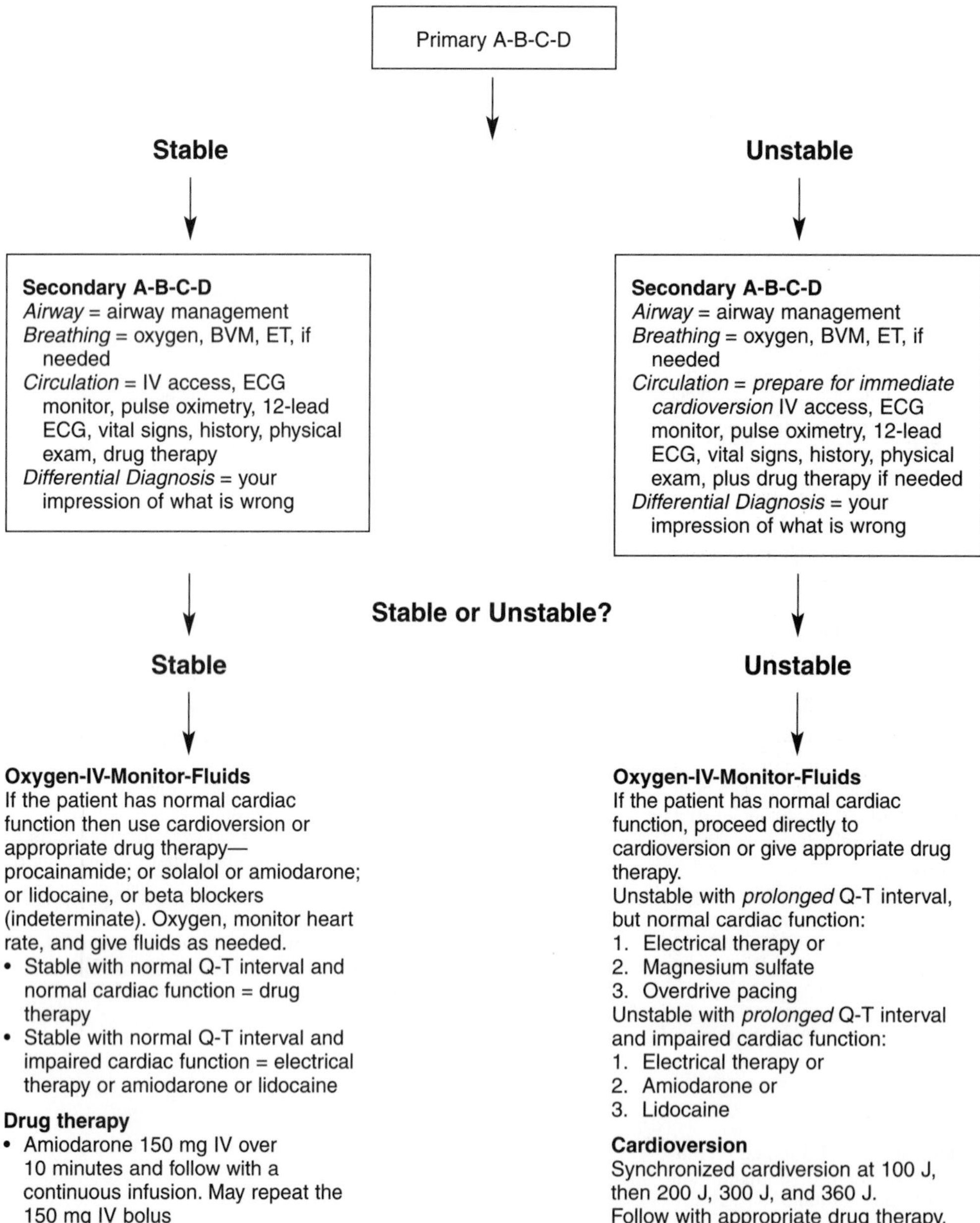
VENTRICULAR TACHYCARDIA
POLYMORPHIC: QRS complexes that are different in shape, size, and duration
Determine the patient's Q-T interval
Primary A-B-C-D
Stable
Unstable
Secondary A-B-C-D
Airway = airway management
Breathing = oxygen, BVM, ET, if needed
Circulation = IV access, ECG monitor, pulse oximetry, 12-lead ECG, vital signs, history, physical exam, drug therapy
Differential Diagnosis = your impression of what is wrong
Secondary A-B-C-D
Airway = airway management
Breathing = oxygen, BVM, ET, if needed
Circulation = prepare for immediate cardioversion IV access, ECG monitor, pulse oximetry, 12-lead ECG, vital signs, history, physical exam, plus drug therapy if needed
Differential Diagnosis = your impression of what is wrong
Stable or Unstable?
Stable
Unstable
Oxygen-IV-Monitor-Fluids
If the patient has normal cardiac function then use cardioversion or appropriate drug therapy—procainamide; or solalol or amiodarone; or lidocaine, or beta blockers (indeterminate). Oxygen, monitor heart rate, and give fluids as needed.
• Stable with normal Q-T interval and normal cardiac function = drug therapy
• Stable with normal Q-T interval and impaired cardiac function = electrical therapy or amiodarone or lidocaine
Drug therapy
• Amiodarone 150 mg IV over 10 minutes and follow with a continuous infusion. May repeat the 150 mg IV bolus
Oxygen-IV-Monitor-Fluids
If the patient has normal cardiac function, proceed directly to cardioversion or give appropriate drug therapy.
Unstable with prolonged Q-T interval, but normal cardiac function:
1. Electrical therapy or
2. Magnesium sulfate
3. Overdrive pacing
Unstable with prolonged Q-T interval and impaired cardiac function:
1. Electrical therapy or
2. Amiodarone or
3. Lidocaine
Cardioversion
Synchronized cardiversion at 100 J, then 200 J, 300 J, and 360 J.
Follow with appropriate drug therapy.

Algorithm 7-2 Ventricular tachycardia (V-tach), polymorphic. (Modified from Aelhert B: *ACLS quick review study guide*, ed 2, St Louis, 2002, Mosby.)

OR

- Procainamide 100 mg IV over 5 minutes with total maximum dose of 17 mg/kg

OR

- Lidocaine 1 to 1.5 mg/kg IV; may repeat at 0.5 to 0.75 mg/kg (half-dose) up to a total of 3 mg/kg

OR

- Esmolol 0.5-mg/kg IV bolus over 1 minute

OR

- Atenolol 5-mg IV bolus over 5 minutes

OR

- Metoprolol 5 mg IV over 2 to 5 minutes

Note: Ventricular tachycardia with hemodynamic collapse should be treated with defibrillation starting at 200 J

Algorithm 7-2, cont'd Ventricular tachycardia (V-tach), polymorphic. (Modified from Aelhert B: *ACLS quick review study guide*, ed 2, St Louis, 2002, Mosby.)

VENTRICULAR FIBRILLATION

Perform Primary A-B-C-D

Airway – ensure open airway
Breathing – give two *slow* breaths
Circulation – chest compressions
Defibrillation – evaluate cardiac rhythm and defibrillate as soon as AED or defibrillator is available

↓

Perform Secondary A-B-C-D

Airway – perform advanced airway management (endotracheal intubation), ensure open airway
Breathing – confirm ET placement (two methods). Provide positive pressure ventilations
Circulation – establish IV access, give appropriate drug therapy
Differential Diagnosis: search for reversible causes and treatment

Defibrillation
- Evaluate cardiac rhythm and defibrillate at 200 J, repeat at 300 J and 360 J as needed, up to three times
- Consider defibrillation after each dosage of drug therapy

Drug Therapy
- ***Epinephrine*** – 1 mg IV or 2 to 2.5 mg ET. May repeat every 3 to 5 minutes

OR

- ***Vasopressin*** – 40 units IV, single dose. Do not repeat

NOTE: If you give vasopressin and want to continue with epinephrine, you must wait 10 to 20 minutes after giving the vasopressin.

Consider Antiarrhythmics

- ☐ ***Amiodarone*** – 300-mg IV bolus (diluted in 20 ml of NS or D5W). May repeat dose at 150-mg IV bolus, diluted
- ☐ ***Lidocaine*** – 1- to 1.5-mg/kg IV bolus. May repeat at 0.5- to 0.75-mg IV bolus up to a total maximum dose of 3 mg/kg
- ☐ ***Procainamide*** – 20 mg/min IV; total dose of 17 mg/kg IV
- ☐ ***Magnesium Sulfate*** – If torsades de pointes or hypomagnesemia is suspected, give 1 to 2 gram IV diluted
- ☐ ***Consider Sodium Bicarbonate*** – 1 mEq/kg IV

Ensure adequate CPR during the arrest except while defibrillation is in process

Algorithm 7-3 Ventricular fibrillation (V-fib) or pulseless ventricular tachycardia (V-tach). (Modified from Aelhert B: *ACLS quick review study guide*, ed 2, St Louis, 2002, Mosby.)

ASYSTOLE

Perform Primary A-B-C-D

Airway – ensure open airway
Breathing – give two *slow* breaths
Circulation – chest compressions
Defibrillation – evaluate cardiac rhythm and go on to secondary survey if V fib is not present
*E*valuate asystole in two leads

↓

Perform Secondary A-B-C-D

Airway – perform advanced airway management (endotracheal intubation), ensure open airway
Breathing – confirm ET placement (two methods). Provide positive pressure ventilations
Circulation – establish IV access, give appropriate drug therapy
Differential Diagnosis: search for reversible causes and treat reversible conditions

↓

Consider immediate transcutaneous pacing – immediate being within the first 10 minutes of arrest

Appropriate drug therapy:

- ☐ ***Epinephrine*** – 1-mg IV bolus; may repeat every 3 to 5 minutes during arrest
- ☐ ***Atrophine*** – 1-mg IV bolus every 3 to 5 minutes during arrest up to a total dose of 0.04 mg/kg
- ☐ ***Consider sodium bicarbonate*** – 1 mEq/kg IV
- ☐ ***Consider terminating the arrest***

Algorithm 7-4 Asystole. (Modified from Aelhert B: *ACLS quick review study guide*, ed 2, St Louis, 2002, Mosby.)

PULSELESS ELECTRICAL ACTIVITY

Perform Primary A-B-C-D

Airway – ensure open airway
Breathing – give two *slow* breaths
Circulation – chest compressions
Defibrillation – evaluate cardiac rhythm and go on to secondary survey if V-fib is not present

↓

Perform Secondary A-B-C-D

Airway – perform advanced airway management (endotracheal intubation), ensure open airway
Breathing – confirm ET placement (two methods). Provide positive pressure ventilations
Circulation – establish IV access, give appropriate drug therapy
Differential Diagnosis: search for reversible causes and treat reversible conditions

↓

Search, identify and treat possible reversible causes:

- ☐ ***H*** – hypoxia
- ☐ ***H*** – hypovolemia
- ☐ ***H*** – heart, acute myocardial infarction, coronary thrombosis
- ☐ ***H*** – hydrogen ion imbalance, acidosis
- ☐ ***H*** – hyperkalemia, electrolyte disturbances
- ☐ ***T*** – tablet, drug overdose
- ☐ ***T*** – thrombosis, pulmonary embolism
- ☐ ***T*** – tension pneumothorax
- ☐ ***T*** – tamponade, cardiac
- ☐ ***T*** – temperature; hyperthermia and hypothermia

Appropriate Drug Therapy:

- ***Epinephrine*** – 1-mg IV bolus; may repeat every 3 to 5 minutes during the arrest
- ***Atropine*** – 1-mg IV bolus if the rate of the rhythm is less than 60 beats per minute; may repeat every 3 to 5 minutes up to a total maximum dose of 0.04 mg/kg
- ***Fluids*** – consider a fluid challenge 250 to 500 ml or normal saline
- ***Sodium bicarbonate*** – 1-mEq/kg IV bolus if acidosis suspected; may repeat 0.5 mEq/kg IV

Consider termination – when all possible causes are exhausted, consider terminating resuscitative efforts

Algorithm 7-5 Pulseless electrical activity (PEA). (Modified from Aelhert B: *ACLS quick review study guide*, ed 2, St Louis, 2002, Mosby.)

Chapter 7 Self-Test

1. Multiple Choice: Which of the following best describes a P wave in a ventricular rhythm:
   a. Absent
   b. Present, but prolonged
   c. Present, but shorter than normal duration
   d. Absent every other complex

2. Multiple Choice: Which of the following best describes a QRS complex in a ventricular rhythm?
   a. Narrow and less than a 0.12-second duration
   b. A duration of 0.06 to 0.10 second and uniform in appearance
   c. Wide and bizarre with a duration longer than 0.12 second
   d. None of the above

3. Multiple Choice: A ventricular rhythm with PVCs usually has a T wave that:
   a. Deflects in the same direction as the QRS complex
   b. Deflects in the opposite direction of the QRS complex
   c. Is absent
   d. None of the above

4. Multiple Choice: When you see a sinus rhythm with PVCs, the PVCs create:
   a. A compensatory pause
   b. A noncompensatory pause
   c. An episode of chest pain
   d. A near-syncopal episode

5. Multiple Choice: PVCs are considered dangerous in a sinus rhythm if
   a. They are frequent (more than three per minute)
   b. They are uniform, and one occurs every 2 to 3 minutes
   c. The PVC is a narrow complex
   d. They are wide and bizarre, they are multifocal, and there are more than six per minute

6. Multiple choice: ____________________ on ____________________ is when a PVC falls every second or third beat.
   a. Bigeminy, quadrigeminy
   b. Bigeminy, compensatory
   c. Compensatory, noncompensatory
   d. Bigeminy, trigeminy

7. Multiple Choice: Three or more PVCs in a row is called:
   a. Ventricular tachycardia
   b. Trigeminy
   c. Ventricular standstill
   d. Ventricular compensation

8. Multiple Choice: V-tach usually has a rate of ________________ to ________________ .
   a. 101 to 250 beats per minute
   b. 101 to 140 beats per minute
   c. 101 to 210 beats per minute
   d. 50 to 100 beats per minute

9. Multiple Choice: A ventricular rhythm is usually:
   a. Irregular
   b. Regular
   c. Chaotic
   d. P-R interval greater than 0.12 second

10. Multiple Choice: A patient with V-tach may experience:
    a. Chest pain
    b. Syncope
    c. Dizziness, anxiety
    d. Seizures due to cerebral ischemia
    e. All of the above

11. Multiple Choice: The pacemaker cells in the Purkinje fibers have an intrinsic firing rate of:
    a. 60 to 100 beats per minute
    b. 30 to 50 beats per minute
    c. 40 to 60 beats per minute
    d. 20 to 40 beats per minute

12. Multiple Choice: The QRS complex represents which of the following electrical activities:
    a. Atrial depolarization
    b. Atrial repolarization
    c. Ventricular depolarization
    d. Ventricular repolarization

13. Multiple Choice: Ventricular diastole refers to which of the following:
    a. A dying heart
    b. Ventricular contraction
    c. Mean diastolic pressure
    d. Ventricular relaxation

14. Multiple Choice: An accelerated idioventricular rhythm usually has a rate of:
    a. More than 100 beats per minute
    b. 80 to 100 beats per minute
    c. 40 to 100 beats per minute
    d. 20 to 40 beats per minute

15. Multiple Choice: Torsades de pointes is recognized by:
    a. P waves that are pointed
    b. "Rounded but small QRS complexes"
    c. "Twisting of the points"
    d. An inverted T wave with a tall point

16. Multiple Choice: The drug of choice for torsades de pointes is:
    a. Lidocaine
    b. Amiodarone
    c. Magnesium sulfate
    d. Procainamide

17. Multiple Choice: In ventricular asystole you will find:
    a. An ECG rhythm but no pulse
    b. Absence of a QRS complex every third or fourth beat
    c. No atrial activity, but a regular ventricular rhythm with no pulse
    d. A flat line on the ECG monitor

18. Multiple Choice: A dysrhythmia that has repetitive series of chaotic waves is:
    a. Ventricular tachycardia
    b. Ventricular fibrillation
    c. A dysrhythmia with PVCs
    d. Pulseless electrical activity

19. Multiple Choice: The P-R interval of an idioventricular rhythm is:
    a. Interrupted every third beat
    b. Irregular
    c. Regular
    d. Absent

20. Multiple Choice: Ventricular complexes that arrive late in the cardiac cycle are:
    a. Premature complexes
    b. Irregular beats
    c. Escape beats
    d. Aberrant beats

21. Multiple Choice: A ventricular complex that is considered a protective mechanism is:
    a. A premature complex
    b. An irregular beat
    c. An escape beat
    d. An aberrant beat

22. Fill in the Blank: An ____________________ on ____________________ is considered a very dangerous type of PVC.

ECG Practice Strips

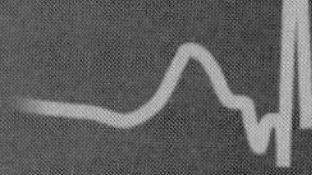

Please calculate the following 15 ECG practice strips

- Determine the rate
- Is the rhythm regular or irregular?
- Measure the P-R interval
- Measure the QRS complex duration
- Check to see if there is a P wave before every QRS complex
- Check to see if there is a QRS complex after every P wave
- Then give your interpretation of the rhythm
- All strips are lead II unless otherwise noted

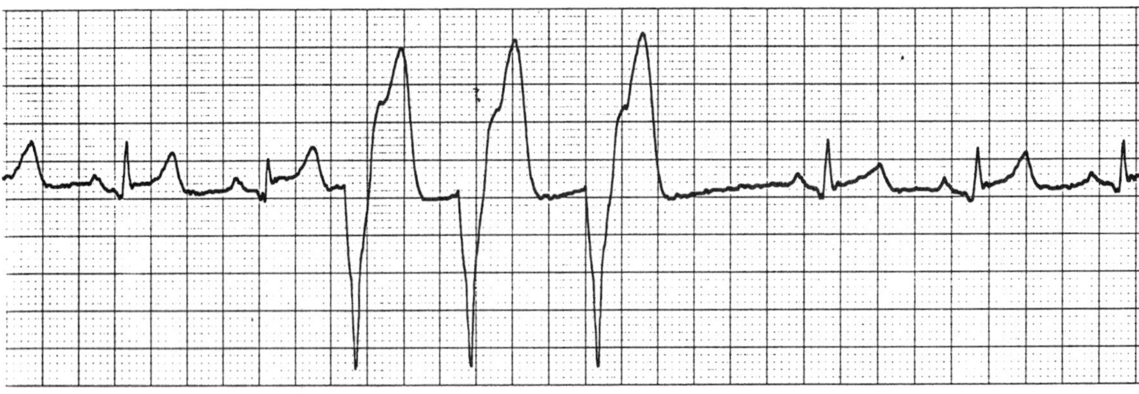

Practice Figure 7-1

Rate: ____________ Rhythm: ____________ P-R interval: ____________ QRS complex: ____________

Is there a P wave before every QRS complex? ____

Is there a QRS complex after every P wave? ____

Interpretation: ____

____

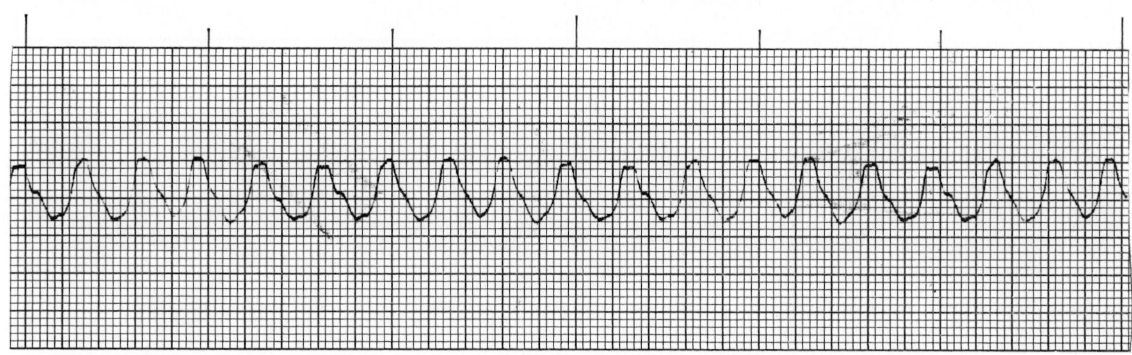

Practice Figure 7-2

Rate: ____________ Rhythm: ____________ P-R interval: ____________ QRS complex: ____________

Is there a P wave before every QRS complex? ____________

Is there a QRS complex after every P wave? ____________

Interpretation: ____________

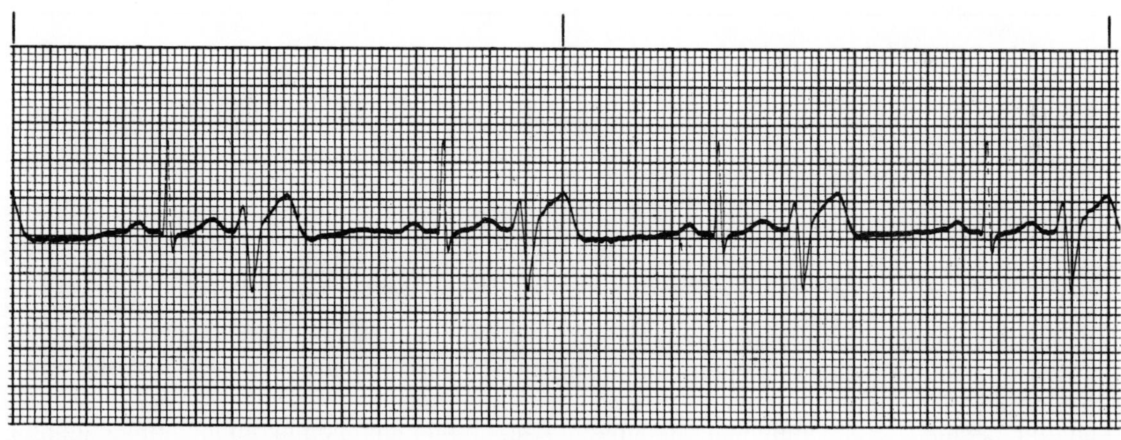

Practice Figure 7-3

Rate: ____________ Rhythm: ____________ P-R interval: ____________ QRS complex: ____________

Is there a P wave before every QRS complex? ____________

Is there a QRS complex after every P wave? ____________

Interpretation: ____________

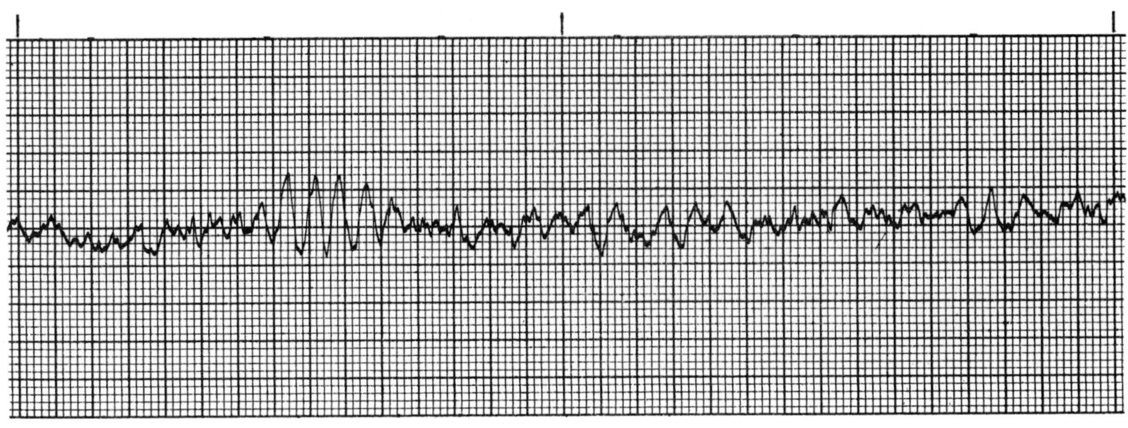

Practice Figure 7-4

Rate: ____________ Rhythm: ____________ P-R interval: ____________ QRS complex: ____________

Is there a P wave before every QRS complex? ____________

Is there a QRS complex after every P wave? ____________

Interpretation: ____________

____

Practice Figure 7-5

Rate: ____________ Rhythm: ____________ P-R interval: ____________ QRS complex: ____________

Is there a P wave before every QRS complex? ____________

Is there a QRS complex after every P wave? ____________

Interpretation: ____________

____

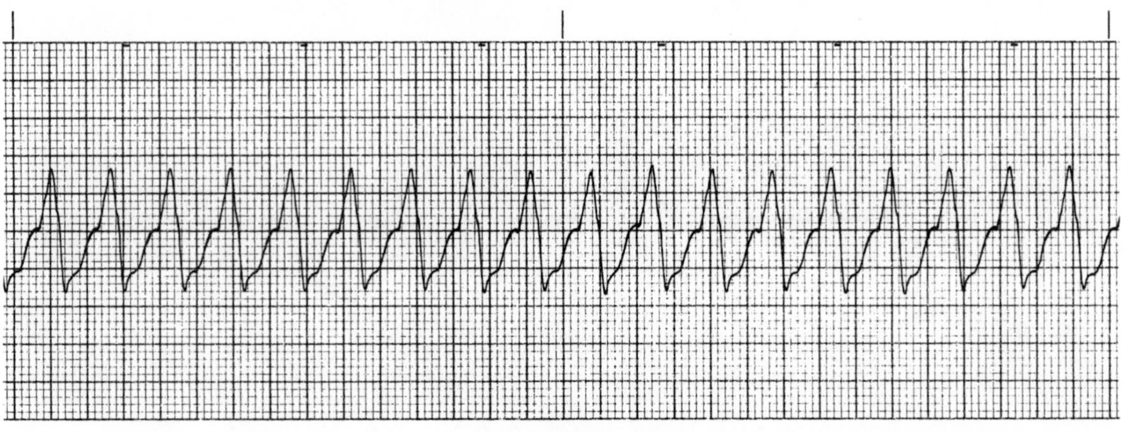

Practice Figure 7-6

Rate: ____________ Rhythm: ____________ P-R interval: ____________ QRS complex: ____________

Is there a P wave before every QRS complex? ____

Is there a QRS complex after every P wave? ____

Interpretation: ____

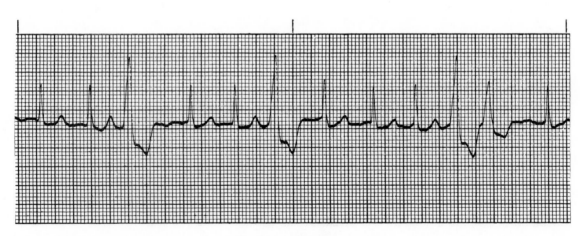

____

Practice Figure 7-7

Rate: ____________ Rhythm: ____________ P-R interval: ____________ QRS complex: ____________

Is there a P wave before every QRS complex? ____

Is there a QRS complex after every P wave? ____

Interpretation: ____

____

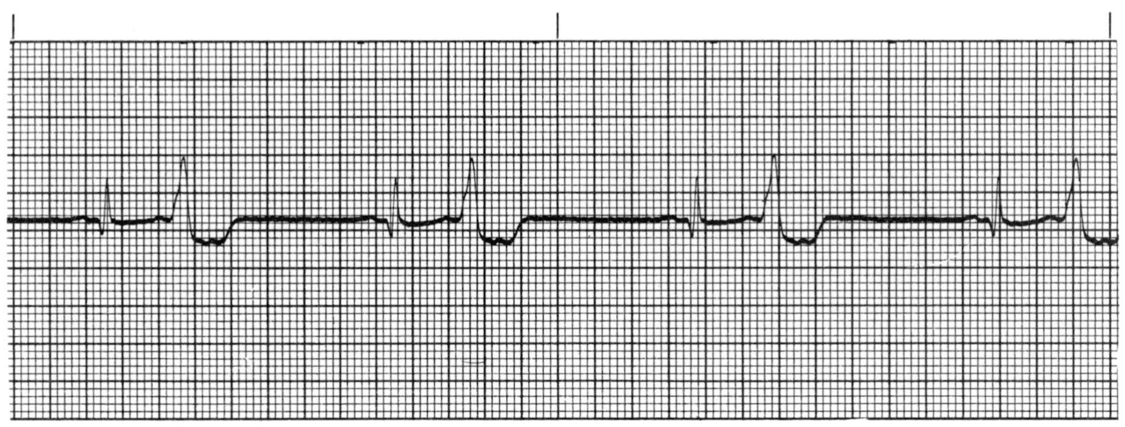

Practice Figure 7-8

Rate: ____________ Rhythm: ____________ P-R interval: ____________ QRS complex: ____________

Is there a P wave before every QRS complex? ____________

Is there a QRS complex after every P wave? ____________

Interpretation: ____________

____

Practice Figure 7-9

Rate: ____________ Rhythm: ____________ P-R interval: ____________ QRS complex: ____________

Is there a P wave before every QRS complex? ____________

Is there a QRS complex after every P wave? ____________

Interpretation: ____________

____

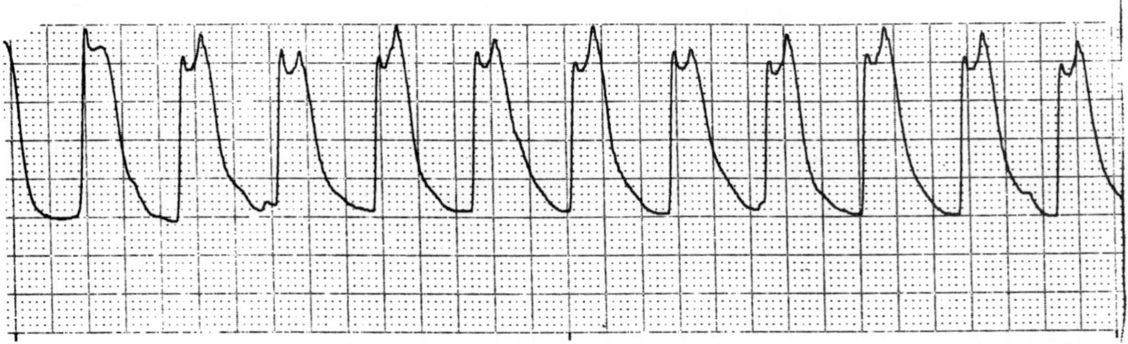

Practice Figure 7-10

Rate: ____________ Rhythm: ____________ P-R interval: ____________ QRS complex: ____________

Is there a P wave before every QRS complex? ____________

Is there a QRS complex after every P wave? ____________

Interpretation: ____________

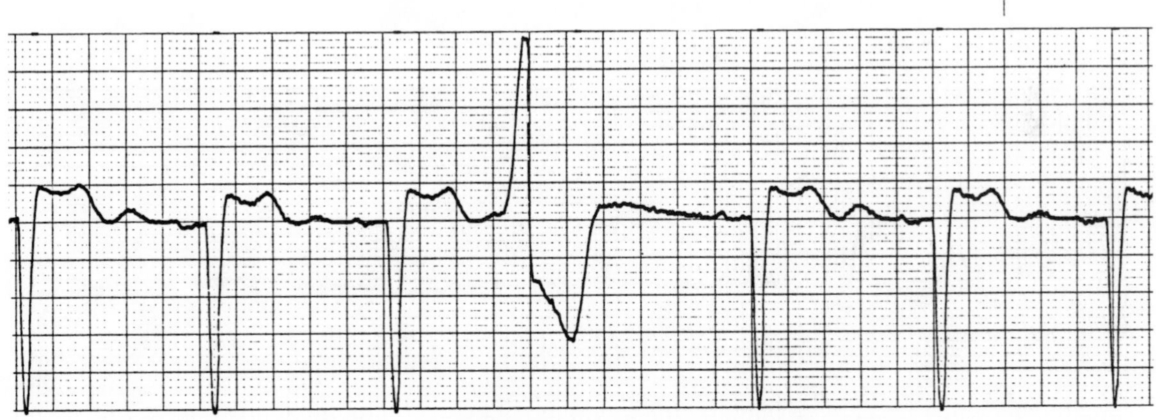

Practice Figure 7-11

Rate: ____________ Rhythm: ____________ P-R interval: ____________ QRS complex: ____________

Is there a P wave before every QRS complex? ____________

Is there a QRS complex after every P wave? ____________

Interpretation: ____________

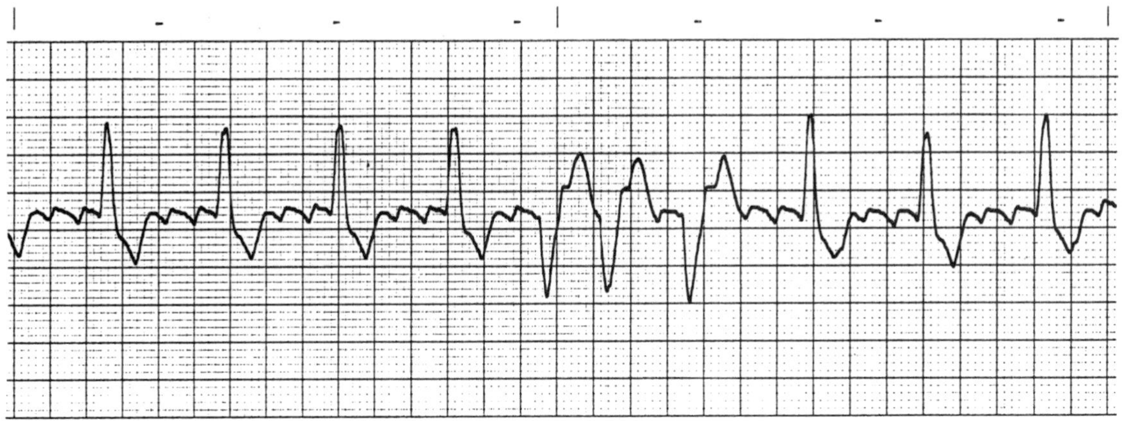

Practice Figure 7-12

Rate: ____________ Rhythm: ____________ P-R interval: ____________ QRS complex: ____________

Is there a P wave before every QRS complex? ____________

Is there a QRS complex after every P wave? ____________

Interpretation: ____________

Practice Figure 7-13

Rate: ____________ Rhythm: ____________ P-R interval: ____________ QRS complex: ____________

Is there a P wave before every QRS complex? ____________

Is there a QRS complex after every P wave? ____________

Interpretation: ____________

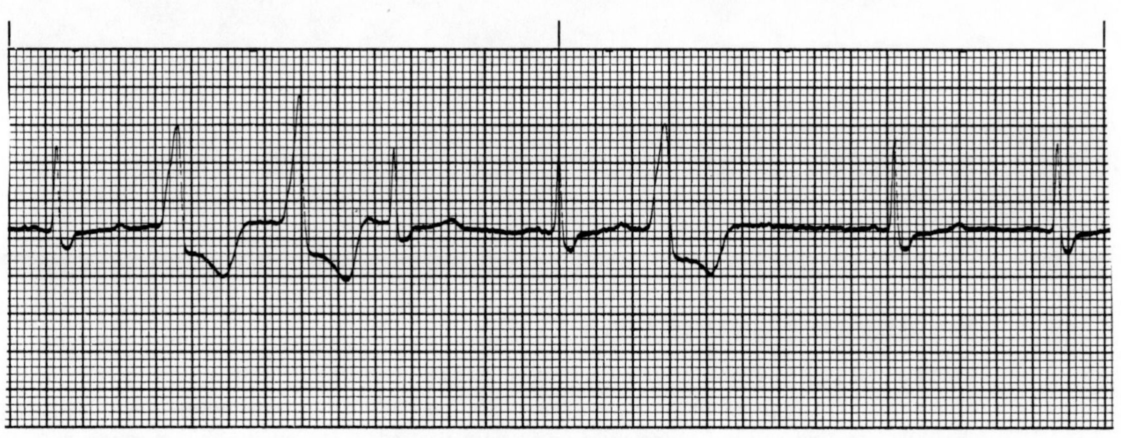

Practice Figure 7-14

Rate: ____________ Rhythm: ____________ P-R interval: ____________ QRS complex: ____________

Is there a P wave before every QRS complex? ____________

Is there a QRS complex after every P wave? ____________

Interpretation: ____________

____

Practice Figure 7-15

Rate: ____________ Rhythm: ____________ P-R interval: ____________ QRS complex: ____________

Is there a P wave before every QRS complex? ____________

Is there a QRS complex after every P wave? ____________

Interpretation: ____________

____

Case Scenarios

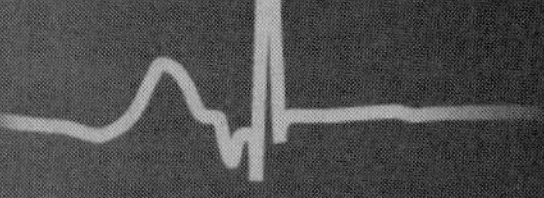

CASE 1

Scenario: (Actual EMS Call)

Your patient is a 38-year-old female sitting in a car at the local gas station. She is complaining of abdominal pain in the mid-epigastric area. She has nausea, but no vomiting. On questioning, she tells you that she had some mild chest pain yesterday, but awoke this morning with the abdominal pain. She thinks it is the flu that has been going around. She is alert, she is oriented ×4, and her skin is pink, warm, and dry. Lung sounds are clear, and vital signs are BP, 110/60; P, 170 and regular; R, 22; and an Sao_2 of 96%. There is nothing in her medical history, and she is not taking any medications. You see the following on the monitor:

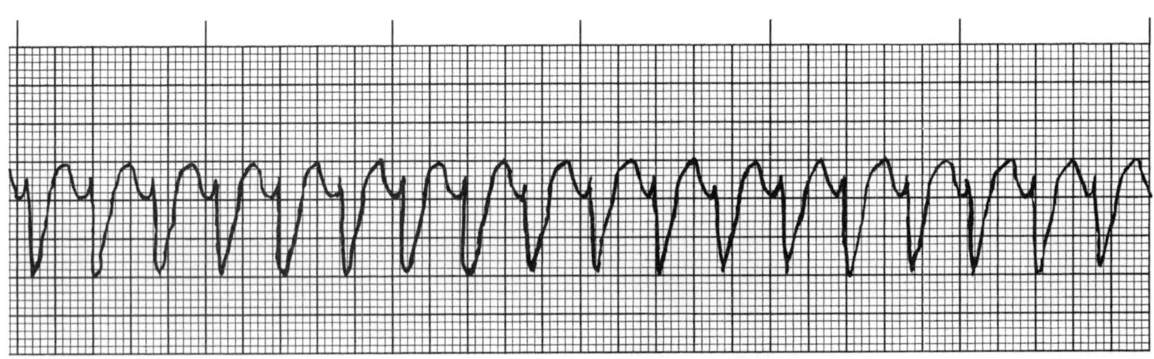

Identify the Rhythm

What is the rate? ______________ What is the rhythm (regular or irregular)? ______________

Is there a P wave before every QRS complex? ______________ Is there a QRS complex after every P wave? ______________

What is the P-R interval? ______________ QRS complex duration? ______________

Interpretation:

____

____

Case 1 Self-Test

In the spaces below give your treatment for the Primary Survey and Secondary Survey, plus the continued care under Oxygen-IV-Monitor-Fluids and Vital Signs. How would you care for this patient, and what orders would you expect from the physician? At the bottom, list your potential diagnosis or impression of what the patient's problem is.

Primary Survey

A.

B.

C.

D.

Secondary Survey

A.

B.

C.

D.

Oxygen-IV-Monitor-Fluids: ______________________________

____

Vital Signs: ______________________________

____

Your Impression: ______________________________

____

CASE 2

Scenario

A car pulls up in front of the emergency department with a 69-year-old male who is unconscious. Your initial survey reveals no respirations and no pulse. His wife tells you quickly that he has a history of two MIs and a bypass operation 5 years ago. She says he has not been feeling well for the past 2 to 3 days and had an upset stomach. You do a quick look with the paddles, and on the monitor you see the following:

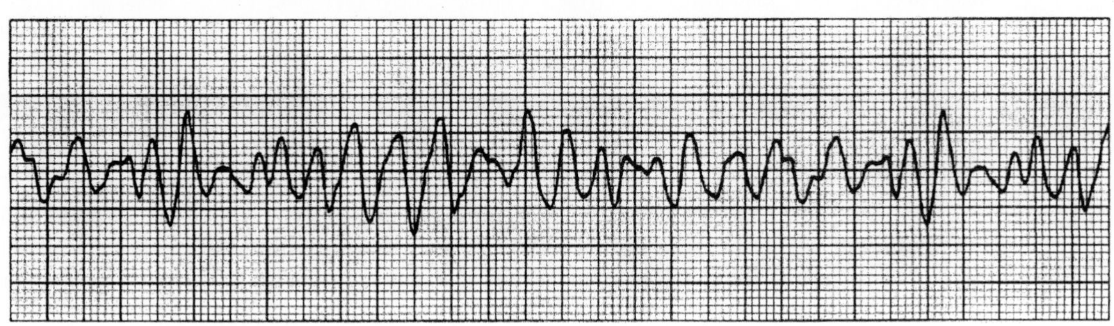

Identify the Rhythm

What is the rate? ______________ What is the rhythm (regular or irregular)? ______________

Is there a P wave before every QRS complex? ______________ Is there a QRS complex after every P wave? ______________

What is the P-R interval? ______________ QRS complex duration? ______________

Interpretation:

____

____

Case 2 Self-Test

In the spaces below give your treatment for the Primary Survey and Secondary Survey, plus the continued care under Oxygen-IV-Monitor-Fluids and Vital Signs. How would you care for this patient, and what orders would you expect from the physician? At the bottom, list your potential diagnosis or impression of what the patient's problem is.

Primary Survey	*Secondary Survey*
A.	A.
B.	B.
C.	C.
D.	D.

Oxygen-IV-Monitor-Fluids: ____

____

Vital Signs: ____

____

Your Impression: ____

____

CASE 3

Scenario

A 68-year-old male collapses at the local golf course. When you arrive, volunteers are performing CPR. His wife tells you that he has not been sick, but does have a history of cardiac disease and also of hypertension. You connect him to the cardiac monitor and see the following on the monitor:

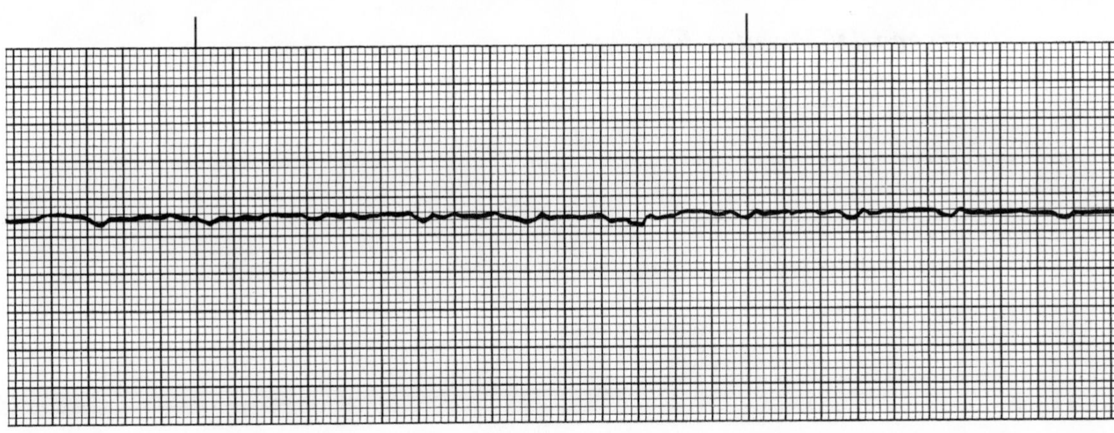

Identify the Rhythm

What is the rate? ______________ What is the rhythm (regular or irregular)? ______________

Is there a P wave before every QRS complex? ______________ Is there a QRS complex after every P wave? ______________

What is the P-R interval? ________________ QRS complex duration? ________________

Interpretation:

____

____

Case 3 Self-Test

In the spaces below give your treatment for the Primary Survey and Secondary Survey, plus the continued care under Oxygen-IV-Monitor-Fluids and Vital Signs. How would you care for this patient, and what orders would you expect from the physician? At the bottom, list your potential diagnosis or impression of what the patient's problem is.

Primary Survey

A.

B.

C.

D.

Secondary Survey

A.

B.

C.

D.

Oxygen-IV-Monitor-Fluids: ______________________________

____

Vital Signs: ______________________________

____

Your Impression: ______________________________

____

CASE 4

Scenario

You are working a busy shift in the emergency department on a hot summer evening. Suddenly someone yells, "He collapsed in the lobby." You find an elderly male, unresponsive and with no vital signs. CPR is initiated immediately, and the monitor shows the following:

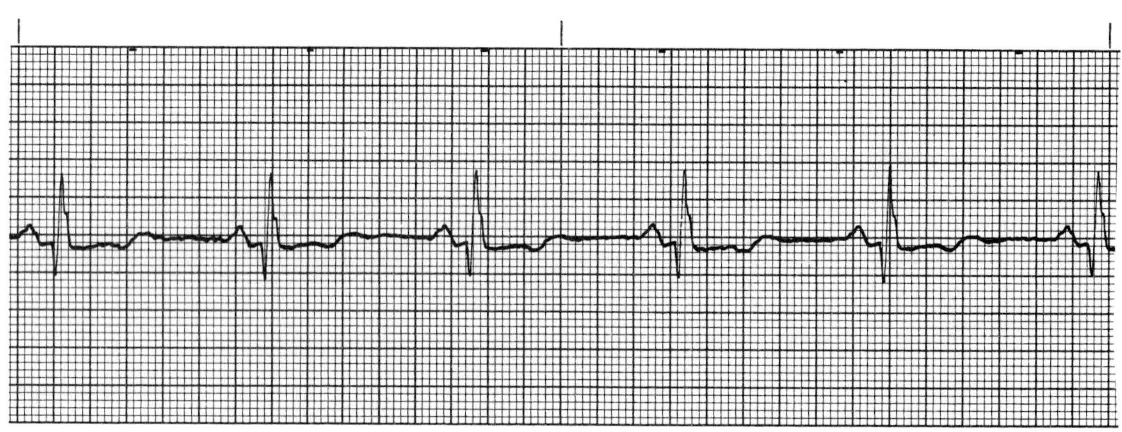

Identify the Rhythm

What is the rate? ____________ What is the rhythm (regular or irregular)? ____________

Is there a P wave before every QRS complex? ____________ Is there a QRS complex after every P wave? ____________

What is the P-R interval? ____________ QRS complex duration? ____________

Interpretation:

____

____

Case 4 Self-Test

In the spaces below give your treatment for the Primary Survey and Secondary Survey, plus the continued care under Oxygen-IV-Monitor-Fluids and Vital Signs. How would you care for this patient, and what orders would you expect from the physician? At the bottom, list your potential diagnosis or impression of what the patient's problem is.

Primary Survey

A.

B.

C.

D.

Secondary Survey

A.

B.

C.

D.

Oxygen-IV-Monitor-Fluids: ______________________________

____

Vital Signs: ______________________________

____

Your Impression: ______________________________

____

8

Pacemaker Rhythms

OBJECTIVES

By the end of this chapter, the student will be able to do the following:

- **Describe the following:**
  - **Various types of pacemakers**
  - **Components of a pacemaker system**
  - **Explain unipolar and bipolar pacing**
  - **Identify primary pacing modes**
  - **Fixed rate and demand pacemakers**
  - **Benefits of AV sequential pacing**
- **Know and understand the following:**
  - **Transcutaneous pacing**
    - **Indications**
    - **Contraindications**
  - **Emergency transvenous pacing**
    - **Indications**
    - **Contraindications**
  - **Indications for permanent pacing**
  - **Complications of pacing**
  - **Waveforms produced on the ECG due to the following:**
    - **Atrial pacing**
    - **Ventricular pacing**
  - **Typical pacemaker spikes**
- **Define and understand the terms *sensitivity, capture, asynchronous,* and *synchronous***

OUTLINE

One of the treatments for many of the dysrhythmias mentioned previously is a cardiac pacemaker. There are a variety of pacemakers available for the physician to use (Box 8-1). But first, what does a pacemaker do? All pacemakers deliver an electrical stimulus through electrodes (external or internal) to the heart. This in turn stimulates depolarization, which causes the myocardium to contract.

Pacemakers are needed when the patient's heart rate is slower than normal. The slower rhythms may produce a decrease in cardiac output causing signs and symptoms of hypotension and resulting in syncope. Initial treatment is drug therapy, and additional treatment may include a pacemaker.

Box 8-1 Types of Pacemakers

Transcutaneous: The electrode is located on the skin of the chest wall and back.
Transvenous: The electrode is introduced through the venous system. The tip of the electrode is placed in the right atrium or ventricle.
Transthoracic: The electrode is inserted through the anterior chest wall into the heart.
Transesophageal: The electrode is placed in the esophagus.
Permanent: The electrode is introduced through or inserted in either the venous system or epicardium.

Transcutaneous pacing is external, noninvasive pacing that delivers the current impulses through the use of electrode pads on the skin of the thorax. *Transvenous pacing* is internal and may be temporary or permanent. With a transvenous pacer, the electrodes are passed through the large central veins to the right side of the heart. This in turn stimulates the endocardium producing ventricular contraction.

COMPONENTS OF PACEMAKERS

A pacemaker consists of the following components: a pulse generator, a pacing lead, and an electrode.

1. *Pulse generator:* This is the power source that contains the battery and controls, which regulate the pacemaker.
2. *Pacing lead:* Pacing lead is the wire used to make contact between the pacemaker and the heart. The exposed portion of the pacing lead is called an *electrode*, which is placed in direct contact with the heart. The pacing lead conducts electrical current from the pulse generator to the patient's heart to produce myocardial contraction.
3. *Electrode tip:* There may be one or two electrode tips called *unipolar* or *bipolar*. These tips may be placed in the endocardium, myocardium, or epicardium.

Unipolar and Bipolar Pacemaker Electrodes

A pacing lead has one or two electrodes at the tip, which is placed in the endocardium, myocardium, or epicardium. The *exposed* part of the pacing lead, the electrode, comes in direct contact with the heart. A unipolar electrode has only one pacing electrode (or exposed portion) at the tip, whereas a bipolar electrode has two pacing electrodes (or exposed portions) near its tip (Figures 8-1 and 8-2).

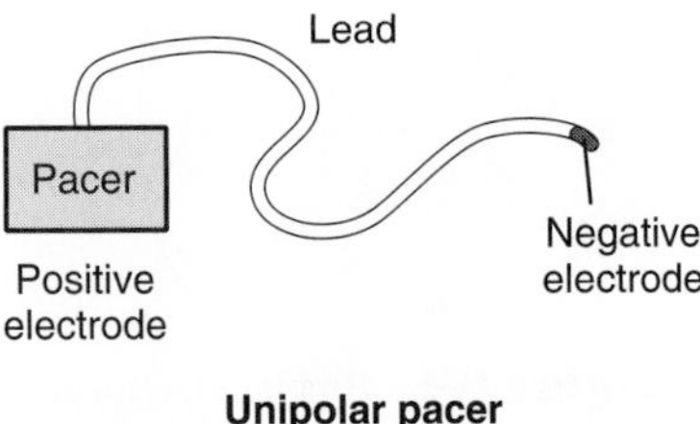

Figure 8-1 Unipolar pacer.

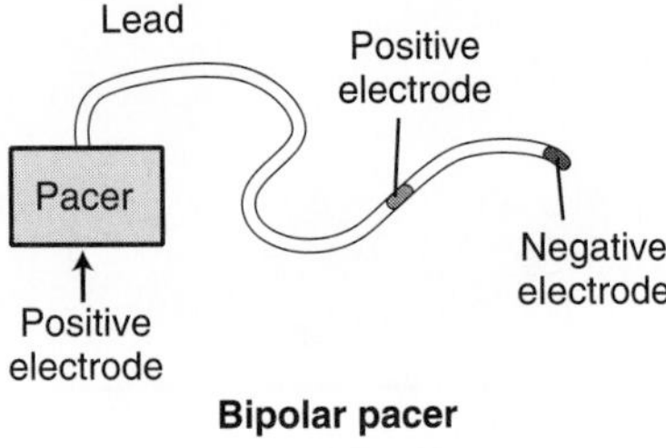

Figure 8-2 Bipolar pacer.

A unipolar system produces larger ECG spikes because of the distance between the positive and negative poles (Figure 8-3). Bipolar systems produce shorter spikes because the two distal electrodes are only a few millimeters apart in the cardiac tissue. The bipolar system is much less susceptible to external electrical interference (Figure 8-4). Permanent pacemakers may be either unipolar or bipolar.

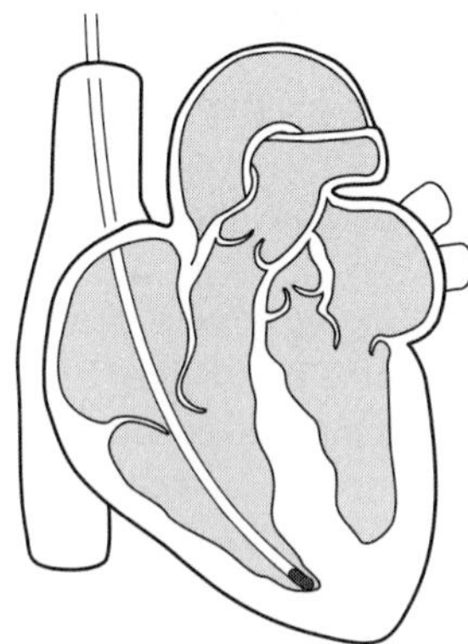

Figure 8-3 Unipolar electrode.

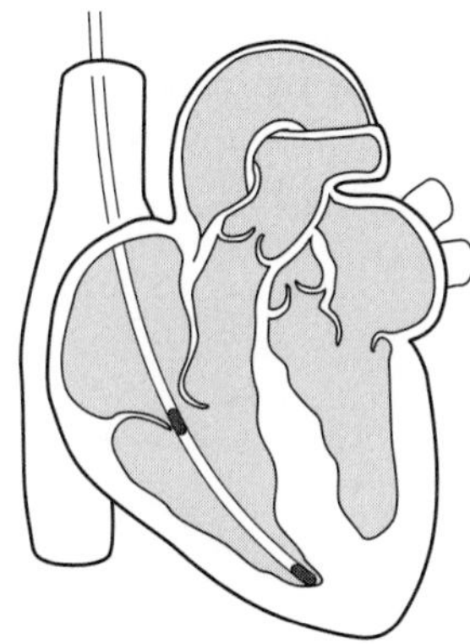

Figure 8-4 Bipolar electrode.

Electrical Output

The pulse generator produces electrical output that is used to stimulate the heart. This is measured in milliamperes (mA).

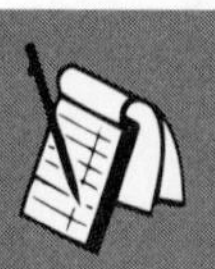

Note

Remember: electricity flows from positive to negative poles.

Hysteresis

Hysteresis is defined as a delay in the effect produced when the forces, which act on a particular body, are changed. Newer pulse generators have this feature that avoids competition between the patient's own heart rate and the pacemaker's stimulated heart rate.

FIXED RATE AND DEMAND PACEMAKERS

A fixed-rate pacemaker unit fires at a preset rate (Box 8-2). This pacemaker continues to stimulate the heart at the preset rate, usually 70 to 80 beats per minute, regardless of the patient's own intrinsic heart rate. One advantage of the fixed-rate pacer is its simple mechanics, which reduce the risk of failure. However, there may be competition between the patient's rhythm and the pacer rhythm. The pacer may fire, causing an impulse to fall during the vulnerable period of the T wave, resulting in V-tach or V-fib.

A demand or synchronous pacemaker fires only when the patient's own heart rate drops below the pacemaker's set rate. This type is programmable; it is usually set at 70 to 72 beats per minute. If the patient's rate drops below the preset rate, the pacemaker discharges, stimulating the heart to contract. Demand pacers that are not programmable have preset voltage level and rate, which are set by the manufacturer.

PACEMAKER CODING

A coding system of pacemakers was developed by the Intersociety Commission for Heart Disease Resources. This system was then revised by the North American Society of Pacing and Electrophysiology (NASPE), in conjunction with the British Pacing Electrophysiology Group (BPEG) (Box 8-3 and Table 8-1).

Box 8-2 Pacemaker Modes

Asynchronous—fixed rate
Synchronous—demand

Box 8-3 Pacemaker Coding System

I: The first letter of the code indicates which chamber of the heart is being paced.
II: The second letter of the code indicates which chamber of the heart the pacemaker senses.
III: The third letter indicates what the response mode is or how the pacemaker generator responds to the sensed event.
IV: The fourth letter indicates the number of programmable functions available.
V: The fifth letter indicates how the pacemaker responds to tachycardia or tachydysrhythmias.

TABLE 8-1 Pacemaker Codes

Chamber Paced	Chamber Sensed	Response Mode	Programmable Functions	Tachydysrhythmia Functions
A = atrium	A = atrium	T= triggers pacing	P = programmable rate, output, or both	P = pacing
V = ventricle	V = ventricle	I = inhibits pacing	M = multiprogammable mode; rate output or sensitivity	S = shock
D = dual chamber	D = dual chamber	D = dual triggers and inhibits pacing	C = communications (telemetry)	D = dual pacing and shock
			R = rate response	
O = none	O = none	O = none	O = none	O = none

PACEMAKER MODES

The letters that designate the pacemaker modes are derived from the codes in Table 8-1. Examples follow.

AAI—The pacemaker has atrial pacing and sensing (**A** = atrial pacing, **A** = atrial sensing, and **I** = inhibits pacing). When the pacer senses atrial activity, pacing is inhibited.

VVI—The pacemaker paces and senses in the ventricle (**V** = ventricular pacing, **V** = ventricular sensing, and **I** = inhibits pacing). When the pacemaker senses ventricular activity, pacing is inhibited. This is one of the most common types of pacemakers used.

VDD—This type of pacemaker senses both the atrium and the ventricle, but paces only the ventricle (**V** = ventricle, **D** = dual chamber, and **D** = dual; triggers and inhibits pacing). When intrinsic atrial activity is sensed, the pacemaker triggers pacing, but when ventricular activity is sensed, pacing is inhibited.

DVI—This type of pacemaker can pace the atrium, the ventricles, or both; however, sensing only takes place in the ventricles (**D** = dual chamber, **V** = ventricle, and **I** = inhibits pacing). When intrinsic ventricular activity is sensed, then pacing is inhibited.

DDD—With this mode, the pacemaker paces and senses in the atrium, the ventricle, or both (**D** = dual chamber, **D** = dual chamber, and **D** = dual, which triggers and inhibits pacing). When it senses activity in either chamber, the pacemaker may inhibit pacing. On the other hand, if it senses activity in the atrium, the pacer may trigger ventricular pacing. This is also known as the *atrioventricular sequential pacemaker*.

An AV sequential pacemaker is a dual-chamber pacer that has one lead placed in the right atrium and one lead placed in the right ventricle. The dual-chambered pacer represents normal cardiac function by first stimulating the right atrium and then the right ventricle on demand. The dual-chambered unit is a DDD pacemaker. Sensing and pacing occur in both chambers separately. If spontaneous atrial depolarization does not occur, the atrial portion discharges, stimulating the atrium to contract. At this point this pacemaker is programmed for a normal P-R interval delay. It simulates this delay in conduction through the AV node (P-R interval). The "created" P-R interval is called an *AV interval*. If no intrinsic ventricular activity is sensed, the ventricular pulse generator is triggered to fire an impulse. The advantage is that the DDD closely follows normal cardiac activity and retains the atrial kick, whereas the disadvantage is that it is more difficult to insert.

When examining paced rhythms on the ECG, specifically note the P wave, its rate, its shape, and its relationship to the QRS complex. Then answer these questions:

- First, is there a pacer spike that indicates pacer stimulus?
- What is the rate of the paced rhythm?
- Is there intrinsic rhythm? If so, what is the rate?
- Is atrial sensing present?
- Did the pacemaker produce atrial capture?
- Is ventricular rate appropriate?
- Did the pacemaker produce ventricular capture?

TRANSCUTANEOUS PACING

Transcutaneous or external pacing involves placing two pacing pads or electrodes on the thorax; one is placed anterior and one posterior. The anterior pad is the negative electrode, placed to the left of the sternum, halfway between the xiphoid process and the left nipple. The posterior pad or positive electrode is placed on the left posterior thorax. This placement allows for defibrillation without removing the pacing pads (Boxes 8-4 and 8-5).

Box 8-4 Indications for Transcutaneous Pacing

Significant bradycardia unresponsive to atropine
Witnessed asystole or asystole of <10 minutes' duration
Used as a temporary measure until a transvenous or permanent pacemaker can be inserted
Complete heart blocks (prehospital EMS)

EMS, Emergency medical services.

Box 8-5 Contraindications to Transcutaneous Pacing

Chest trauma
Flail chest
Hypothermia
Children who weigh <15 kg, in which case pediatric pacing electrodes must be used

TRANSVENOUS AND PERMANENT PACEMAKERS

Indications for transvenous and permanent pacemakers differ from those of transcutaneous pacemakers (Boxes 8-6 and 8-7).

COMPLICATIONS OF PACING

Failure to Pace

Failure to pace occurs when the pacemaker *fails to discharge an electrical impulse* or when it *fails to deliver the correct number of impulses per minute*. This is evident by pacemaker spikes

Box 8-6 Emergency Transvenous Pacing

Unstable bradycardia accompanied by chest pain, hypotension, or pulmonary edema
Complete AV block
Symptomatic second-degree AV blocks
Symptomatic sick sinus syndrome
Permanent pacemaker failure
Symptomatic atrial fibrillation with a slow ventricular rate
Bradycardias with escape rhythms not responding to drug therapy
Tachycardias not responding to drug therapy

AV, Atrioventricular.

Box 8-7 Indications for Permanent Pacemakers

Intermittent or permanent complete AV block
Sinus node dysfunction
Intermittent or permanent second-degree AV block, Mobitz II

AV, Atrioventricular.

not followed by P waves (atrial electrode) or pacemaker spikes not followed by QRS complexes (ventricular electrode). Signs and symptoms include hypotension, chest pain, bradycardia, and syncope (Table 8-2).

Table 8-2 Failure to Pace

Possible Causes	Interventions
Lead is displaced or broken	Replace or reposition the lead
Battery failure or circuit failure	Replace battery, generator, or lead
Broken lead-generator connection	Repair connection
Electromagnetic interference	Remove source of interference

Failure to Capture

Failure to capture is the *inability of the pacemaker stimulus to depolarize the myocardium* and allow for ventricular contraction. Again, this may be recognized by pacer spikes not followed by P waves, or pacer spikes not followed by QRS complexes, depending on which chamber the pacemaker is located in. Signs and symptoms of failure to capture include fatigue, hypotension, and bradycardia (Table 8-3).

TABLE 8-3 Failure to Capture

Possible Causes	Interventions
Pacer voltage too low	Increase voltage (milliamperes)
Battery is dead	Replace battery
Electrode tip out of position	Reposition the tip
Lead wire is broken	Replace lead wire
Scar tissue at electrode tip	Prepare patient for surgery
Perforation of myocardium by lead wire	Reposition lead wire
MI at lead wire	

MI, Myocardial infarction.

Failure to Sense

Under normal conditions the pacemaker senses and recognizes intrinsic electrical activity resulting in no discharge from the pacemaker. Failure to sense is evident when the pacemaker *fails to recognize normal myocardial depolarization*. The pacemaker fires, and this malfunction is evident by pacer spikes too close to the patient's own QRS complexes. This may result in pacer spikes that fall on T waves (R on T) or even competition between the pacemaker and the patient's own rhythm. Signs and symptoms include palpitations, skipped beats, pacer spikes where they should not be, and V-tach (Table 8-4).

TABLE 8-4 Failure to Sense

Possible Causes	Interventions
Battery failure	Replace battery
Lead wire is broken	Replace lead wire
Displacement of electrode tip	Reposition electrode
	Reposition patient on the patient's left side
Edema or fibrosis at tip	Increase sensitivity setting
Antidysrhythmic medications	Readjust patient's medications

Oversensing

Oversensing is a definite malfunction that occurs when there is an *inappropriate sensing of electrical signals*. This may occur when atrial pacers mistakenly sense ventricular activity or when a pacer mistakes a T wave for a QRS complex. Signs and symptoms include pacemaker spikes when the rate is slower than the set rate or no paced beats when the pacemaker's set rate is greater than the patient's spontaneous rate (Table 8-5).

TABLE 8-5 Oversensing

Possible Causes	Interventions
Electromagnetic interference	Test with magnet
Sensing T waves or atrial P waves	Insert bipolar lead
Sensitivity set too high	Decrease sensitivity

PACEMAKER COMPLICATIONS

Pacemaker complications are listed in Box 8-8.

Box 8-8 Pacemaker Complications

Transcutaneous Pacemaker

Pain from electrical stimulation
Tissue damage
Failure to recognize that the pacer is not capturing

Transvenous Pacemaker

Pneumothorax
Bleeding
Infection
Myocardial infarction
Electrode displacement
Hematoma at insertion site
Perforation of right ventricle
Perforation of right vena cava
Cardiac dysrhythmias
Pneumothorax

Permanent Pacemaker Implantation Procedure Complications

Air embolism
Cardiac dysrhythmias
Pneumothorax
Bleeding

Permanent Pacemaker: Long-Term Complications

Congestive heart failure
Pacemaker-induced dysrhythmias
Infection
Perforation of right ventricle
Electrode displacement

ANALYZING THE PACEMAKER RHYTHM

Analyzing the pacemaker rhythm needs to be conducted in an organized manner. The following provides one method of analysis:

1. Is there an intrinsic rhythm (patient's own)?
   What is the ventricular rate? Is the rhythm regular or irregular?
   Are there P waves present? Is there a P wave before every QRS complex?
   Are there QRS complexes present? Is there a QRS complex after every P wave?
2. Is there paced activity? Is the paced activity atrial? Ventricular? Both? (Figures 8-5, 8-6, and 8-7)
3. Evaluate any escape interval—the length of time between the patient's last beat and the first paced beat
4. Analyze the ECG strip for any of the pacemaker malfunctions such as:
   a. Failure to capture
   b. Failure to pace
   c. Failure to sense
   d. Oversensing

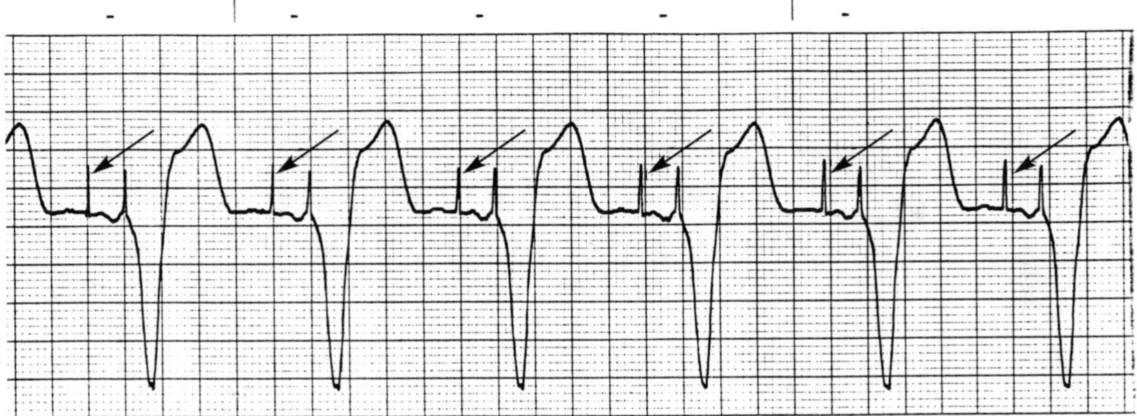

Figure 8-5 Atrial pacing.

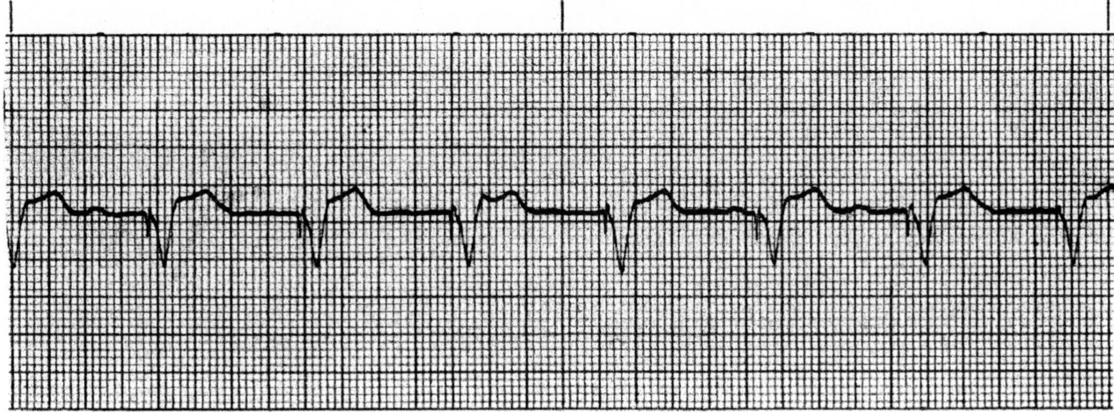

Figure 8-6 Ventricular pacing.

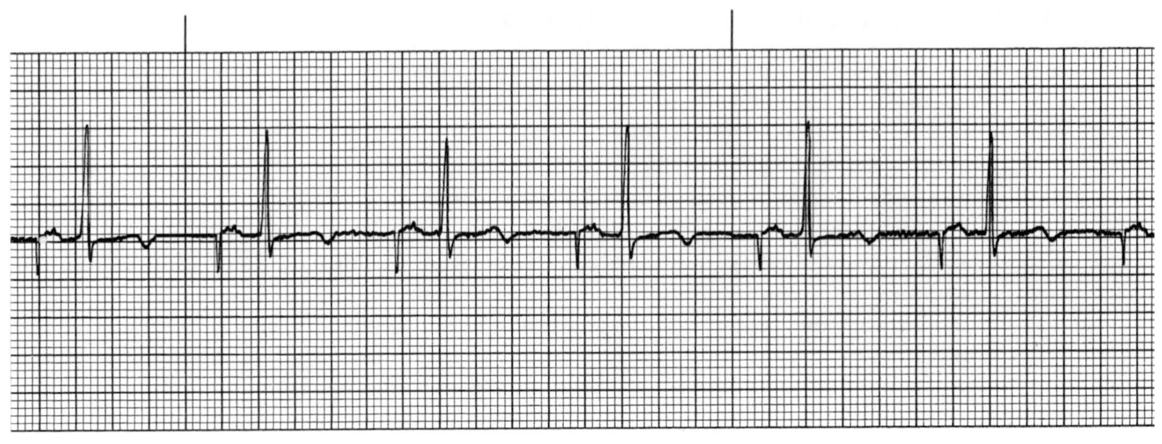

Figure 8-7 Typical pacemaker spikes.

Chapter 8 Self-Test

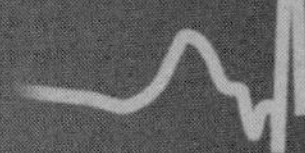

1. Fill in the Blank: Which type of pacer has the electrode located on the skin of the chest wall and back?

   ____

2. Multiple Choice: When the electrode is inserted through the venous system with the tip in the right atrium, it is known as:
   a. Transcutaneous
   b. Transthoracic
   c. Permanent
   d. Transvenous

3. Multiple Choice: When the electrode is located either in the venous system or in the epicardium, it is known as:
   a. Transcutaneous
   b. Transthoracic
   c. Permanent
   d. Transvenous

4. Multiple Choice: A device that has a power source, contains the battery, and controls and regulates the pacemaker is known as the:
   a. Transesophageal
   b. Power source
   c. Pulse generator
   d. Pacing lead

5. True or False: The electrode tip may be placed in the epicardium, the myocardium, or the endocardium.

6. True or False: The pacing lead is a wire used to make contact between the pacemaker and the heart and may have one or two electrode tips.

7. Multiple Choice: A pacing lead with one exposed tip is:
   a. Unipolar
   b. Bipolar
   c. A negative electrode
   d. A positive electrode

8. True or False: A unipolar system produces larger ECG spikes because of the distance between the positive and negative poles.

9. True or False: The unipolar pacer system is less susceptible to external electrical interference than the bipolar system because there is only one exposed tip.

10. True or False: Electricity flows from the negative pole toward the positive pole.

11. Fill in the Blank: Electrical output produced by the polar generator is measured in ________________ .

12. Multiple Choice: Which of the following is true regarding a fixed-rate pacer?
    a. It fires at a preset rate
    b. It is synchronous
    c. It is programmable and usually set at a rate of 70 to 72 beats per minute
    d. None of the above

13. True or False: The first letter of the coding system indicates which chamber of the heart is being paced.

14. True or False: The fourth letter of the code indicates which chamber of the heart the pacemaker senses.

15. Multiple Choice: The S in the code stands for:
    a. Septum
    b. Set rate
    c. Shock
    d. Synchronous

16. Multiple Choice: Which of the following accurately defines the term *AAI*?
    a. *A* = atrial sensing, *A* = atrial pacing, *I* = inhibits pacing
    b. *A* = atrial pacing, *A* = atrial sensing, *I* = inhibits pacing
    c. Both of the above
    d. None of the above

17. Multiple Choice: The AV sequential pacemaker:
    a. Has one lead placed in the right atrium and one lead placed in the left ventricle
    b. Has one lead in the right ventricle only
    c. Has one lead placed in the right atrium and one lead placed in the right ventricle
    d. Is unipolar

18. Fill in the Blank: List three indications for transcutaneous pacing:

    ____

    ____

    ____

19. Fill in the Blank: List three contraindications for transcutaneous pacing:

    ____

    ____

    ____

20. Fill in the Blank: List five indications for emergency transvenous pacing:

____

____

____

____

21. Match the following complications of pacing with their definitions:

______________________________ Failure to pace

______________________________ Failure to capture

______________________________ Failure to sense

______________________________ Oversensing

a. This is the inability of the pacemaker stimulus to depolarize the myocardium and allow for ventricular contraction.
b. This occurs when there is an inappropriate sensing of electrical signals.
c. This occurs when the pacemaker fails to discharge an electrical impulse or when it fails to deliver the correct number of impulses per minute.
d. This occurs when the pacemaker fails to recognize myocardial depolarization.

22. Fill in the Blank: Name two complications of transcutaneous pacing:

____

____

23. Fill in the Blank: List five complications of a transvenous pacemaker:

____

____

____

____

____

24. Fill in the Blank: Name three serious permanent pacemaker implantation procedure complications:

____

____

____

25. Fill in the Blank: List three long-term complications of a permanent pacemaker:

____

____

____

ECG Practice Strips

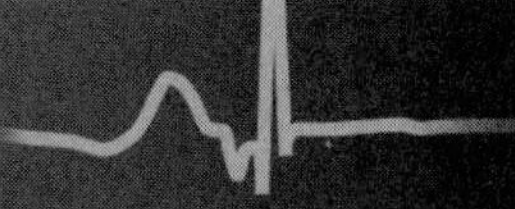

Please calculate the following 15 ECG practice strips:

- Determine the rate.
- Is the rhythm regular or irregular?
- Measure the P-R interval.
- Measure the QRS complex duration.
- Check to see if there is a P wave *before* every QRS complex.
- Check to see if there is a QRS complex *after* every P wave.
- Then give your interpretation of the rhythm.
- All strips are lead II unless otherwise noted.

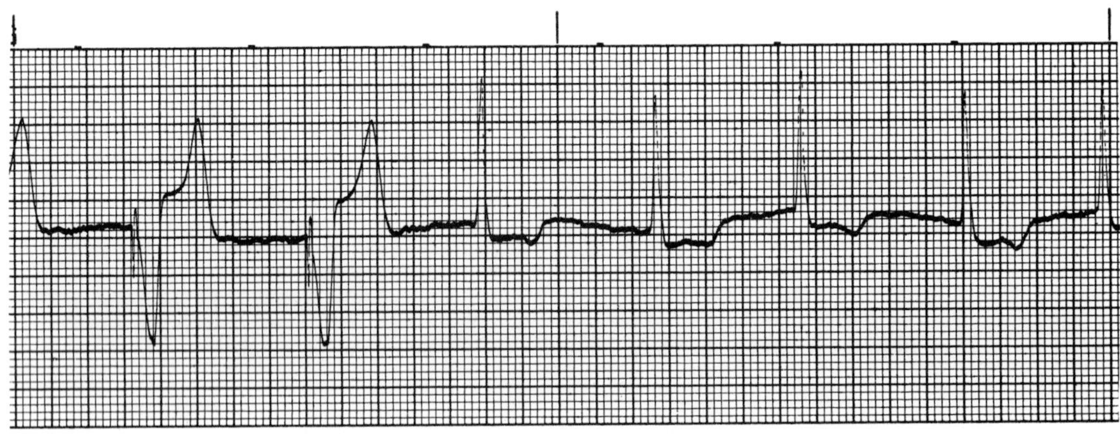

Practice Figure 8-1

Rate: ____________ Rhythm: ____________ P-R interval: ____________ QRS complex: ____________

Is there a P wave before every QRS complex? ____________

Is there a QRS complex after every P wave? ____________

Interpretation: ____________

____

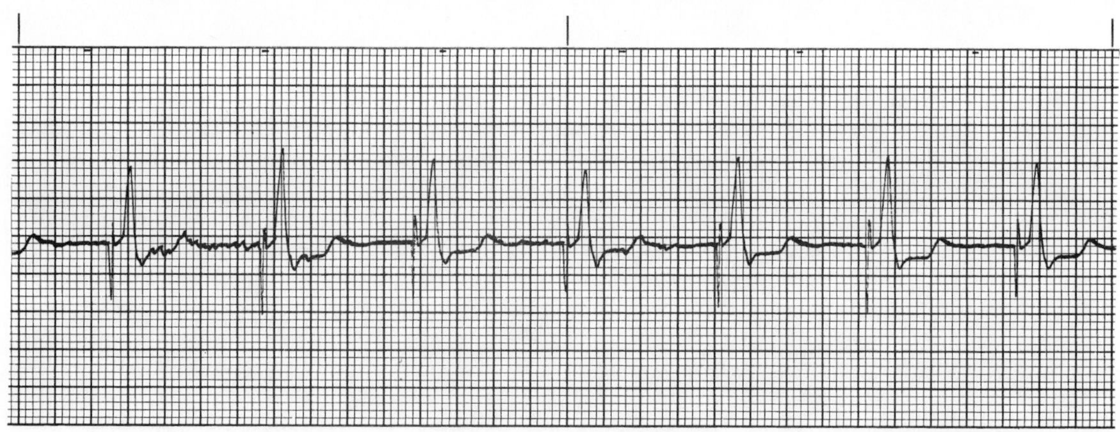

Practice Figure 8-2

Rate: ____________ Rhythm: ____________ P-R interval: ____________ QRS complex: ____________

Is there a P wave before every QRS complex? ____________

Is there a QRS complex after every P wave? ____________

Interpretation: ____________

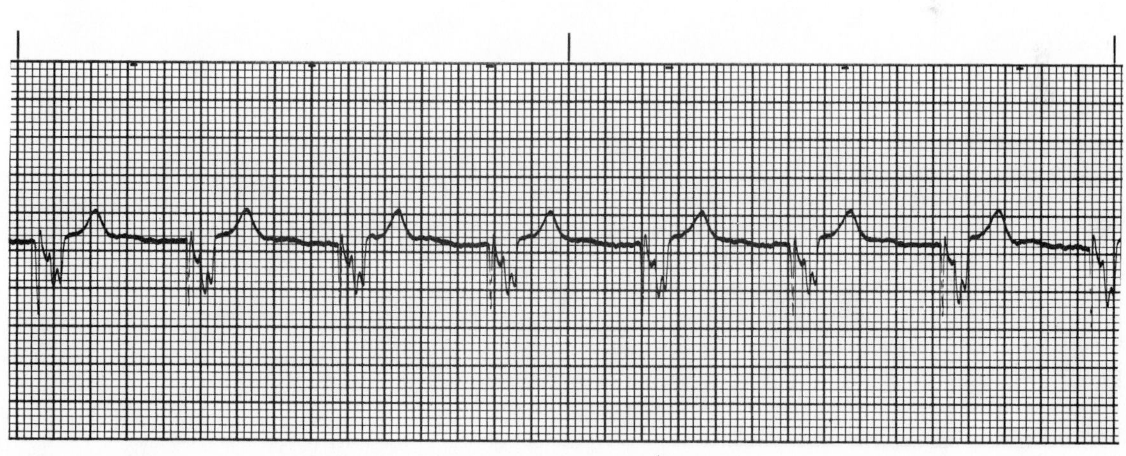

Practice Figure 8-3

Rate: ____________ Rhythm: ____________ P-R interval: ____________ QRS complex: ____________

Is there a P wave before every QRS complex? ____________

Is there a QRS complex after every P wave? ____________

Interpretation: ____________

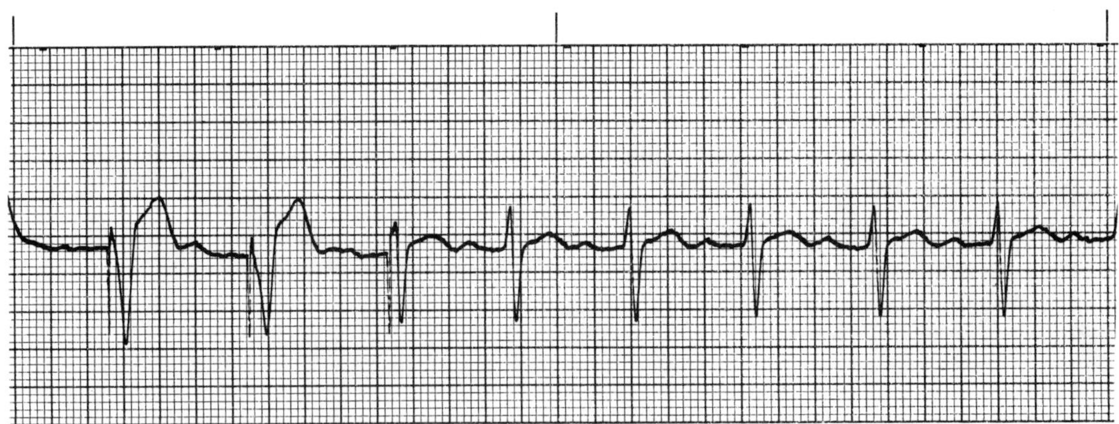

Practice Figure 8-4

Rate: ____________ Rhythm: ____________ P-R interval: ____________ QRS complex: ____________

Is there a P wave before every QRS complex? ____________

Is there a QRS complex after every P wave? ____________

Interpretation: ____________

____

Practice Figure 8-5

Rate: ____________ Rhythm: ____________ P-R interval: ____________ QRS complex: ____________

Is there a P wave before every QRS complex? ____________

Is there a QRS complex after every P wave? ____________

Interpretation: ____________

____

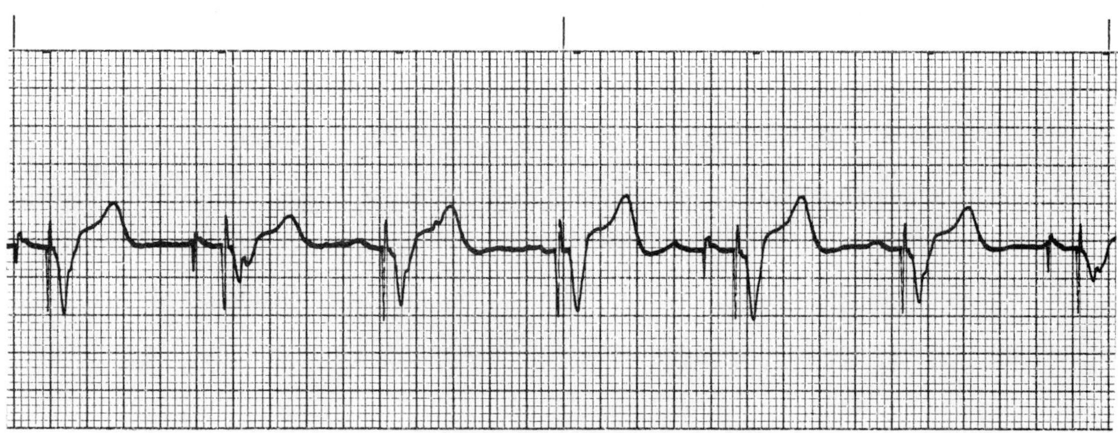

Practice Figure 8-6

Rate: ____________ Rhythm: ____________ P-R interval: ____________ QRS complex: ____________

Is there a P wave before every QRS complex? ____________

Is there a QRS complex after every P wave? ____________

Interpretation: ____________

____

Practice Figure 8-7

Rate: ____________ Rhythm: ____________ P-R interval: ____________ QRS complex: ____________

Is there a P wave before every QRS complex? ____________

Is there a QRS complex after every P wave? ____________

Interpretation: ____________

____

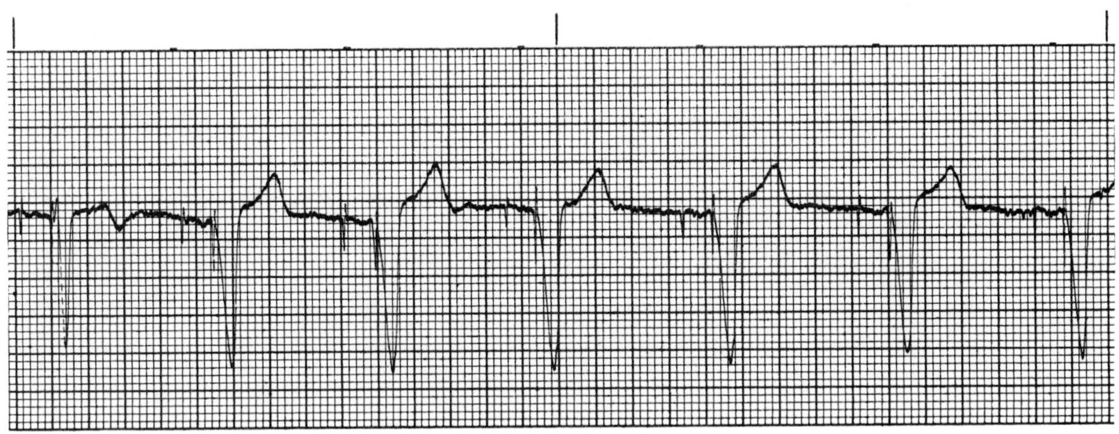

Practice Figure 8-8

Rate: ____________ Rhythm: ____________ P-R interval: ____________ QRS complex: ____________

Is there a P wave before every QRS complex? ______________________________

Is there a QRS complex after every P wave? ______________________________

Interpretation: ______________________________

____

Practice Figure 8-9

Rate: ____________ Rhythm: ____________ P-R interval: ____________ QRS complex: ____________

Is there a P wave before every QRS complex? ______________________________

Is there a QRS complex after every P wave? ______________________________

Interpretation: ______________________________

____

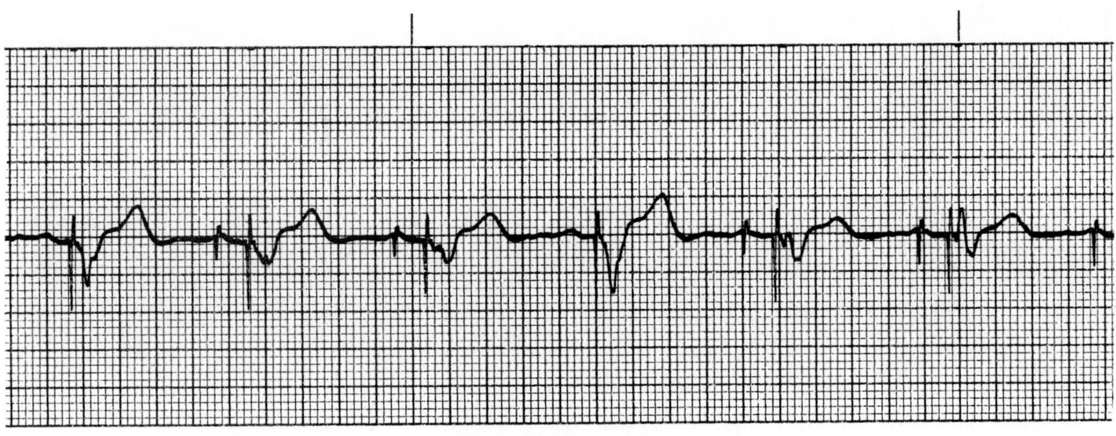

Practice Figure 8-10

Rate: ____________ Rhythm: ____________ P-R interval: ____________ QRS complex: ____________

Is there a P wave before every QRS complex? ____________

Is there a QRS complex after every P wave? ____________

Interpretation: ____________

____

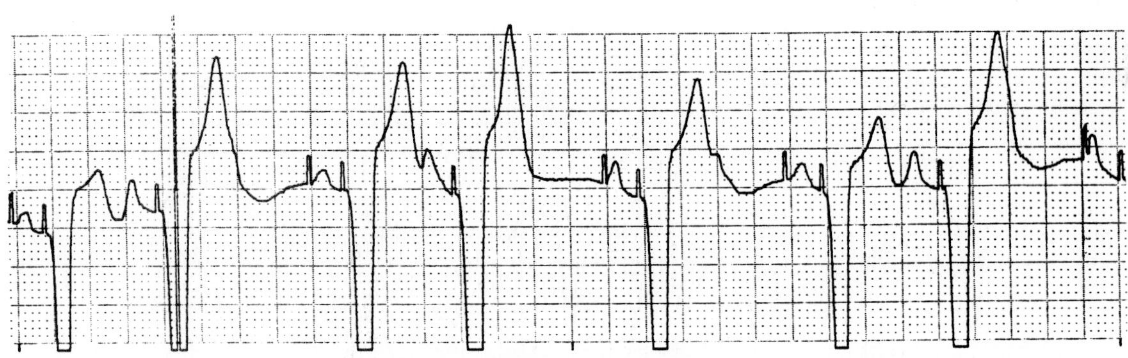

Practice Figure 8-11

Rate: ____________ Rhythm: ____________ P-R interval: ____________ QRS complex: ____________

Is there a P wave before every QRS complex? ____________

Is there a QRS complex after every P wave? ____________

Interpretation: ____________

____

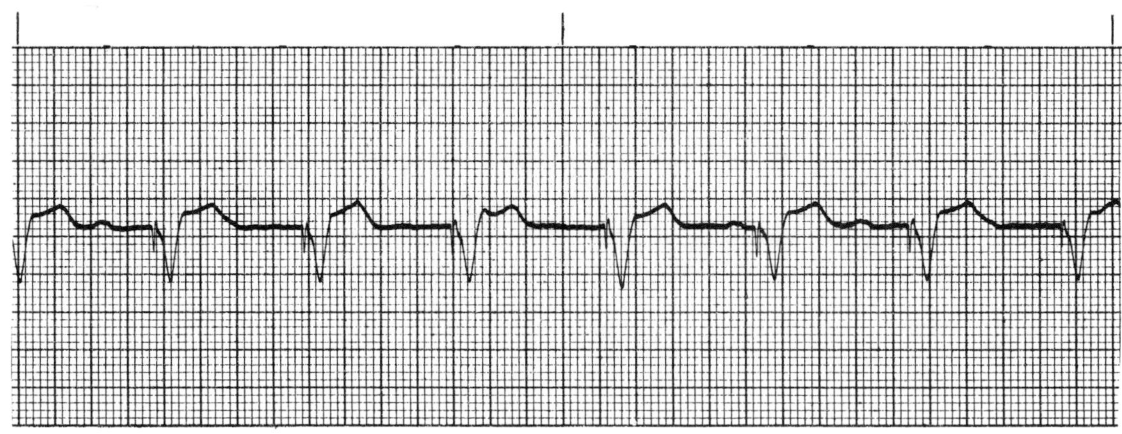

Practice Figure 8-12

Rate: ____________ Rhythm: ____________ P-R interval: ____________ QRS complex: ____________

Is there a P wave before every QRS complex? ____________

Is there a QRS complex after every P wave? ____________

Interpretation: ____________

____

Practice Figure 8-13

Rate: ____________ Rhythm: ____________ P-R interval: ____________ QRS complex: ____________

Is there a P wave before every QRS complex? ____________

Is there a QRS complex after every P wave? ____________

Interpretation: ____________

____

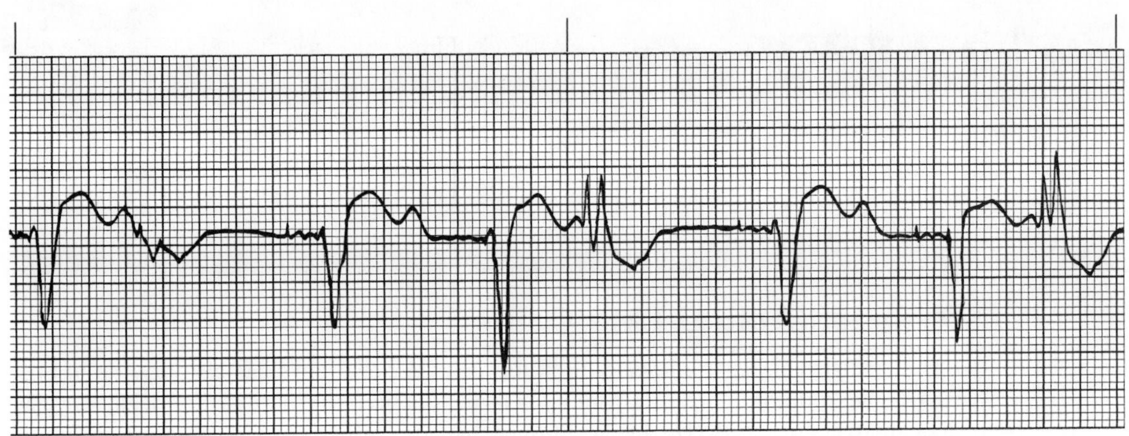

Practice Figure 8-14

Rate: ____________ Rhythm: ____________ P-R interval: ____________ QRS complex: ____________

Is there a P wave before every QRS complex? ____

Is there a QRS complex after every P wave? ____

Interpretation: ____

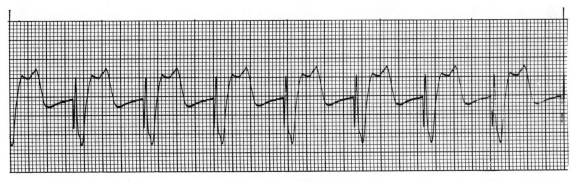

____

Practice Figure 8-15

Rate: ____________ Rhythm: ____________ P-R interval: ____________ QRS complex: ____________

Is there a P wave before every QRS complex? ____

Is there a QRS complex after every P wave? ____

Interpretation: ____

____

Case Scenarios

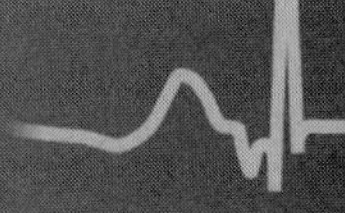

CASE 1

Scenario: (Actual EMS Call)

A man complains of being unusually tired for the past 2 to 3 days. He also says he has been having slight shortness of breath. He tells you he has not been ill otherwise and denies any chest pain or shortness of breath. His medical history includes an MI 8 years ago, a pacemaker, and hypertension. He had some slight problems with fluid 5 years ago that resulted in ankle swelling and slight shortness of breath; he was given furosemide and has been fine ever since. His other medications include nitro SL, Lanoxin, and HCTZ (hydrochlorothiazide). He is alert and oriented ×4, and his skin is pale but warm and dry. Lungs are clear. Vitals signs are BP, 94/60; P, 45; and R, 24. You see the following on the monitor:

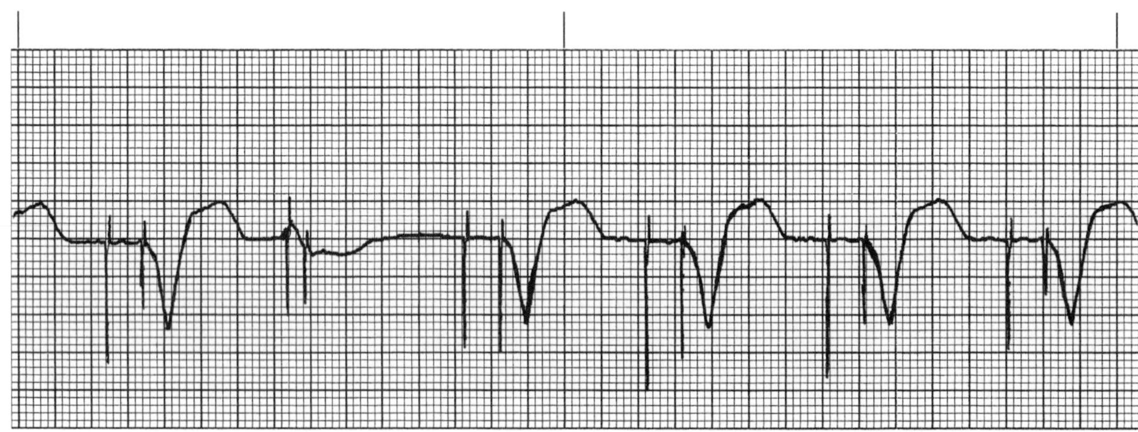

Identify the Rhythm

What is the rate? ______________ What is the rhythm (regular or irregular)? ______________

Is there a P wave before every QRS complex? ______________ Is there a QRS complex after every P wave? ______________

What is the P-R interval? ________________ QRS complex duration? ________________

Interpretation:

____

____

Case 1 Self-Test

In the spaces below give your treatment for the Primary Survey and Secondary Survey, plus the continued care under Oxygen-IV-Monitor-Fluids and Vital Signs. How would you care for this patient, and what orders would you expect from the physician? At the bottom, list your potential diagnosis or impression of what the patient's problem is.

Primary Survey

A.

B.

C.

D.

Secondary Survey

A.

B.

C.

D.

Oxygen-IV-Monitor-Fluids: ______________________________

____

Vital Signs: ______________________________

____

Your Impression: ______________________________

____

CASE 2

Scenario

The family of a 69-year-old male brings him into the emergency department because he had an episode of syncope after eating dinner on Christmas Day. He is awake, alert, and oriented as to time, place, and person at present. He denies any chest pain and has not been ill recently. He does tell you he was in a minor motor vehicle accident last evening in which he was rear-ended by another car. He was wearing a seat belt. He had no injuries, was checked out in the emergency department on the other side of town, and was discharged. His medical history includes an MI 6 years ago, an insertion of a pacemaker, arthritis, and hypertension. His medications are NTG SL, as needed; Vioxx; and Bumex. He takes one baby aspirin per day. His vital signs are BP, 112/58; P, 50 and irregular; R, 20; and $Sao_2 = 96\%$. His skin is pale, warm, and dry. You see the following on the monitor:

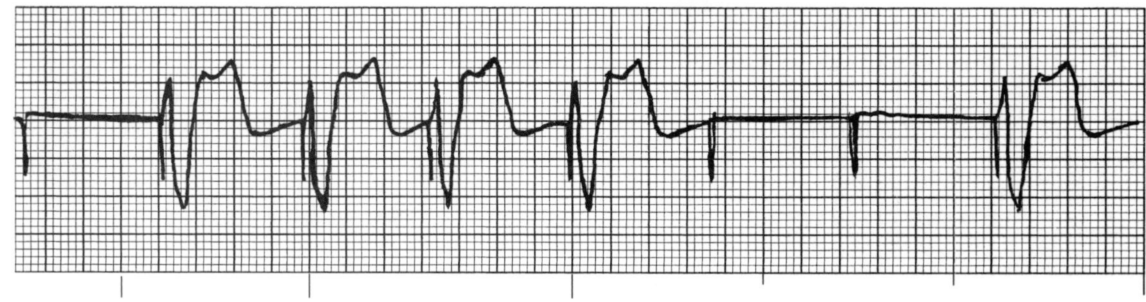

Identify the Rhythm

What is the rate? ____________ What is the rhythm (regular or irregular)? ____________

Is there a P wave before every QRS complex? ____________ Is there a QRS complex after every P wave? ____________

What is the P-R interval? ____________ QRS complex duration? ____________

Interpretation:

____

____

Case 2 Self-Test

In the spaces below give your treatment for the Primary Survey and Secondary Survey, plus the continued care under Oxygen-IV-Monitor-Fluids and Vital Signs. How would you care for this patient, and what orders would you expect from the physician? At the bottom, list your potential diagnosis or impression of what the patient's problem is.

Primary Survey

A.

B.

C.

D.

Secondary Survey

A.

B.

C.

D.

Oxygen-IV-Monitor-Fluids: ____

____

Vital Signs: ____

____

Your Impression: ____

____

CASE 3

Scenario

Your local EMS brings in a 71-year-old male who has had several episodes of being light-headed and dizzy today. According to his family his last syncopal episode lasted 2 minutes. At present he is alert and oriented ×4. He does have a history of angina, stomach ulcers, diabetes that is controlled by diet, COPD, and a pacemaker. His medications are Nitro SL as needed and cimetidine. His vital signs are BP, 106/54; P, 80 and irregular; R, 18; and Sao_2 = 94%. His skin is pale, cool, and dry. You see the following rhythm on the monitor:

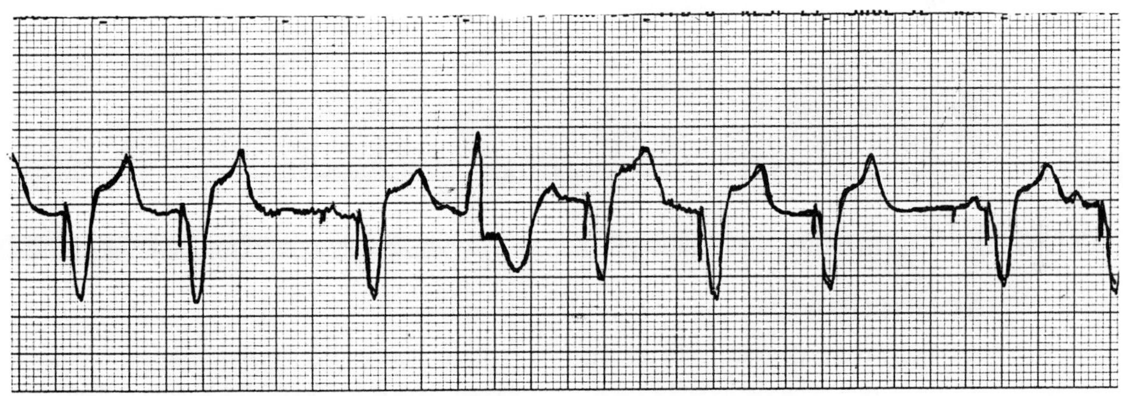

Identify the Rhythm

What is the rate? ______________ What is the rhythm (regular or irregular)? ______________

Is there a P wave before every QRS complex? ______________ Is there a QRS complex after every P wave? ______________

What is the P-R interval? ______________ QRS complex duration? ______________

Interpretation:

____

____

Case 3 Self-Test

In the spaces below give your treatment for the Primary Survey and Secondary Survey, plus the continued care under Oxygen-IV-Monitor-Fluids and Vital Signs. How would you care for this patient, and what orders would you expect from the physician? At the bottom, list your potential diagnosis or impression of what the patient's problem is.

Primary Survey	*Secondary Survey*
A.	A.
B.	B.
C.	C.
D.	D.

Oxygen-IV-Monitor-Fluids: ______________________________

____

Vital Signs: ______________________________

____

Your Impression: ______________________________

____

CASE 4

Scenario

A 54-year-old male walks into the emergency department and complains of heart palpitations. He has a history of a pacemaker insertion 7 years ago because he was having vasovagal bradycardia associated with episodes of syncope. He has had no problems since. There is nothing else in his medical history, and he is not taking any medications. He is alert and oriented ×4, and his skin is pink, warm, and dry. His vital signs are BP, 110/68; P, 72 and irregular; R, 22; and $Sao_2 = 97\%$. You see the following on the ECG monitor:

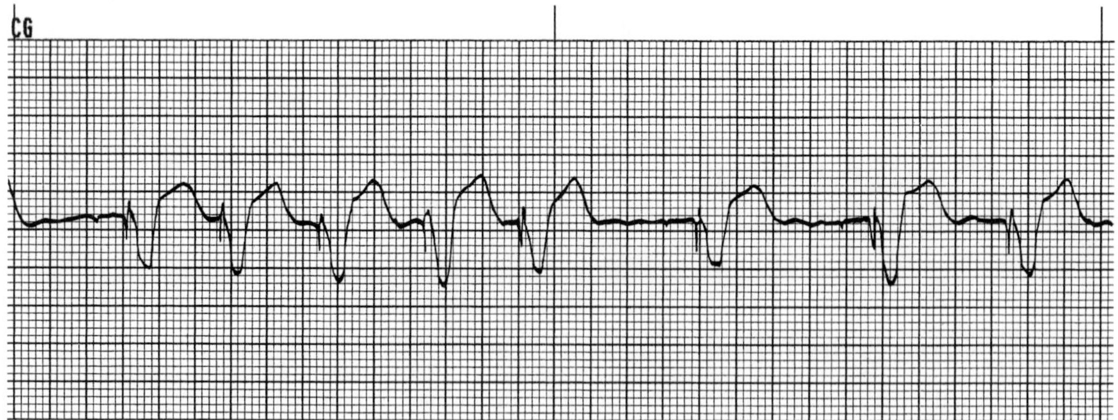

Identify the Rhythm

What is the rate? ____________ What is the rhythm (regular or irregular)? ____________

Is there a P wave before every QRS complex? ____________ Is there a QRS complex after every P wave? ____________

What is the P-R interval? ____________ QRS complex duration? ____________

Interpretation:

____

____

Case 4 Self-Test

In the spaces below give your treatment for the Primary Survey and Secondary Survey, plus the continued care under Oxygen-IV-Monitor-Fluids and Vital Signs. How would you care for this patient, and what orders would you expect from the physician? At the bottom, list your potential diagnosis or impression of what the patient's problem is.

Primary Survey

A.

B.

C.

D.

Secondary Survey

A.

B.

C.

D.

Oxygen-IV-Monitor-Fluids: ____

____

Vital Signs: ____

____

Your Impression: ____

____

9

Practice Rhythms

Please calculate the following ECG practice strips:

- Determine the rate.
- Is the rhythm regular or irregular?
- Measure the P-R interval.
- Measure the QRS complex duration.
- Check to see if there is a P wave *before* every QRS complex.
- Check to see if there is a QRS complex *after* every P wave.
- Then give your interpretation of the rhythm.
- All strips are lead II unless otherwise noted.

Answers appear in the Appendix.

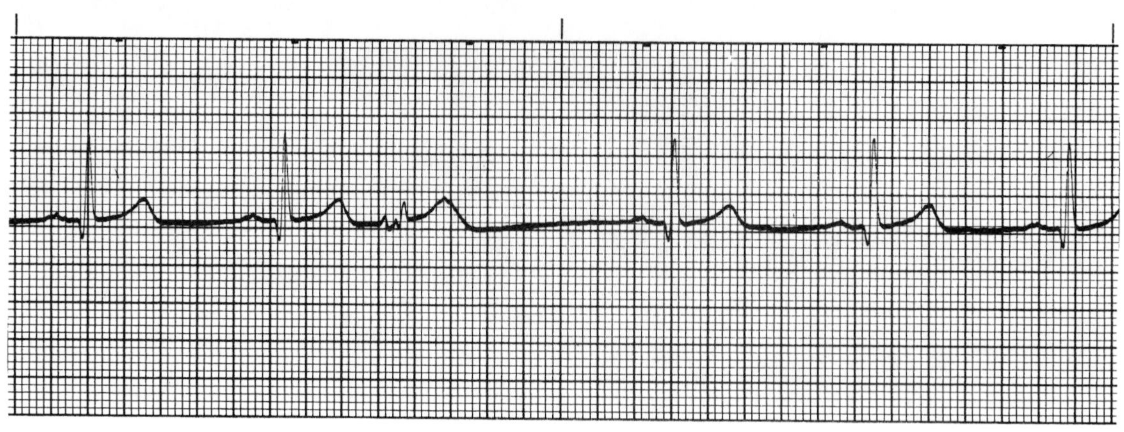

Practice Figure 9-1

Rate: __________ Rhythm: __________ P-R interval: __________ QRS complex: __________

Is there a P wave before every QRS complex? __________

Is there a QRS complex after every P wave? __________

Interpretation: __________

____

Practice Figure 9-2

Rate: __________ Rhythm: __________ P-R interval: __________ QRS complex: __________

Is there a P wave before every QRS complex? __________

Is there a QRS complex after every P wave? __________

Interpretation: __________

____

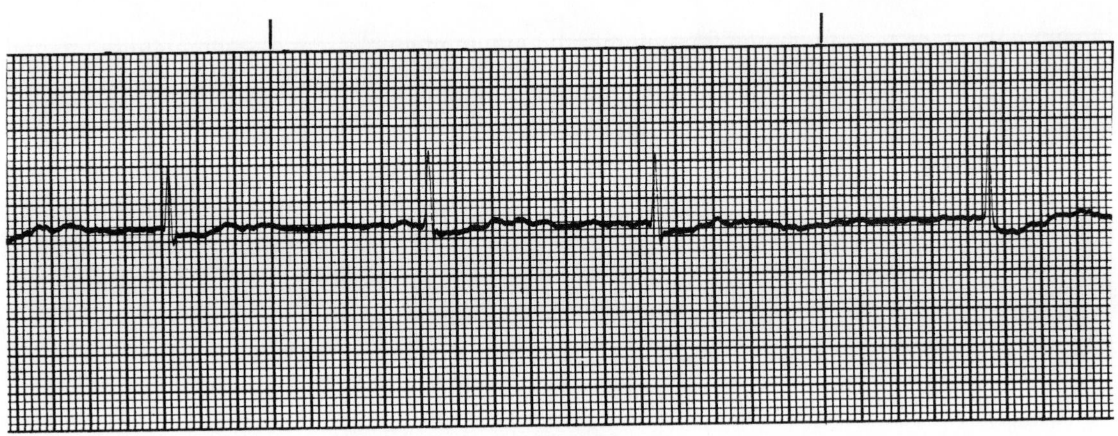

Practice Figure 9-3

Rate: ____________ Rhythm: ____________ P-R interval: ____________ QRS complex: ____________

Is there a P wave before every QRS complex? ____________

Is there a QRS complex after every P wave? ____________

Interpretation: ____________

____

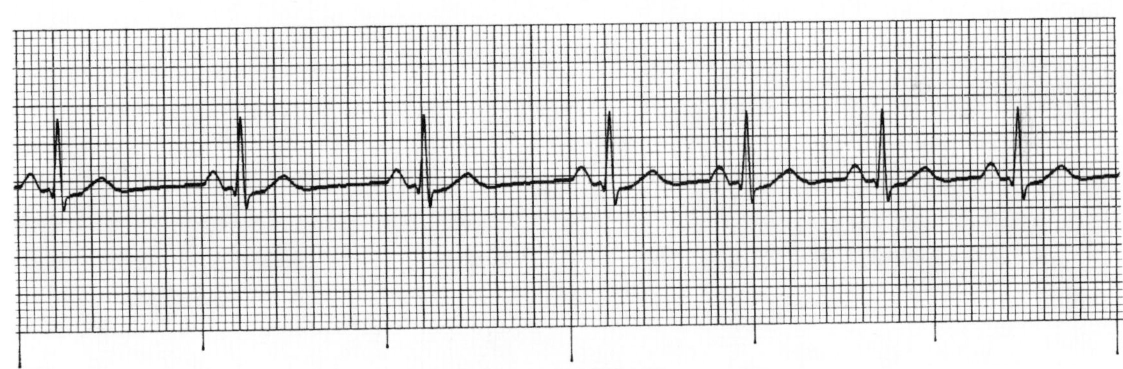

Practice Figure 9-4

Rate: ____________ Rhythm: ____________ P-R interval: ____________ QRS complex: ____________

Is there a P wave before every QRS complex? ____________

Is there a QRS complex after every P wave? ____________

Interpretation: ____________

____

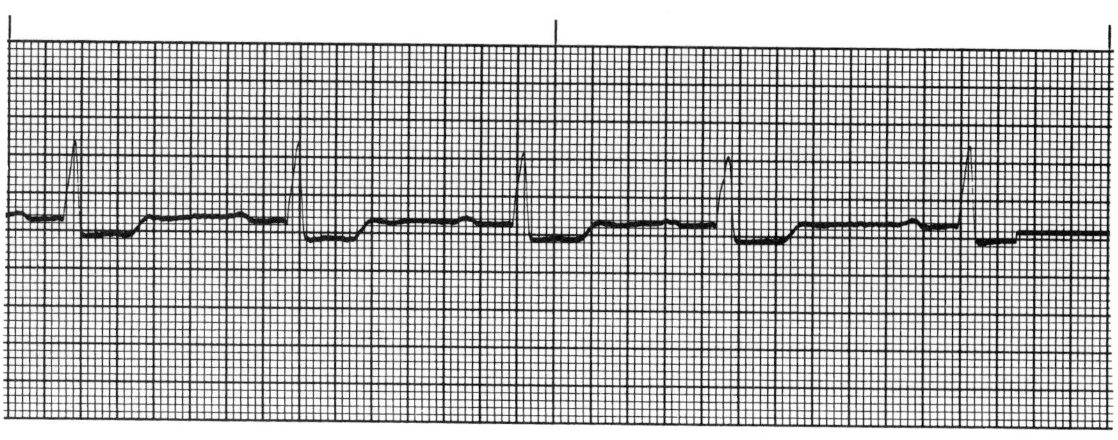

Practice Figure 9-5

Rate: ____________ Rhythm: ____________ P-R interval: ____________ QRS complex: ____________

Is there a P wave before every QRS complex? ____

Is there a QRS complex after every P wave? ____

Interpretation: ____

____

Practice Figure 9-6

Rate: ____________ Rhythm: ____________ P-R interval: ____________ QRS complex: ____________

Is there a P wave before every QRS complex? ____

Is there a QRS complex after every P wave? ____

Interpretation: ____

____

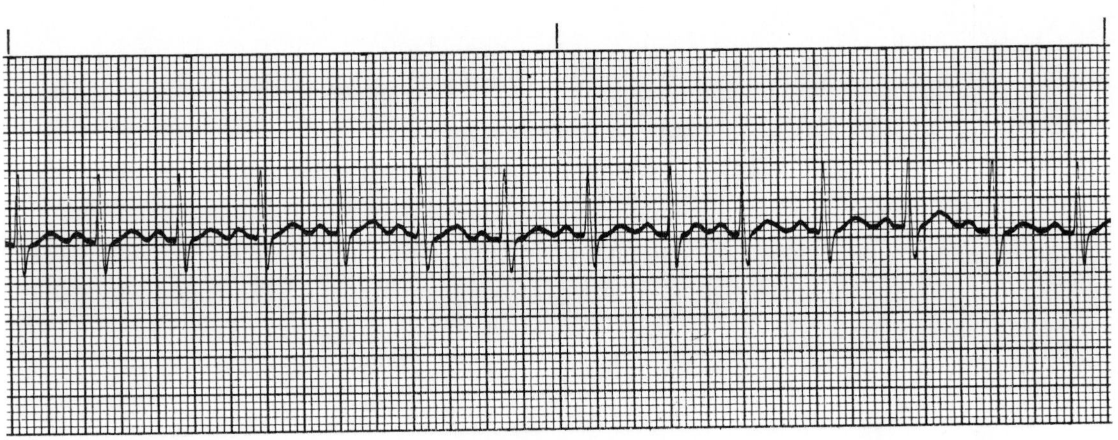

Practice Figure 9-7

Rate: ____________ Rhythm: ____________ P-R interval: ____________ QRS complex: ____________

Is there a P wave before every QRS complex? ____

Is there a QRS complex after every P wave? ____

Interpretation: ____

____

Practice Figure 9-8

Rate: ____________ Rhythm: ____________ P-R interval: ____________ QRS complex: ____________

Is there a P wave before every QRS complex? ____

Is there a QRS complex after every P wave? ____

Interpretation: ____

____

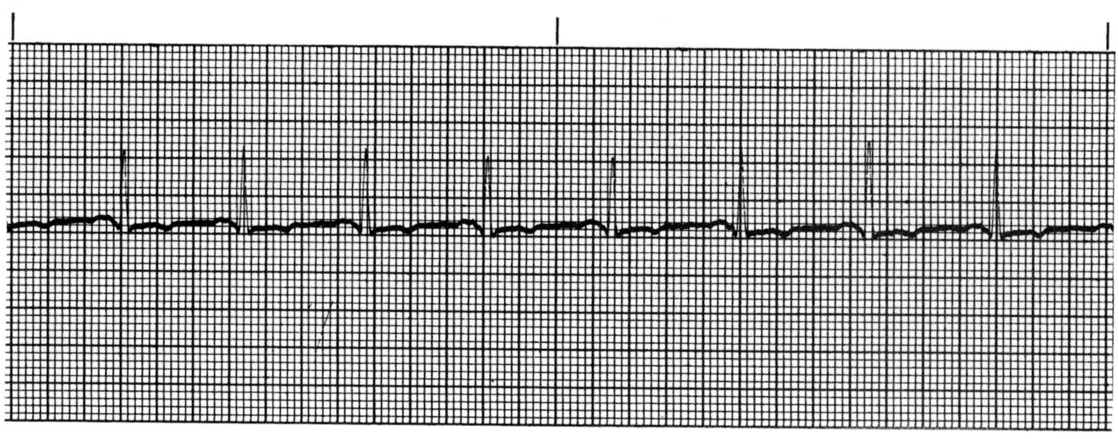

Practice Figure 9-9

Rate: ____________ Rhythm: ____________ P-R interval: ____________ QRS complex: ____________

Is there a P wave before every QRS complex? ____________

Is there a QRS complex after every P wave? ____________

Interpretation: ____________

Practice Figure 9-10

Rate: ____________ Rhythm: ____________ P-R interval: ____________ QRS complex: ____________

Is there a P wave before every QRS complex? ____________

Is there a QRS complex after every P wave? ____________

Interpretation: ____________

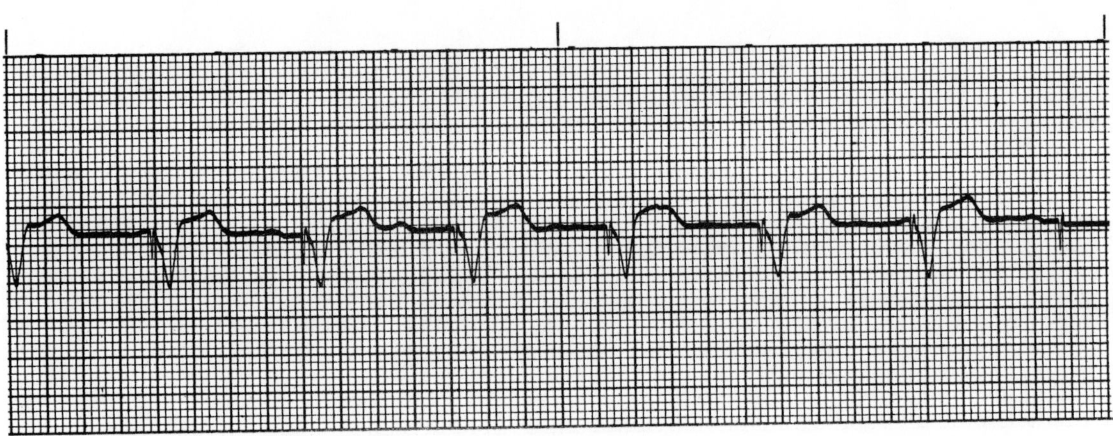

Practice Figure 9-11

Rate: ____________ Rhythm: ____________ P-R interval: ____________ QRS complex: ____________

Is there a P wave before every QRS complex? ____

Is there a QRS complex after every P wave? ____

Interpretation: ____

____

Practice Figure 9-12

Rate: ____________ Rhythm: ____________ P-R interval: ____________ QRS complex: ____________

Is there a P wave before every QRS complex? ____

Is there a QRS complex after every P wave? ____

Interpretation: ____

____

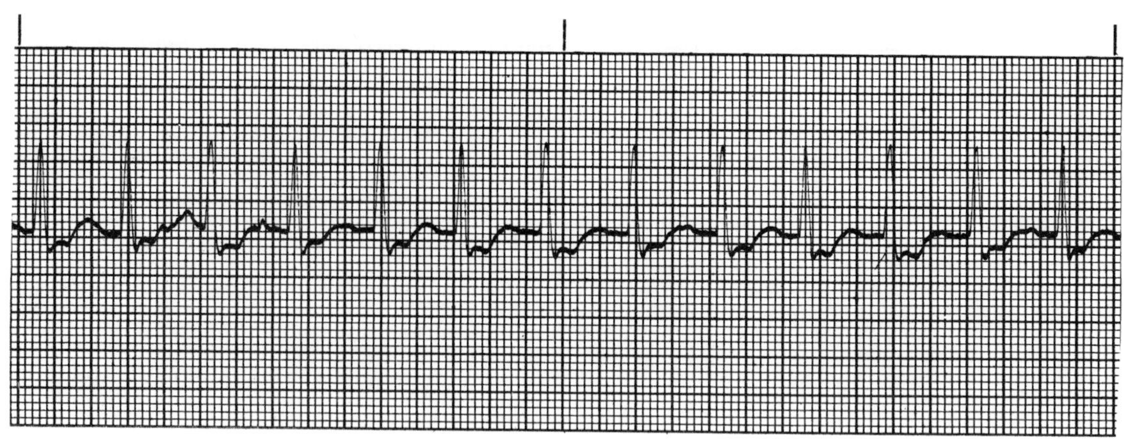

Practice Figure 9-13

Rate: ____________ Rhythm: ____________ P-R interval: ____________ QRS complex: ____________

Is there a P wave before every QRS complex? ____________

Is there a QRS complex after every P wave? ____________

Interpretation: ____________

Practice Figure 9-14

Rate: ____________ Rhythm: ____________ P-R interval: ____________ QRS complex: ____________

Is there a P wave before every QRS complex? ____________

Is there a QRS complex after every P wave? ____________

Interpretation: ____________

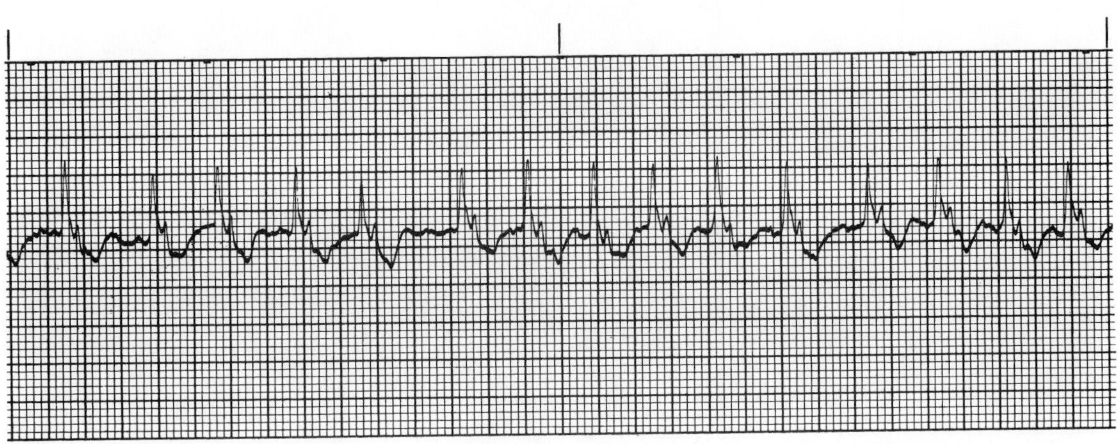

Practice Figure 9-15

Rate: ____________ Rhythm: ____________ P-R interval: ____________ QRS complex: ____________

Is there a P wave before every QRS complex? ____________

Is there a QRS complex after every P wave? ____________

Interpretation: ____________

____

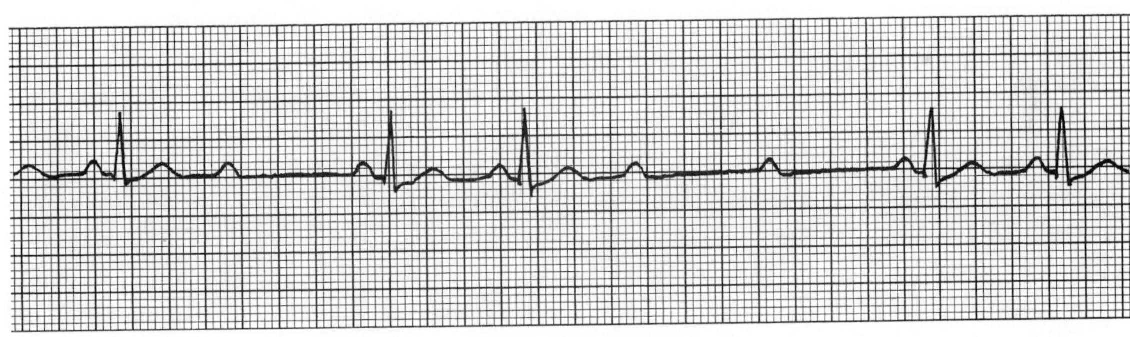

Practice Figure 9-16

Rate: ____________ Rhythm: ____________ P-R interval: ____________ QRS complex: ____________

Is there a P wave before every QRS complex? ____________

Is there a QRS complex after every P wave? ____________

Interpretation: ____________

____

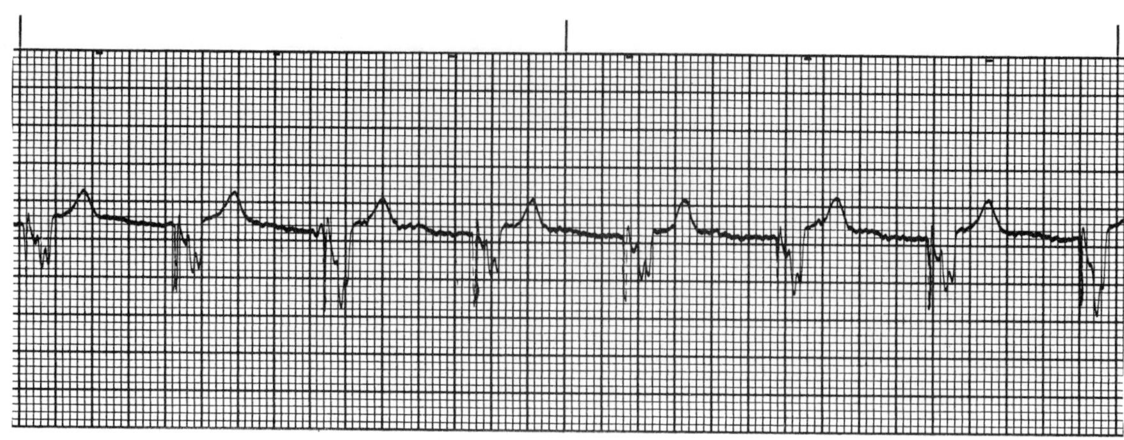

Practice Figure 9-17

Rate: ____________ Rhythm: ____________ P-R interval: ____________ QRS complex: ____________

Is there a P wave before every QRS complex? ____________

Is there a QRS complex after every P wave? ____________

Interpretation: ____________

____

Practice Figure 9-18

Rate: ____________ Rhythm: ____________ P-R interval: ____________ QRS complex: ____________

Is there a P wave before every QRS complex? ____________

Is there a QRS complex after every P wave? ____________

Interpretation: ____________

____

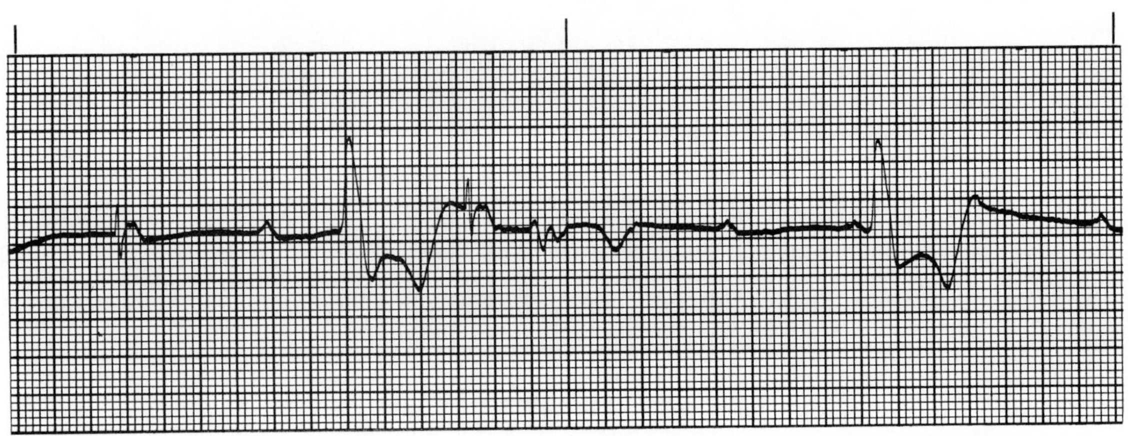

Practice Figure 9-19

Rate: ____________ Rhythm: ____________ P-R interval: ____________ QRS complex: ____________

Is there a P wave before every QRS complex? ____

Is there a QRS complex after every P wave? ____

Interpretation: ____

____

Practice Figure 9-20

Rate: ____________ Rhythm: ____________ P-R interval: ____________ QRS complex: ____________

Is there a P wave before every QRS complex? ____

Is there a QRS complex after every P wave? ____

Interpretation: ____

____

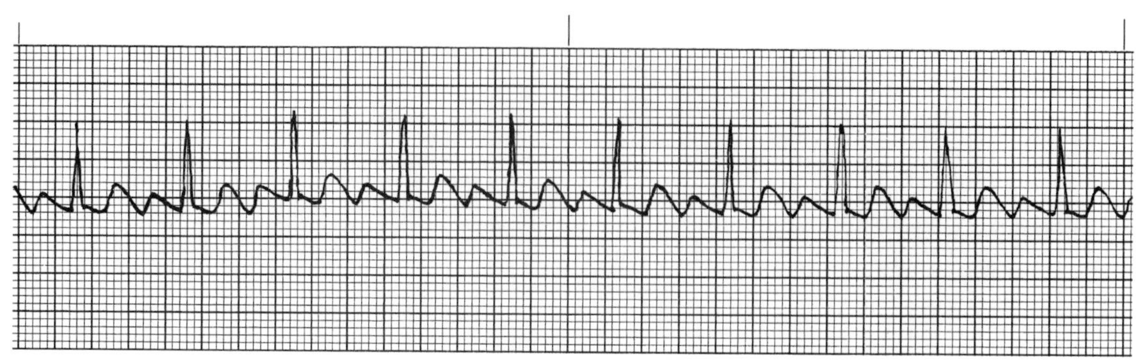

Practice Figure 9-21

Rate: ____________ Rhythm: ____________ P-R interval: ____________ QRS complex: ____________

Is there a P wave before every QRS complex? ____________

Is there a QRS complex after every P wave? ____________

Interpretation: ____________

Practice Figure 9-22

Rate: ____________ Rhythm: ____________ P-R interval: ____________ QRS complex: ____________

Is there a P wave before every QRS complex? ____________

Is there a QRS complex after every P wave? ____________

Interpretation: ____________

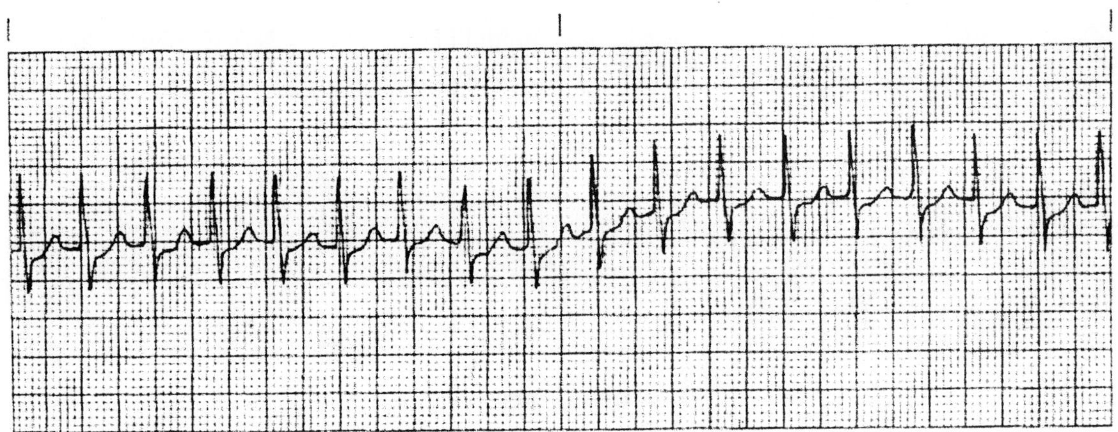

Practice Figure 9-23

Rate: ____________ Rhythm: ____________ P-R interval: ____________ QRS complex: ____________

Is there a P wave before every QRS complex? ____

Is there a QRS complex after every P wave? ____

Interpretation: ____

____

Practice Figure 9-24

Rate: ____________ Rhythm: ____________ P-R interval: ____________ QRS complex: ____________

Is there a P wave before every QRS complex? ____

Is there a QRS complex after every P wave? ____

Interpretation: ____

____

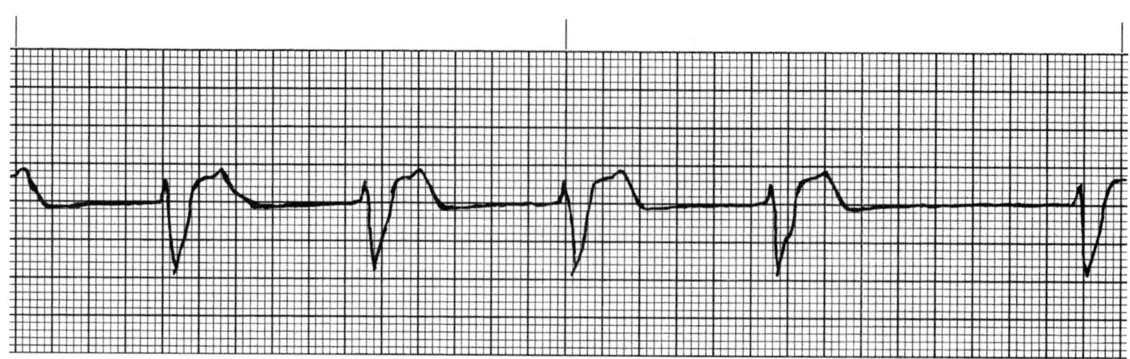

Practice Figure 9-25

Rate: ____________ Rhythm: ____________ P-R interval: ____________ QRS complex: ____________

Is there a P wave before every QRS complex? ____________

Is there a QRS complex after every P wave? ____________

Interpretation: ____________

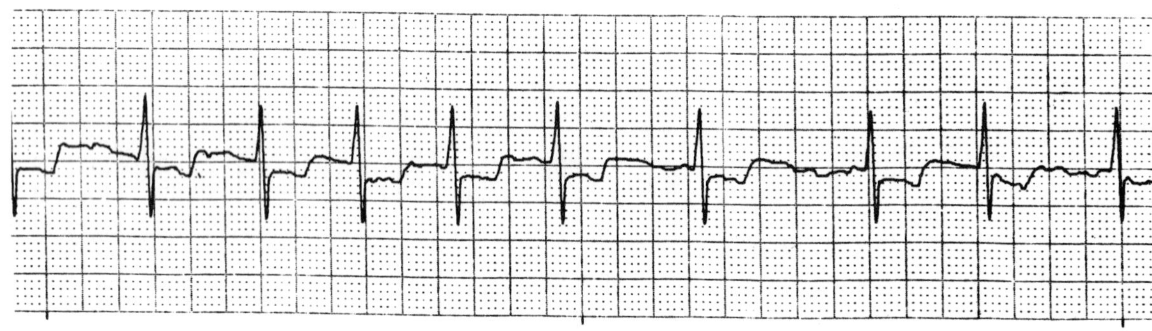

Practice Figure 9-26

Rate: ____________ Rhythm: ____________ P-R interval: ____________ QRS complex: ____________

Is there a P wave before every QRS complex? ____________

Is there a QRS complex after every P wave? ____________

Interpretation: ____________

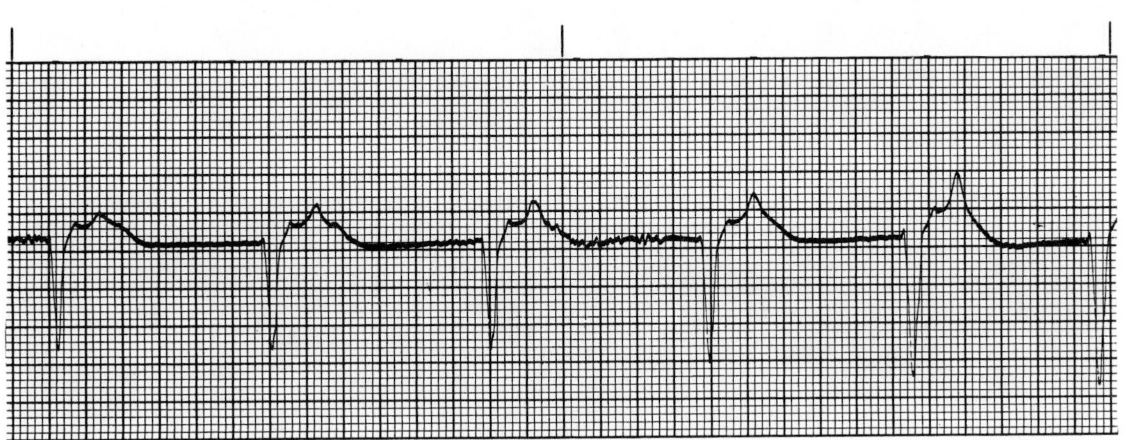

Practice Figure 9-27

Rate: ____________ Rhythm: ____________ P-R interval: ____________ QRS complex: ____________

Is there a P wave before every QRS complex? ____________

Is there a QRS complex after every P wave? ____________

Interpretation: ____________

Practice Figure 9-28

Rate: ____________ Rhythm: ____________ P-R interval: ____________ QRS complex: ____________

Is there a P wave before every QRS complex? ____________

Is there a QRS complex after every P wave? ____________

Interpretation: ____________

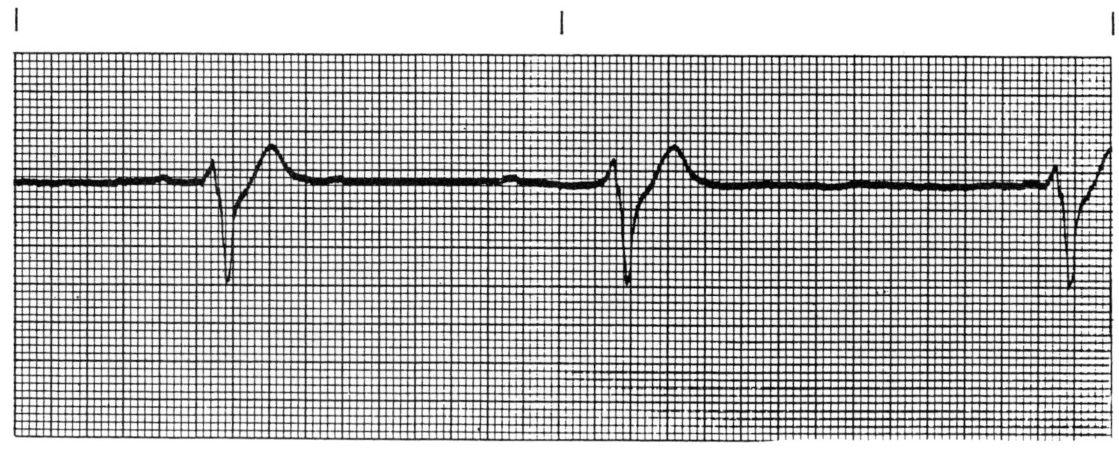

Practice Figure 9-29

Rate: ____________ Rhythm: ____________ P-R interval: ____________ QRS complex: ____________

Is there a P wave before every QRS complex? ____________

Is there a QRS complex after every P wave? ____________

Interpretation: ____________

____

Practice Figure 9-30

Rate: ____________ Rhythm: ____________ P-R interval: ____________ QRS complex: ____________

Is there a P wave before every QRS complex? ____________

Is there a QRS complex after every P wave? ____________

Interpretation: ____________

____

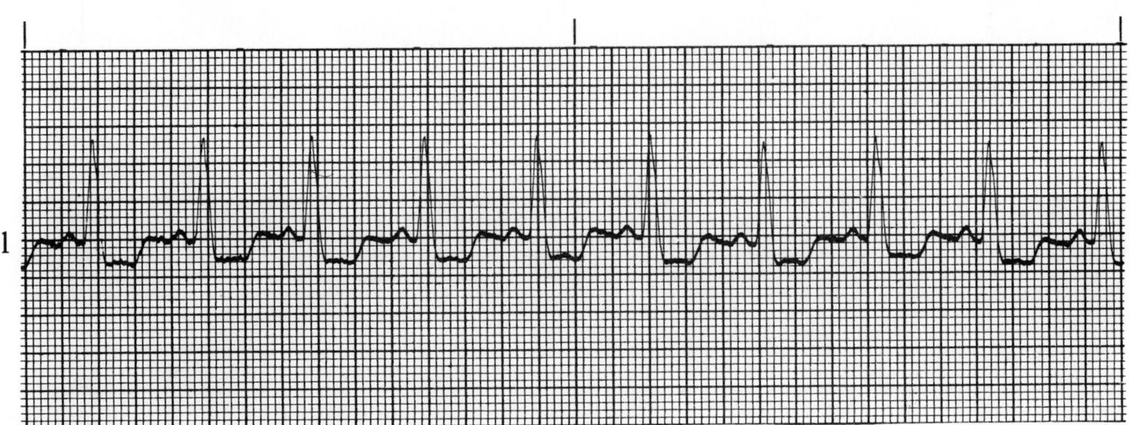

Practice Figure 9-31

Rate: ____________ Rhythm: ____________ P-R interval: ____________ QRS complex: ____________

Is there a P wave before every QRS complex? ____

Is there a QRS complex after every P wave? ____

Interpretation: ____

____

Practice Figure 9-32

Rate: ____________ Rhythm: ____________ P-R interval: ____________ QRS complex: ____________

Is there a P wave before every QRS complex? ____

Is there a QRS complex after every P wave? ____

Interpretation: ____

____

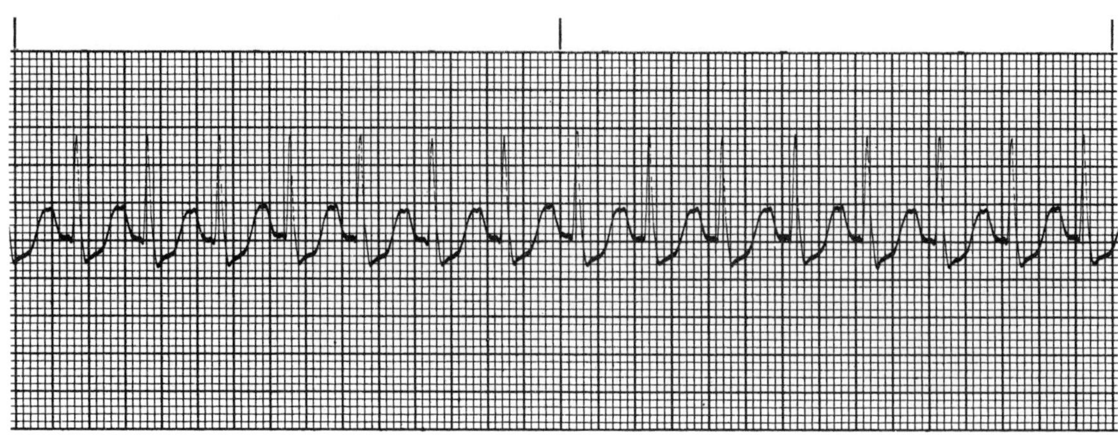

Practice Figure 9-33

Rate: ____________ Rhythm: ____________ P-R interval: ____________ QRS complex: ____________

Is there a P wave before every QRS complex? ____________

Is there a QRS complex after every P wave? ____________

Interpretation: ____________

____

Practice Figure 9-34

Rate: ____________ Rhythm: ____________ P-R interval: ____________ QRS complex: ____________

Is there a P wave before every QRS complex? ____________

Is there a QRS complex after every P wave? ____________

Interpretation: ____________

____

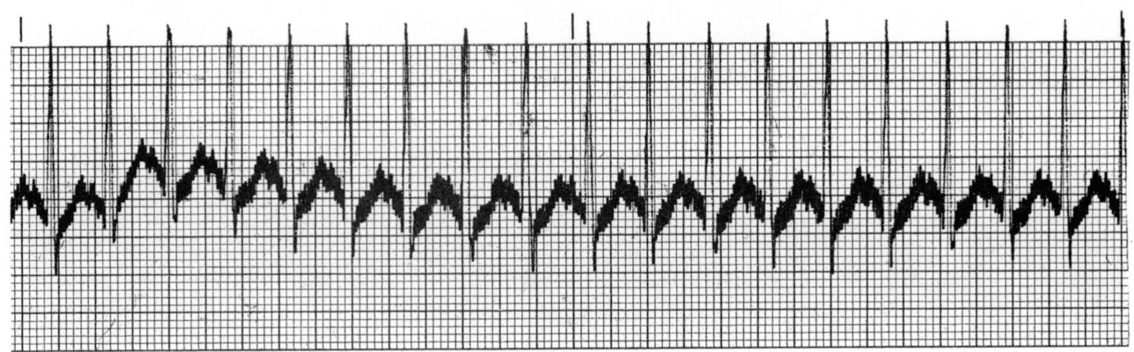

Practice Figure 9-35

Rate: ____________ Rhythm: ____________ P-R interval: ____________ QRS complex: ____________

Is there a P wave before every QRS complex? ____________

Is there a QRS complex after every P wave? ____________

Interpretation: ____________

____

Practice Figure 9-36

Rate: ____________ Rhythm: ____________ P-R interval: ____________ QRS complex: ____________

Is there a P wave before every QRS complex? ____________

Is there a QRS complex after every P wave? ____________

Interpretation: ____________

____

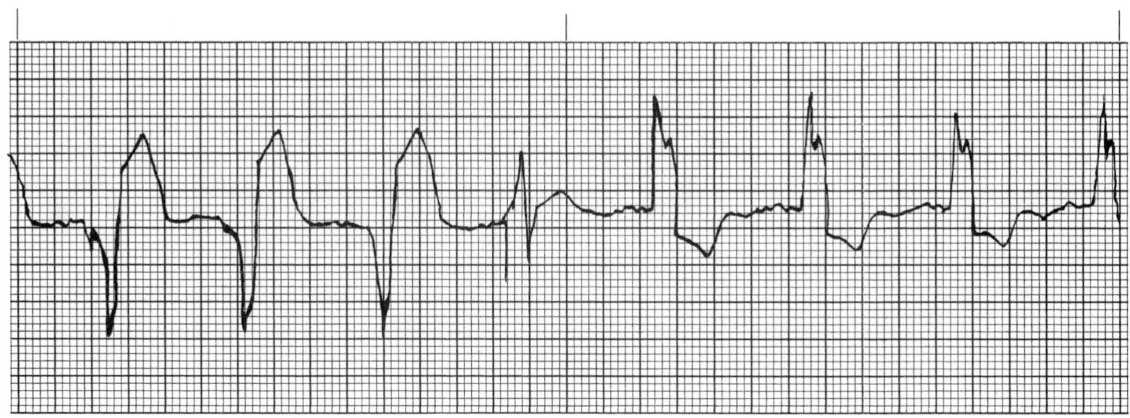

Practice Figure 9-37

Rate: ____________ Rhythm: ____________ P-R interval: ____________ QRS complex: ____________

Is there a P wave before every QRS complex? ____________

Is there a QRS complex after every P wave? ____________

Interpretation: ____________

____

Practice Figure 9-38

Rate: ____________ Rhythm: ____________ P-R interval: ____________ QRS complex: ____________

Is there a P wave before every QRS complex? ____________

Is there a QRS complex after every P wave? ____________

Interpretation: ____________

____

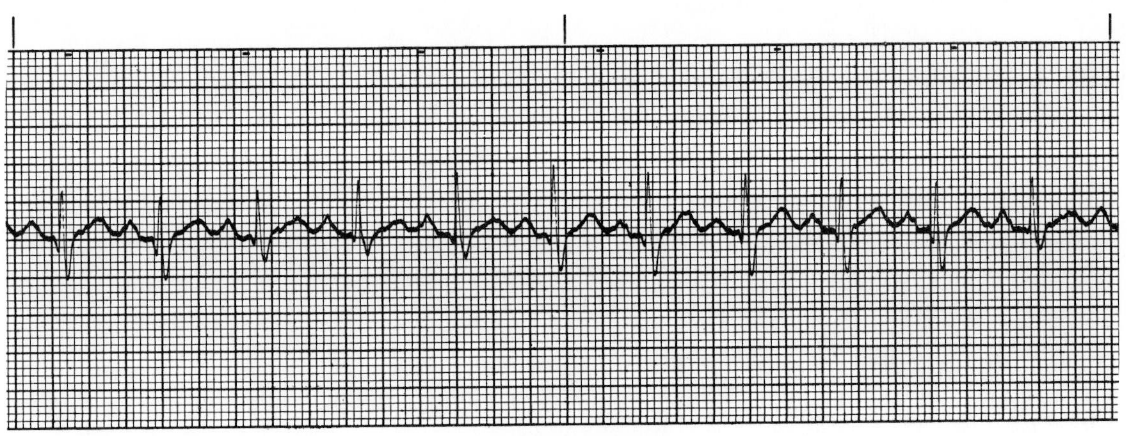

Practice Figure 9-39

Rate: ____________ Rhythm: ____________ P-R interval: ____________ QRS complex: ____________

Is there a P wave before every QRS complex? ____________

Is there a QRS complex after every P wave? ____________

Interpretation: ____________

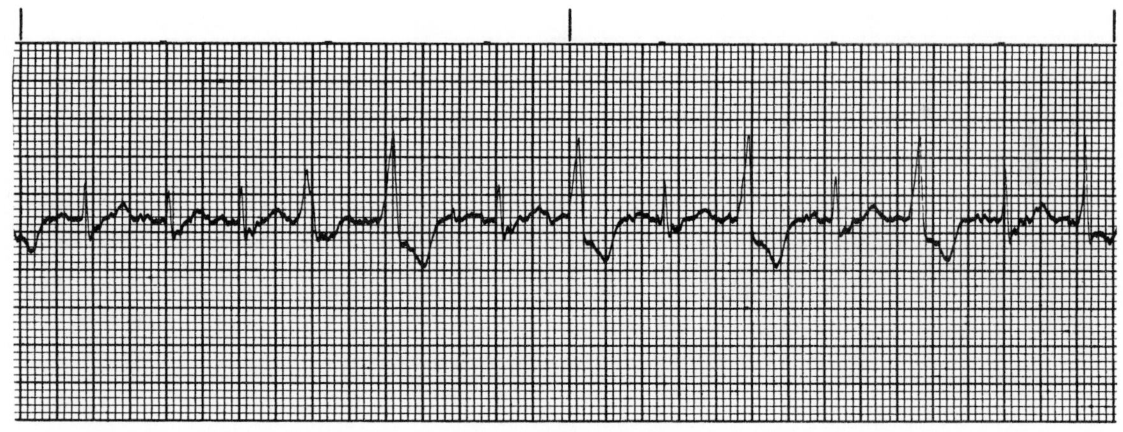

Practice Figure 9-40

Rate: ____________ Rhythm: ____________ P-R interval: ____________ QRS complex: ____________

Is there a P wave before every QRS complex? ____________

Is there a QRS complex after every P wave? ____________

Interpretation: ____________

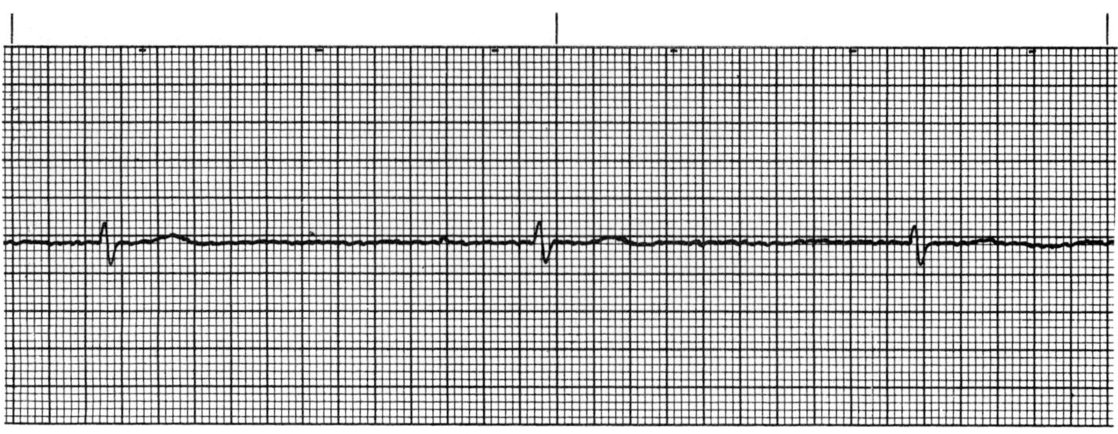

Practice Figure 9-41

Rate: ____________ Rhythm: ____________ P-R interval: ____________ QRS complex: ____________

Is there a P wave before every QRS complex? ________________________________

Is there a QRS complex after every P wave? ________________________________

Interpretation: ____

____

Practice Figure 9-42

Rate: ____________ Rhythm: ____________ P-R interval: ____________ QRS complex: ____________

Is there a P wave before every QRS complex? ________________________________

Is there a QRS complex after every P wave? ________________________________

Interpretation: ____

____

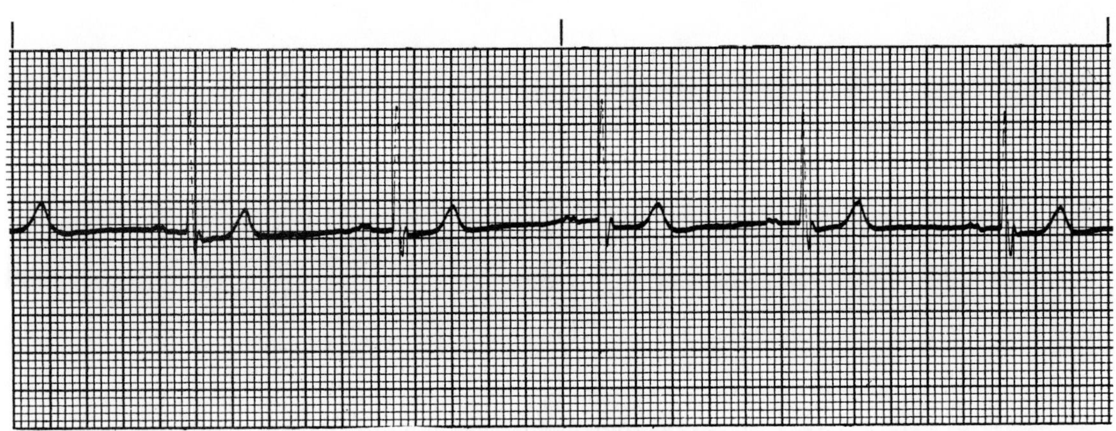

Practice Figure 9-43

Rate: ____________ Rhythm: ____________ P-R interval: ____________ QRS complex: ____________

Is there a P wave before every QRS complex? ____________

Is there a QRS complex after every P wave? ____________

Interpretation: ____________

Practice Figure 9-44

Rate: ____________ Rhythm: ____________ P-R interval: ____________ QRS complex: ____________

Is there a P wave before every QRS complex? ____________

Is there a QRS complex after every P wave? ____________

Interpretation: ____________

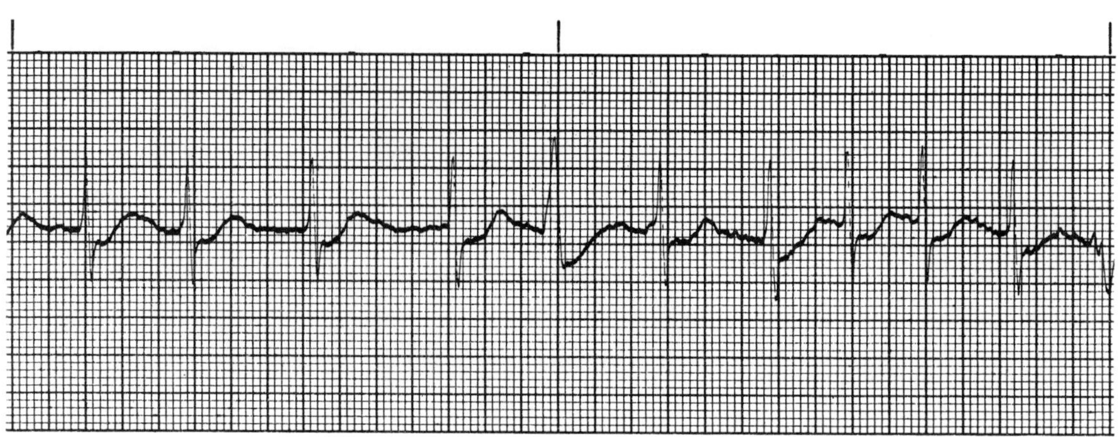

Practice Figure 9-45

Rate: ____________ Rhythm: ____________ P-R interval: ____________ QRS complex: ____________

Is there a P wave before every QRS complex? ____________

Is there a QRS complex after every P wave? ____________

Interpretation: ____________

____

Practice Figure 9-46

Rate: ____________ Rhythm: ____________ P-R interval: ____________ QRS complex: ____________

Is there a P wave before every QRS complex? ____________

Is there a QRS complex after every P wave? ____________

Interpretation: ____________

____

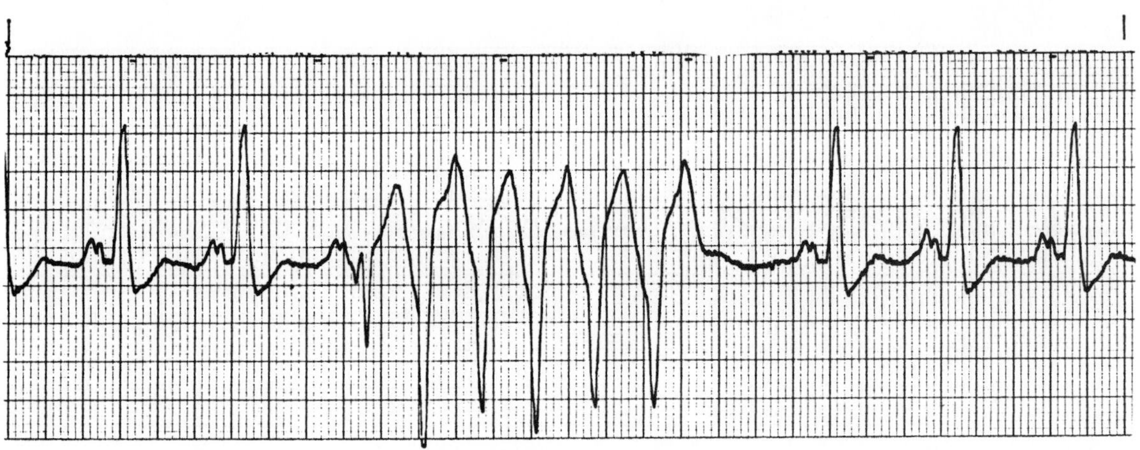

Practice Figure 9-47

Rate: ____________ Rhythm: ____________ P-R interval: ____________ QRS complex: ____________

Is there a P wave before every QRS complex? ____________

Is there a QRS complex after every P wave? ____________

Interpretation: ____________

____

Practice Figure 9-48

Rate: ____________ Rhythm: ____________ P-R interval: ____________ QRS complex: ____________

Is there a P wave before every QRS complex? ____________

Is there a QRS complex after every P wave? ____________

Interpretation: ____________

____

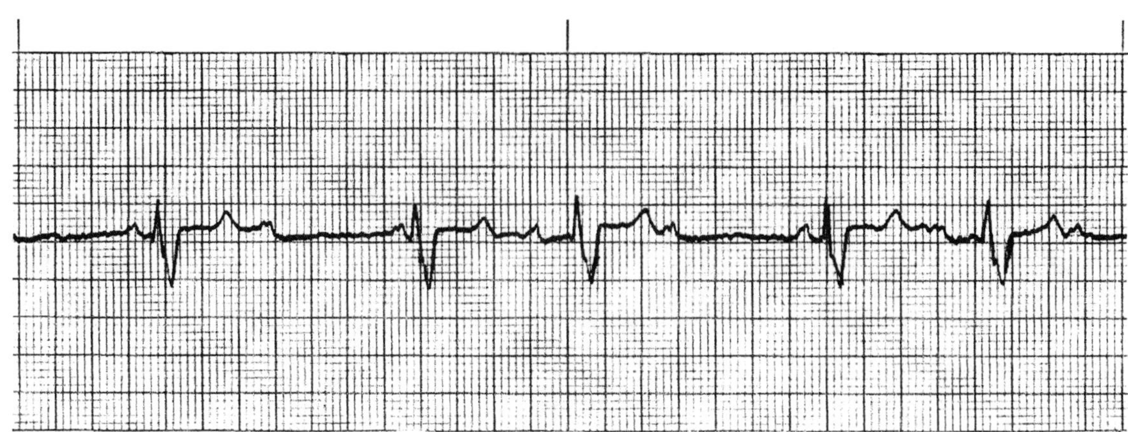

Practice Figure 9-49

Rate: ____________ Rhythm: ____________ P-R interval: ____________ QRS complex: ____________

Is there a P wave before every QRS complex? ____________

Is there a QRS complex after every P wave? ____________

Interpretation: ____________

____

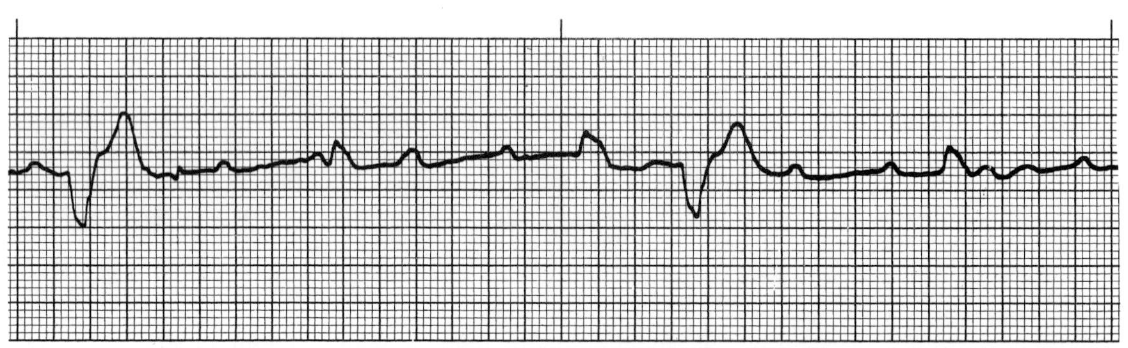

Practice Figure 9-50

Rate: ____________ Rhythm: ____________ P-R interval: ____________ QRS complex: ____________

Is there a P wave before every QRS complex? ____________

Is there a QRS complex after every P wave? ____________

Interpretation: ____________

____

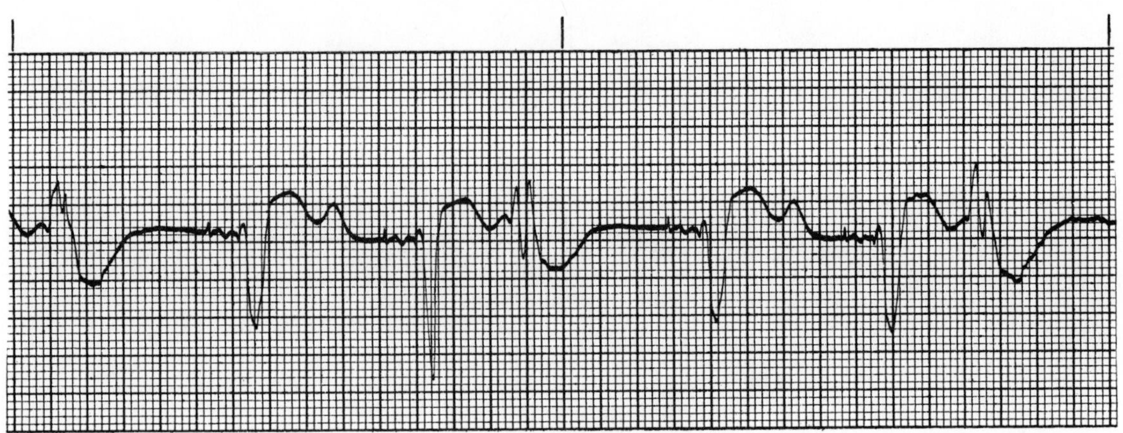

Practice Figure 9-51

Rate: __________ Rhythm: __________ P-R interval: __________ QRS complex: __________

Is there a P wave before every QRS complex? __________

Is there a QRS complex after every P wave? __________

Interpretation: __________

Practice Figure 9-52

Rate: __________ Rhythm: __________ P-R interval: __________ QRS complex: __________

Is there a P wave before every QRS complex? __________

Is there a QRS complex after every P wave? __________

Interpretation: __________

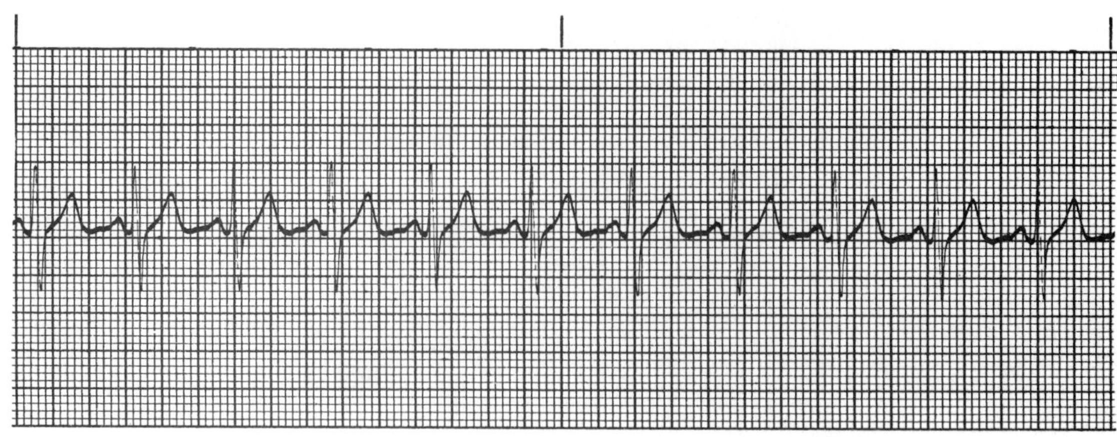

Practice Figure 9-53

Rate: ____________ Rhythm: ____________ P-R interval: ____________ QRS complex: ____________

Is there a P wave before every QRS complex? ____________

Is there a QRS complex after every P wave? ____________

Interpretation: ____________

Practice Figure 9-54

Rate: ____________ Rhythm: ____________ P-R interval: ____________ QRS complex: ____________

Is there a P wave before every QRS complex? ____________

Is there a QRS complex after every P wave? ____________

Interpretation: ____________

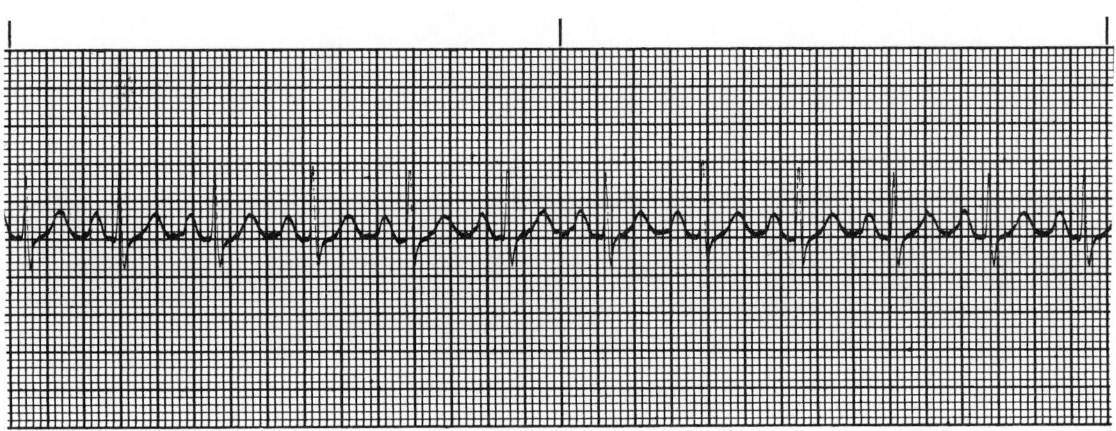

Practice Figure 9-55

Rate: ____________ Rhythm: ____________ P-R interval: ____________ QRS complex: ____________

Is there a P wave before every QRS complex? ____________

Is there a QRS complex after every P wave? ____________

Interpretation: ____________

____

Practice Figure 9-56

Rate: ____________ Rhythm: ____________ P-R interval: ____________ QRS complex: ____________

Is there a P wave before every QRS complex? ____________

Is there a QRS complex after every P wave? ____________

Interpretation: ____________

____

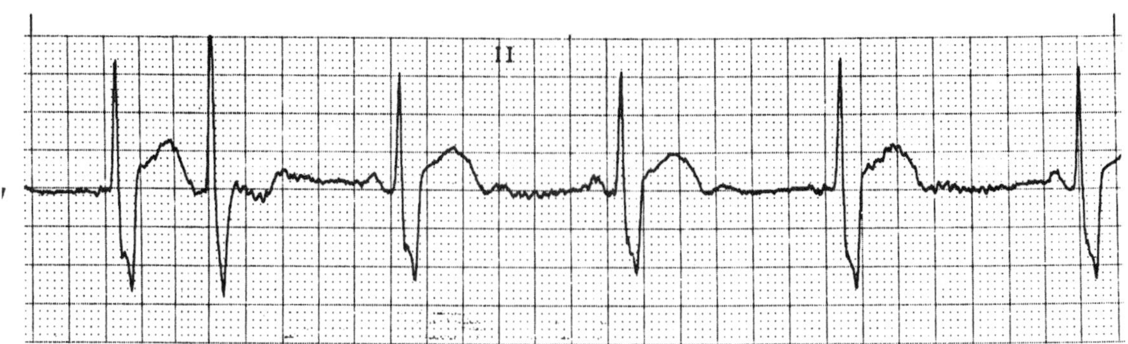

Practice Figure 9-57

Rate: ____________ Rhythm: ____________ P-R interval: ____________ QRS complex: ____________

Is there a P wave before every QRS complex? ____________

Is there a QRS complex after every P wave? ____________

Interpretation: ____________

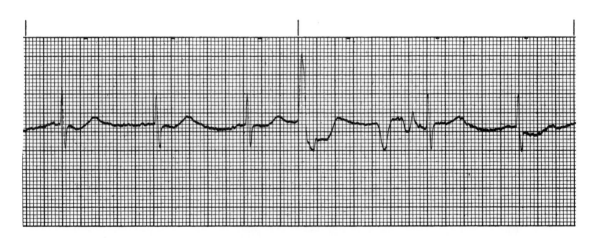

____

Practice Figure 9-58

Rate: ____________ Rhythm: ____________ P-R interval: ____________ QRS complex: ____________

Is there a P wave before every QRS complex? ____________

Is there a QRS complex after every P wave? ____________

Interpretation: ____________

____

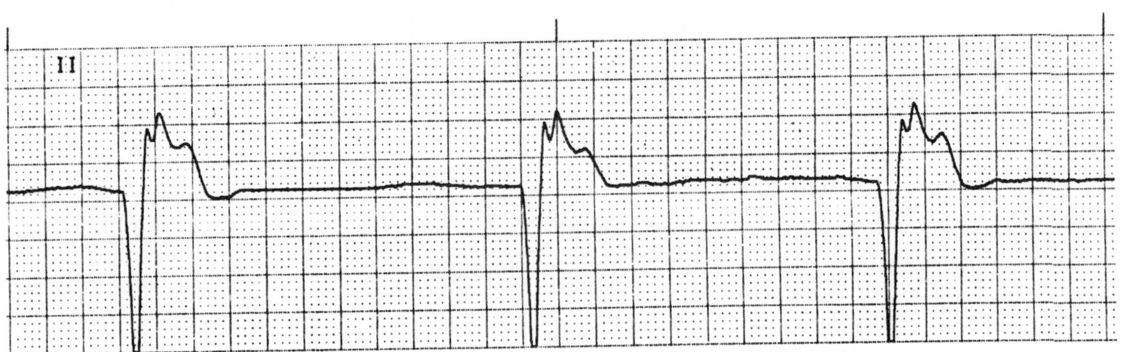

Practice Figure 9-59

Rate: ____________ Rhythm: ____________ P-R interval: ____________ QRS complex: ____________

Is there a P wave before every QRS complex? ____________

Is there a QRS complex after every P wave? ____________

Interpretation: ____________

____

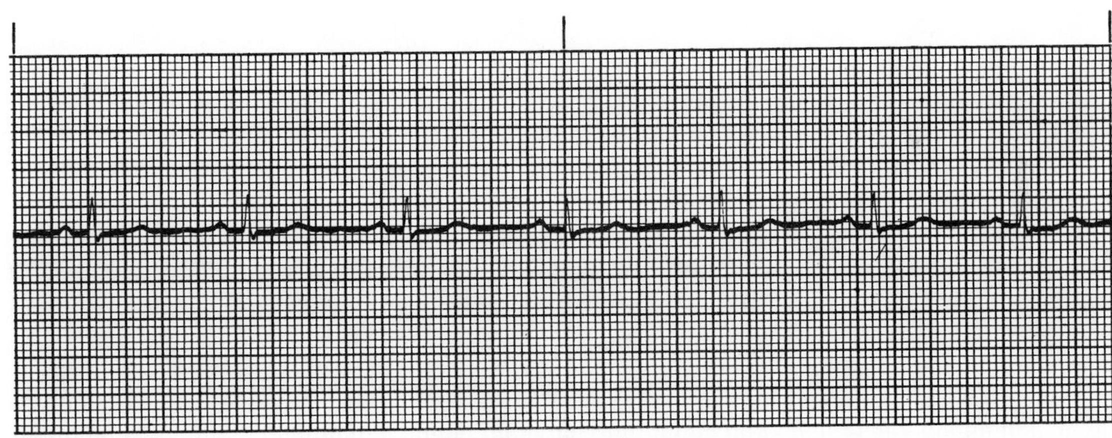

Practice Figure 9-60

Rate: ____________ Rhythm: ____________ P-R interval: ____________ QRS complex: ____________

Is there a P wave before every QRS complex? ____________

Is there a QRS complex after every P wave? ____________

Interpretation: ____________

____

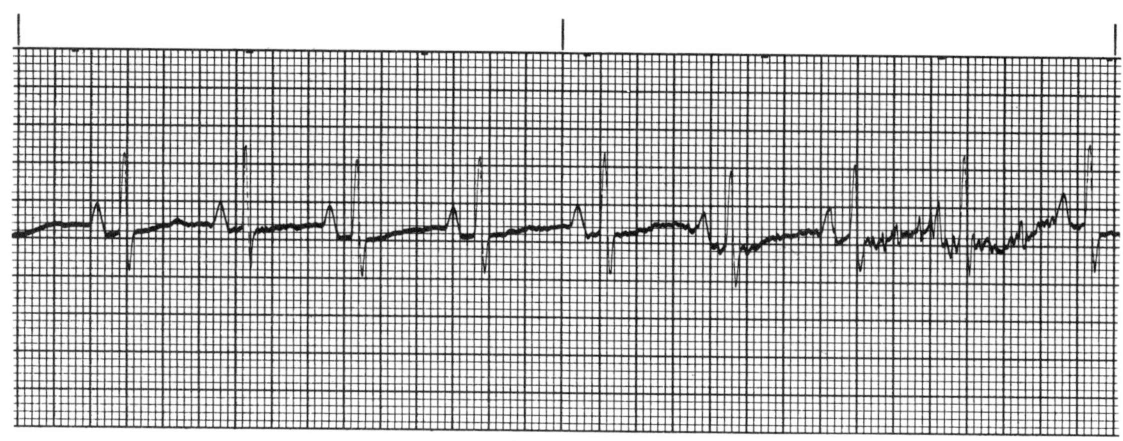

Practice Figure 9-61

Rate: ____________ Rhythm: ____________ P-R interval: ____________ QRS complex: ____________

Is there a P wave before every QRS complex? ____

Is there a QRS complex after every P wave? ____

Interpretation: ____

____

Practice Figure 9-62

Rate: ____________ Rhythm: ____________ P-R interval: ____________ QRS complex: ____________

Is there a P wave before every QRS complex? ____

Is there a QRS complex after every P wave? ____

Interpretation: ____

____

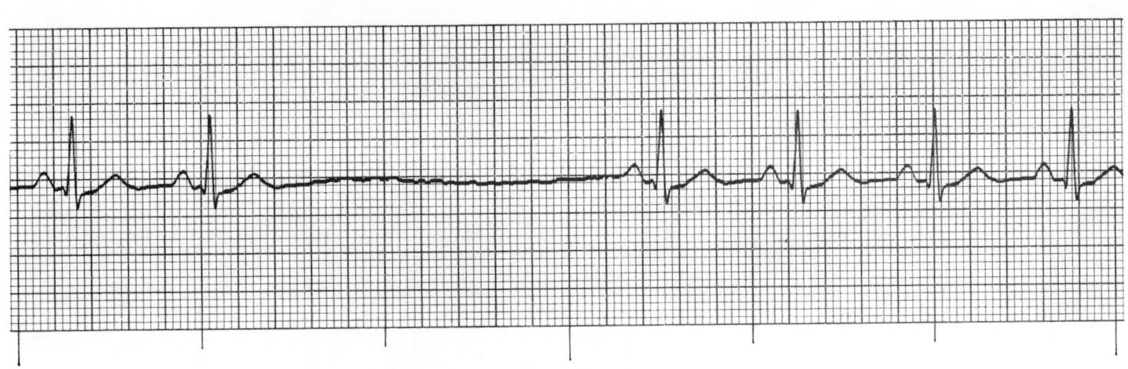

Practice Figure 9-63

Rate: ____________ Rhythm: ____________ P-R interval: ____________ QRS complex: ____________

Is there a P wave before every QRS complex? ____________

Is there a QRS complex after every P wave? ____________

Interpretation: ____________

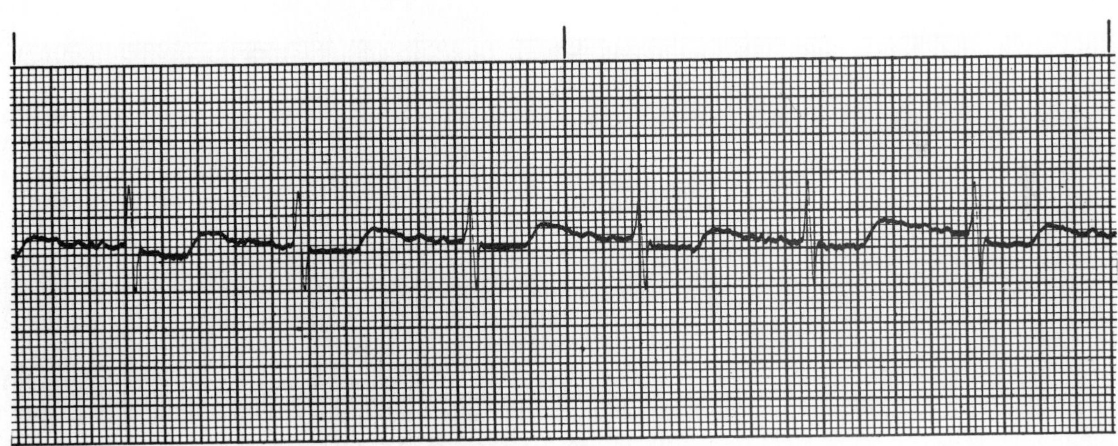

Practice Figure 9-64

Rate: ____________ Rhythm: ____________ P-R interval: ____________ QRS complex: ____________

Is there a P wave before every QRS complex? ____________

Is there a QRS complex after every P wave? ____________

Interpretation: ____________

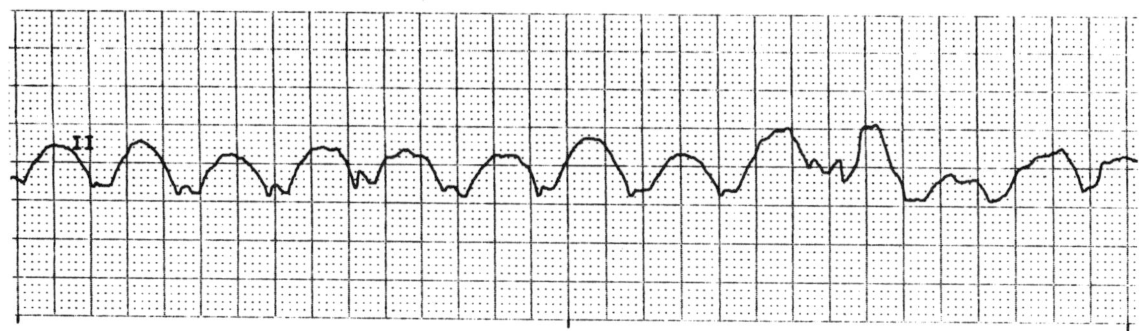

Practice Figure 9-65

Rate: ____________ Rhythm: ____________ P-R interval: ____________ QRS complex: ____________

Is there a P wave before every QRS complex? ____________

Is there a QRS complex after every P wave? ____________

Interpretation: ____________

____

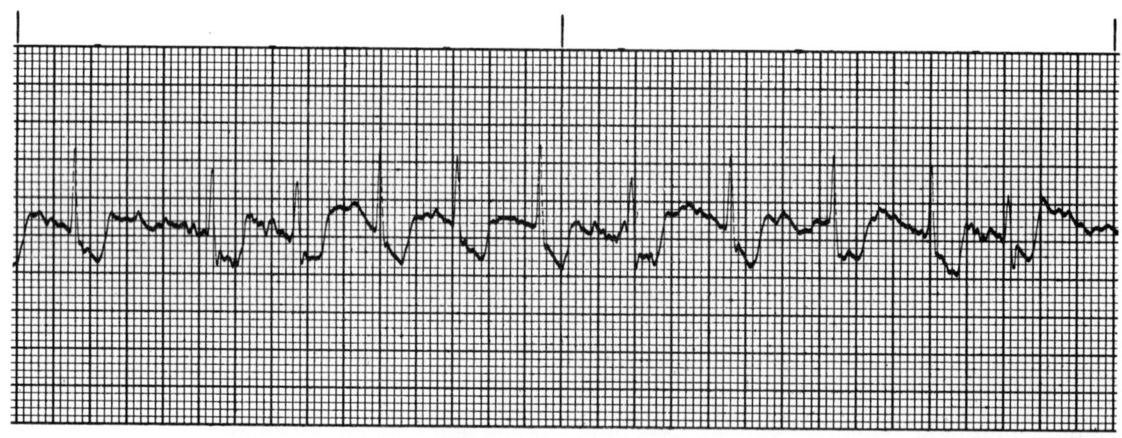

Practice Figure 9-66

Rate: ____________ Rhythm: ____________ P-R interval: ____________ QRS complex: ____________

Is there a P wave before every QRS complex? ____________

Is there a QRS complex after every P wave? ____________

Interpretation: ____________

____

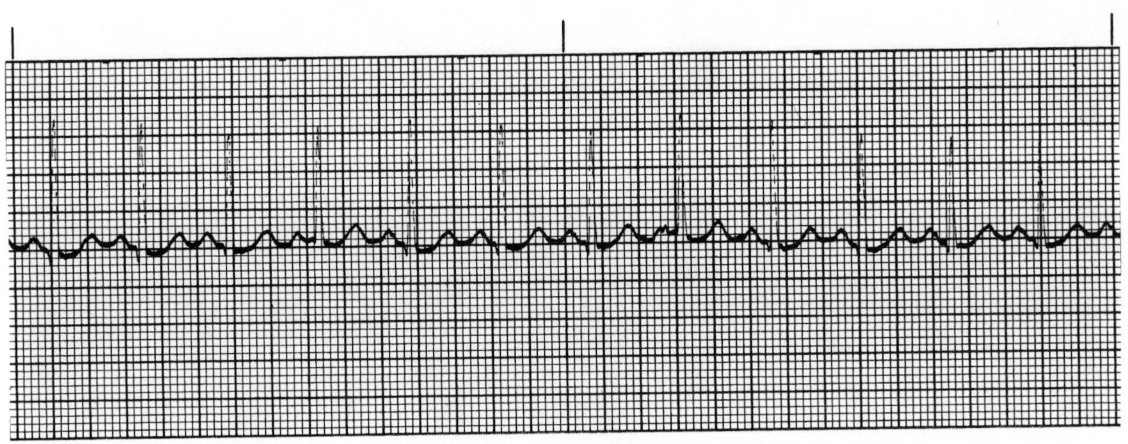

Practice Figure 9-67

Rate: ____________ Rhythm: ____________ P-R interval: ____________ QRS complex: ____________

Is there a P wave before every QRS complex? ____________

Is there a QRS complex after every P wave? ____________

Interpretation: ____________

____

Practice Figure 9-68

Rate: ____________ Rhythm: ____________ P-R interval: ____________ QRS complex: ____________

Is there a P wave before every QRS complex? ____________

Is there a QRS complex after every P wave? ____________

Interpretation: ____________

____

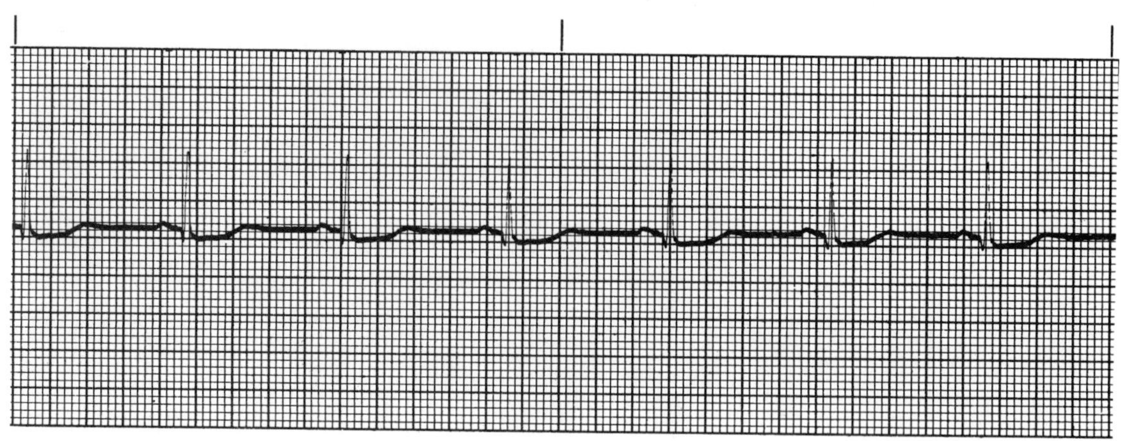

Practice Figure 9-69

Rate: ____________ Rhythm: ____________ P-R interval: ____________ QRS complex: ____________

Is there a P wave before every QRS complex? ____________

Is there a QRS complex after every P wave? ____________

Interpretation: ____________

____

Practice Figure 9-70

Rate: ____________ Rhythm: ____________ P-R interval: ____________ QRS complex: ____________

Is there a P wave before every QRS complex? ____________

Is there a QRS complex after every P wave? ____________

Interpretation: ____________

____

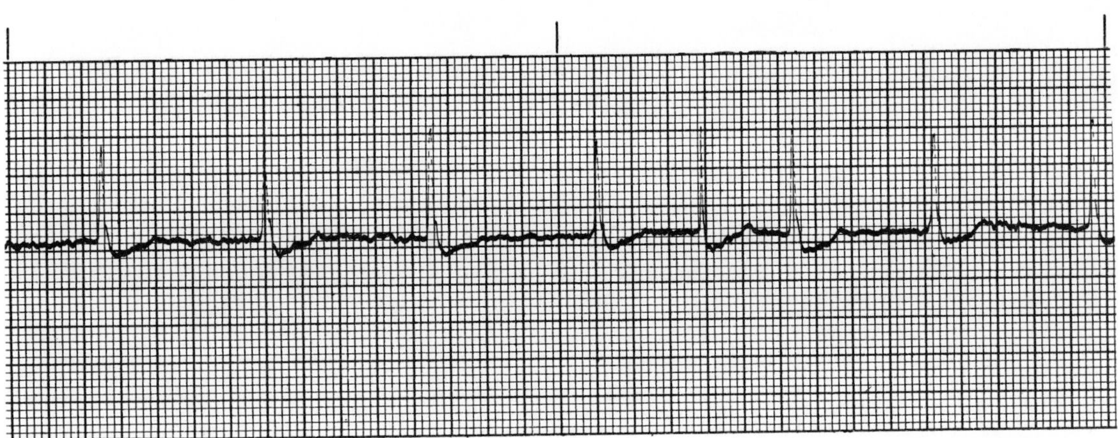

Practice Figure 9-71

Rate: ____________ Rhythm: ____________ P-R interval: ____________ QRS complex: ____________

Is there a P wave before every QRS complex? ____________

Is there a QRS complex after every P wave? ____________

Interpretation: ____________

____

Practice Figure 9-72

Rate: ____________ Rhythm: ____________ P-R interval: ____________ QRS complex: ____________

Is there a P wave before every QRS complex? ____________

Is there a QRS complex after every P wave? ____________

Interpretation: ____________

____

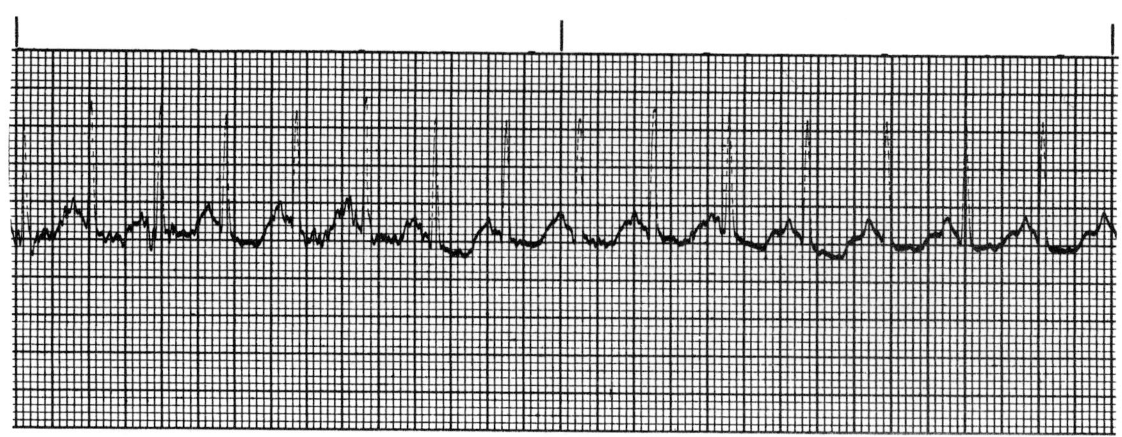

Practice Figure 9-73

Rate: ____________ Rhythm: ____________ P-R interval: ____________ QRS complex: ____________

Is there a P wave before every QRS complex? ____________

Is there a QRS complex after every P wave? ____________

Interpretation: ____________

Practice Figure 9-74

Rate: ____________ Rhythm: ____________ P-R interval: ____________ QRS complex: ____________

Is there a P wave before every QRS complex? ____________

Is there a QRS complex after every P wave? ____________

Interpretation: ____________

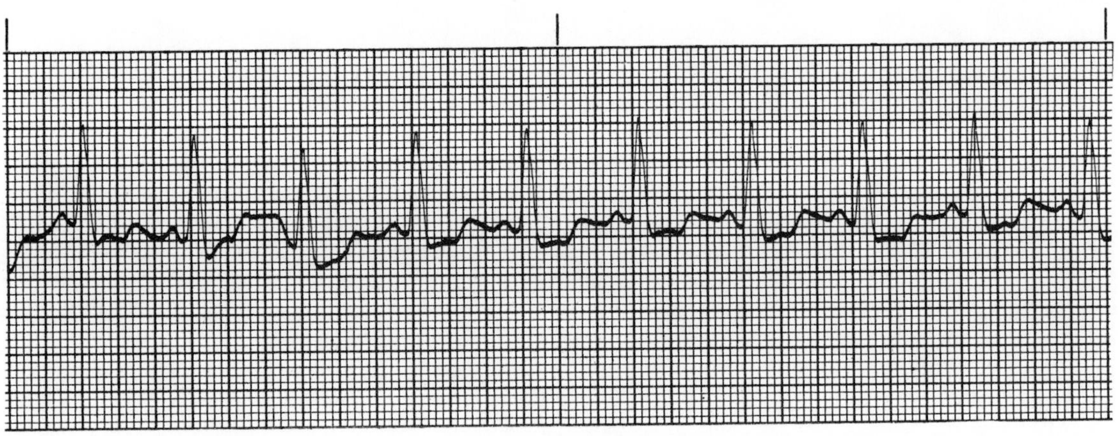

Practice Figure 9-75

Rate: ____________ Rhythm: ____________ P-R interval: ____________ QRS complex: ____________

Is there a P wave before every QRS complex? ____________

Is there a QRS complex after every P wave? ____________

Interpretation: ____________

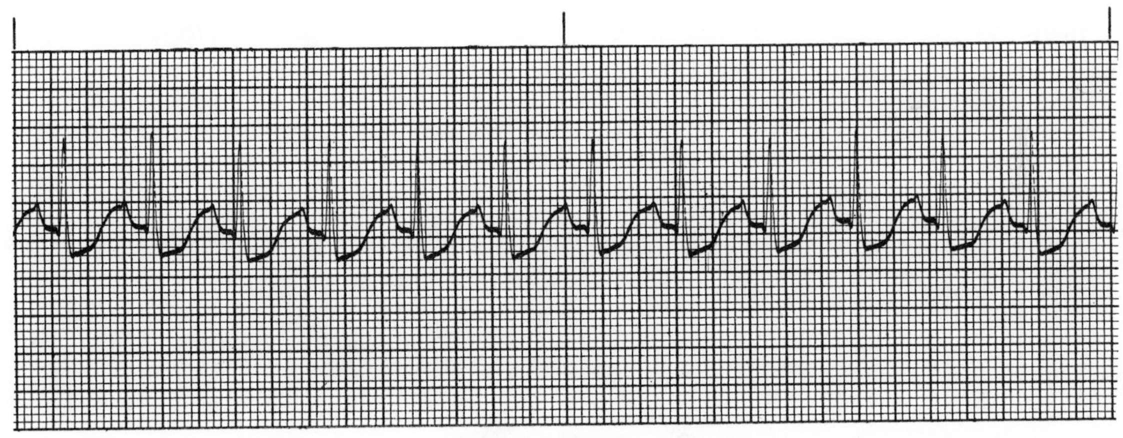

Practice Figure 9-76

Rate: ____________ Rhythm: ____________ P-R interval: ____________ QRS complex: ____________

Is there a P wave before every QRS complex? ____________

Is there a QRS complex after every P wave? ____________

Interpretation: ____________

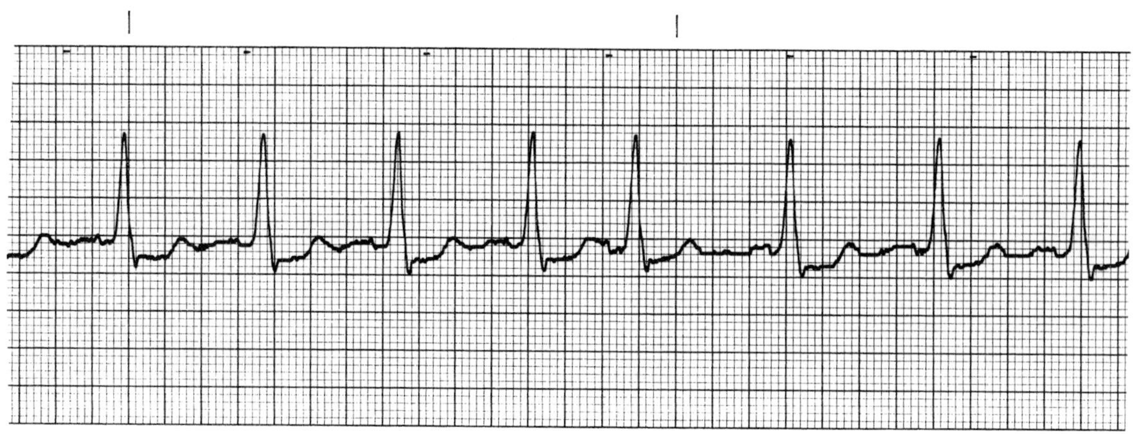

Practice Figure 9-77

Rate: ____________ Rhythm: ____________ P-R interval: ____________ QRS complex: ____________

Is there a P wave before every QRS complex? ____

Is there a QRS complex after every P wave? ____

Interpretation: ____

____

Practice Figure 9-78

Rate: ____________ Rhythm: ____________ P-R interval: ____________ QRS complex: ____________

Is there a P wave before every QRS complex? ____

Is there a QRS complex after every P wave? ____

Interpretation: ____

____

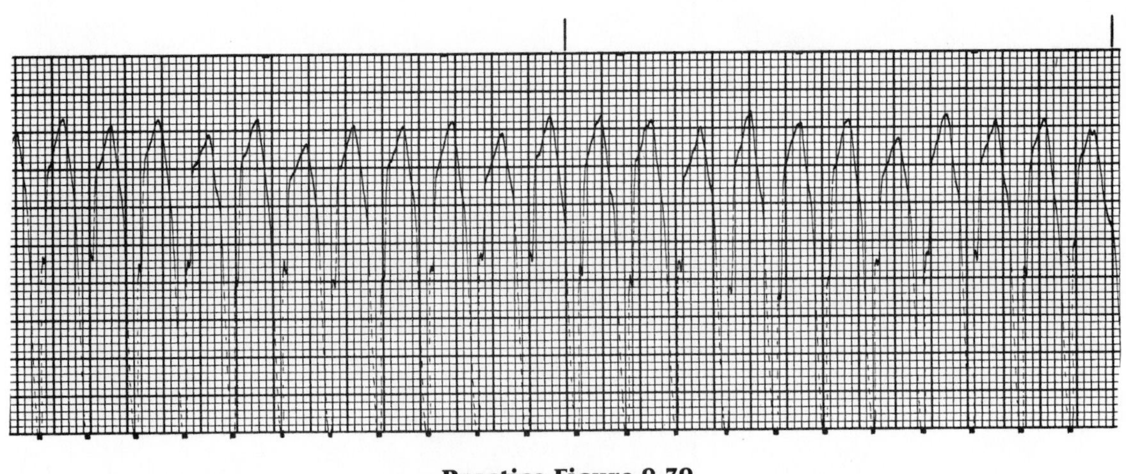

Practice Figure 9-79

Rate: ____________ Rhythm: ____________ P-R interval: ____________ QRS complex: ____________

Is there a P wave before every QRS complex? ____________________________

Is there a QRS complex after every P wave? ____________________________

Interpretation: ____________________________

____

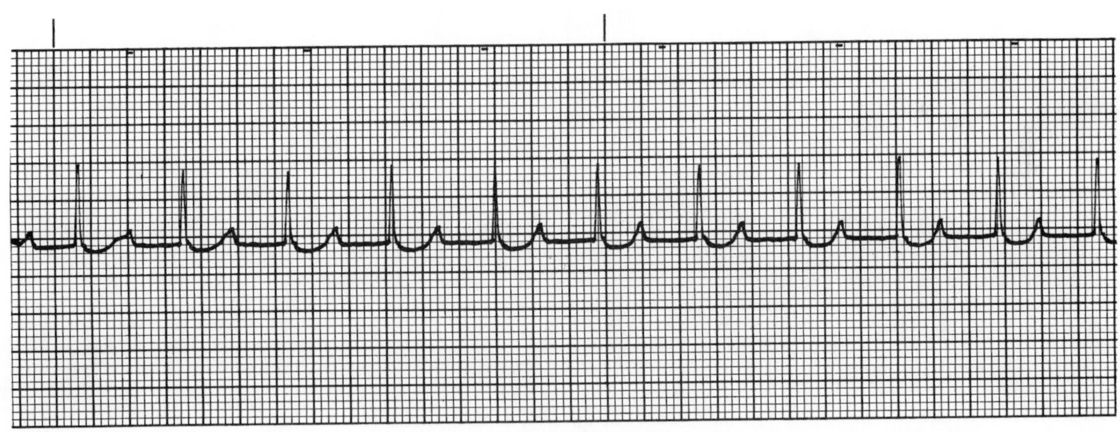

Practice Figure 9-80

Rate: ____________ Rhythm: ____________ P-R interval: ____________ QRS complex: ____________

Is there a P wave before every QRS complex? ____________________________

Is there a QRS complex after every P wave? ____________________________

Interpretation: ____________________________

____

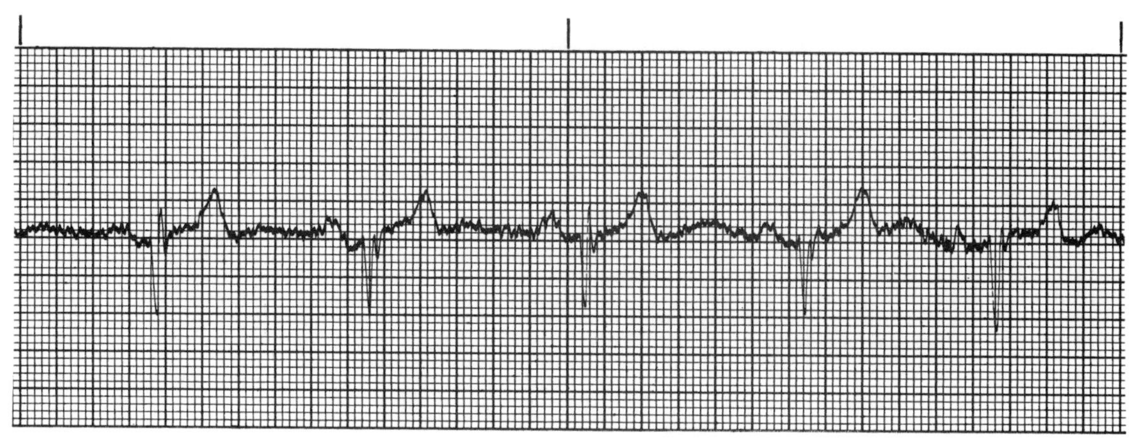

Practice Figure 9-81

Rate: ____________ Rhythm: ____________ P-R interval: ____________ QRS complex: ____________

Is there a P wave before every QRS complex? ____________

Is there a QRS complex after every P wave? ____________

Interpretation: ____________

____

Practice Figure 9-82

Rate: ____________ Rhythm: ____________ P-R interval: ____________ QRS complex: ____________

Is there a P wave before every QRS complex? ____________

Is there a QRS complex after every P wave? ____________

Interpretation: ____________

____

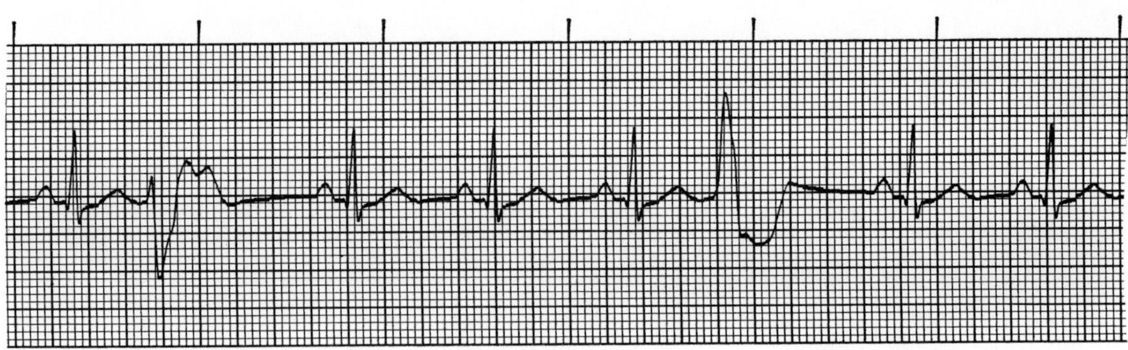

Practice Figure 9-83

Rate: __________ Rhythm: __________ P-R interval: __________ QRS complex: __________

Is there a P wave before every QRS complex? __________

Is there a QRS complex after every P wave? __________

Interpretation: __________

Practice Figure 9-84

Rate: __________ Rhythm: __________ P-R interval: __________ QRS complex: __________

Is there a P wave before every QRS complex? __________

Is there a QRS complex after every P wave? __________

Interpretation: __________

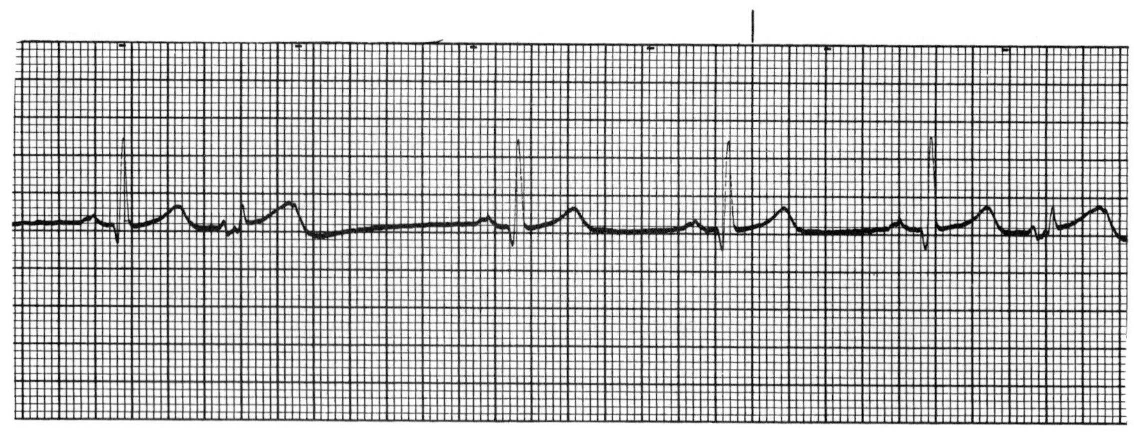

Practice Figure 9-85

Rate: ____________ Rhythm: ____________ P-R interval: ____________ QRS complex: ____________

Is there a P wave before every QRS complex? ____________

Is there a QRS complex after every P wave? ____________

Interpretation: ____________

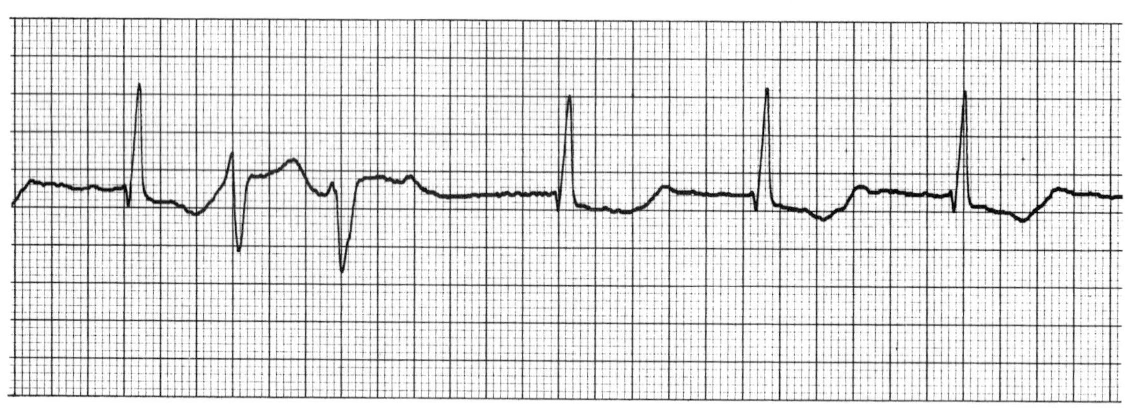

Practice Figure 9-86

Rate: ____________ Rhythm: ____________ P-R interval: ____________ QRS complex: ____________

Is there a P wave before every QRS complex? ____________

Is there a QRS complex after every P wave? ____________

Interpretation: ____________

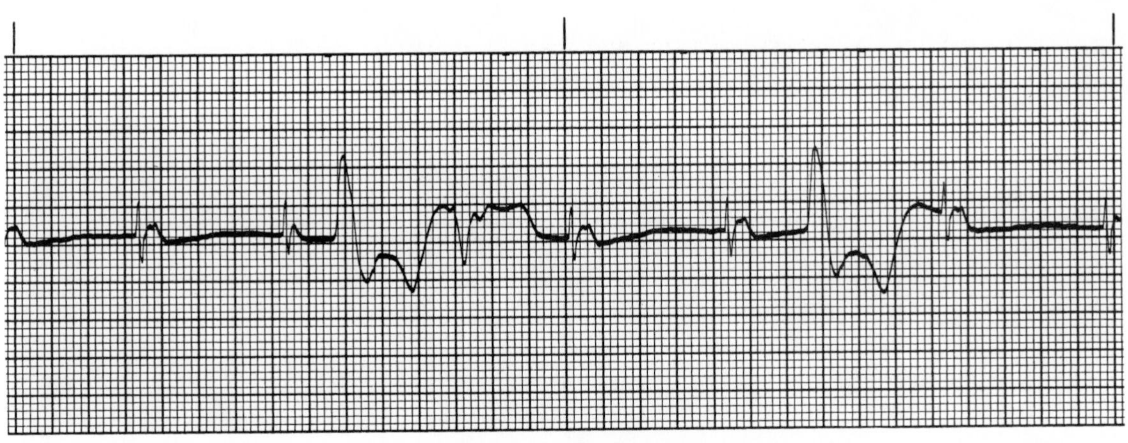

Practice Figure 9-87

Rate: ____________ Rhythm: ____________ P-R interval: ____________ QRS complex: ____________

Is there a P wave before every QRS complex? ____________

Is there a QRS complex after every P wave? ____________

Interpretation: ____________

____

Practice Figure 9-88

Rate: ____________ Rhythm: ____________ P-R interval: ____________ QRS complex: ____________

Is there a P wave before every QRS complex? ____________

Is there a QRS complex after every P wave? ____________

Interpretation: ____________

____

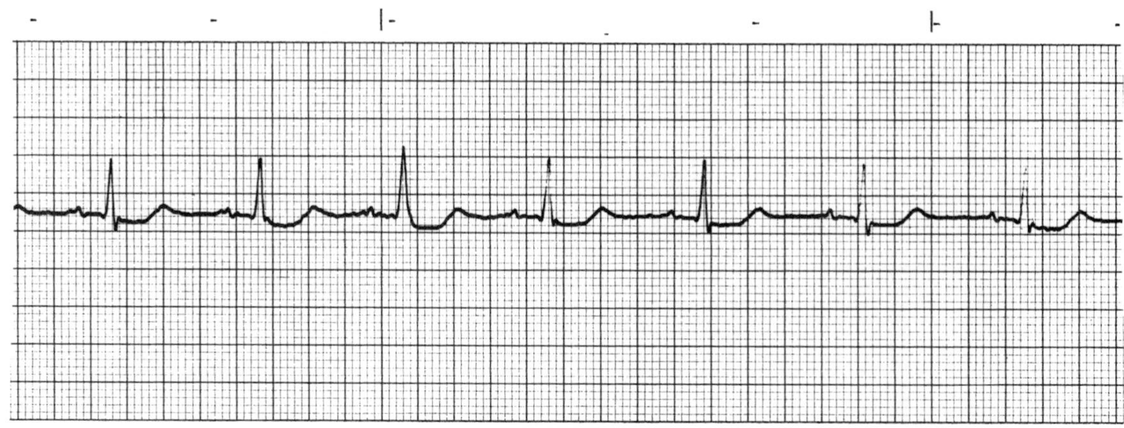

Practice Figure 9-89

Rate: ____________ Rhythm: ____________ P-R interval: ____________ QRS complex: ____________

Is there a P wave before every QRS complex? ____________

Is there a QRS complex after every P wave? ____________

Interpretation: ____________

____

Practice Figure 9-90

Rate: ____________ Rhythm: ____________ P-R interval: ____________ QRS complex: ____________

Is there a P wave before every QRS complex? ____________

Is there a QRS complex after every P wave? ____________

Interpretation: ____________

____

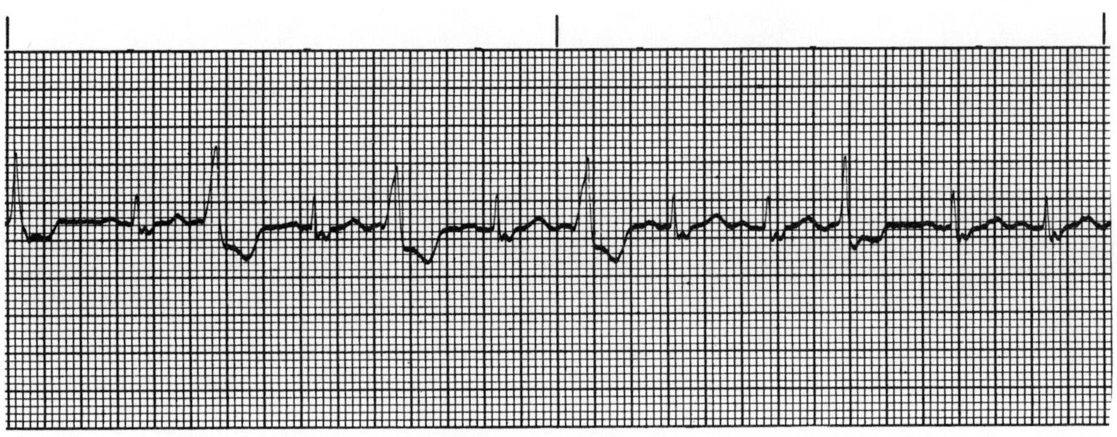

Practice Figure 9-91

Rate: ____________ Rhythm: ____________ P-R interval: ____________ QRS complex: ____________

Is there a P wave before every QRS complex? ____________

Is there a QRS complex after every P wave? ____________

Interpretation: ____________

Practice Figure 9-92

Rate: ____________ Rhythm: ____________ P-R interval: ____________ QRS complex: ____________

Is there a P wave before every QRS complex? ____________

Is there a QRS complex after every P wave? ____________

Interpretation: ____________

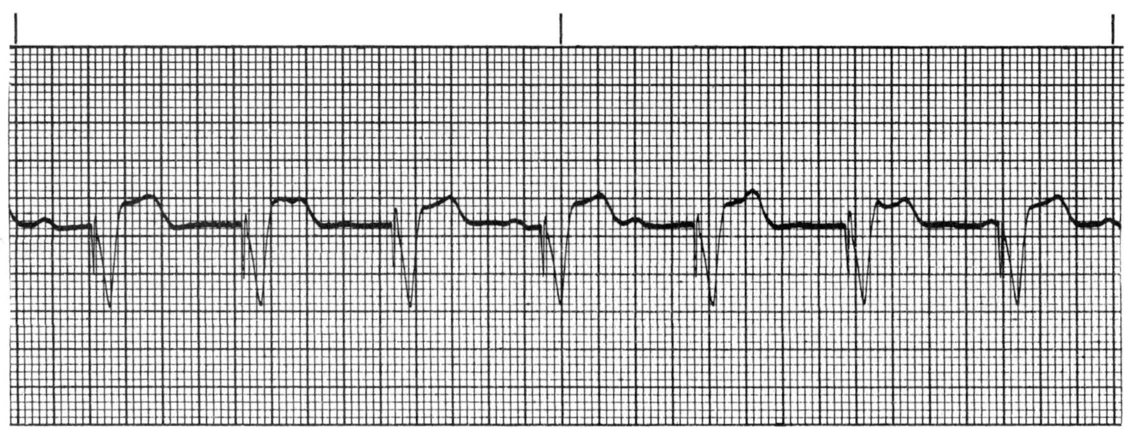

Practice Figure 9-93

Rate: ____________ Rhythm: ____________ P-R interval: ____________ QRS complex: ____________

Is there a P wave before every QRS complex? ____________

Is there a QRS complex after every P wave? ____________

Interpretation: ____________

Practice Figure 9-94

Rate: ____________ Rhythm: ____________ P-R interval: ____________ QRS complex: ____________

Is there a P wave before every QRS complex? ____________

Is there a QRS complex after every P wave? ____________

Interpretation: ____________

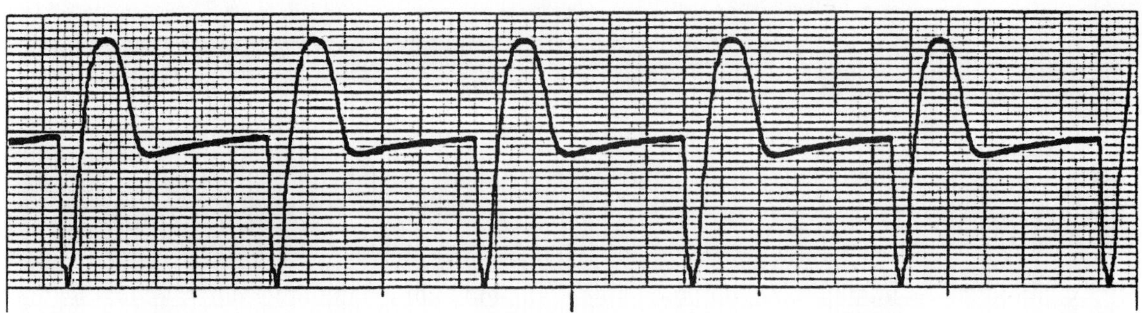

Practice Figure 9-95

Rate: ____________ Rhythm: ____________ P-R interval: ____________ QRS complex: ____________

Is there a P wave before every QRS complex? ____________

Is there a QRS complex after every P wave? ____________

Interpretation: ____________

____

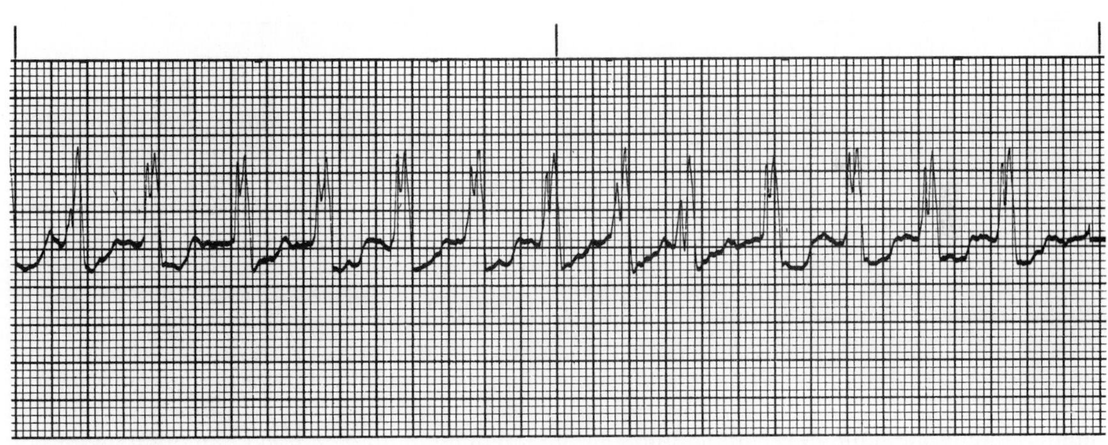

Practice Figure 9-96

Rate: ____________ Rhythm: ____________ P-R interval: ____________ QRS complex: ____________

Is there a P wave before every QRS complex? ____________

Is there a QRS complex after every P wave? ____________

Interpretation: ____________

____

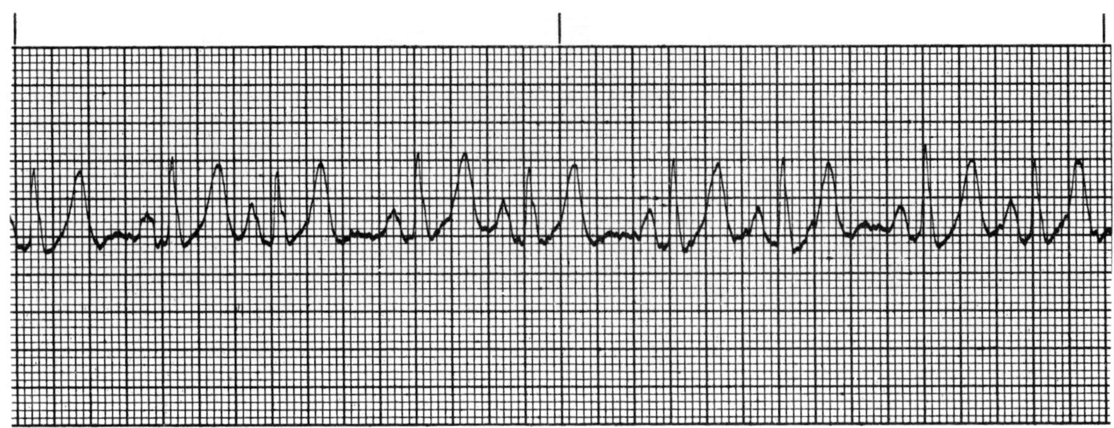

Practice Figure 9-97

Rate: ____________ Rhythm: ____________ P-R interval: ____________ QRS complex: ____________

Is there a P wave before every QRS complex? ____________

Is there a QRS complex after every P wave? ____________

Interpretation: ____________

____

Practice Figure 9-98

Rate: ____________ Rhythm: ____________ P-R interval: ____________ QRS complex: ____________

Is there a P wave before every QRS complex? ____________

Is there a QRS complex after every P wave? ____________

Interpretation: ____________

____

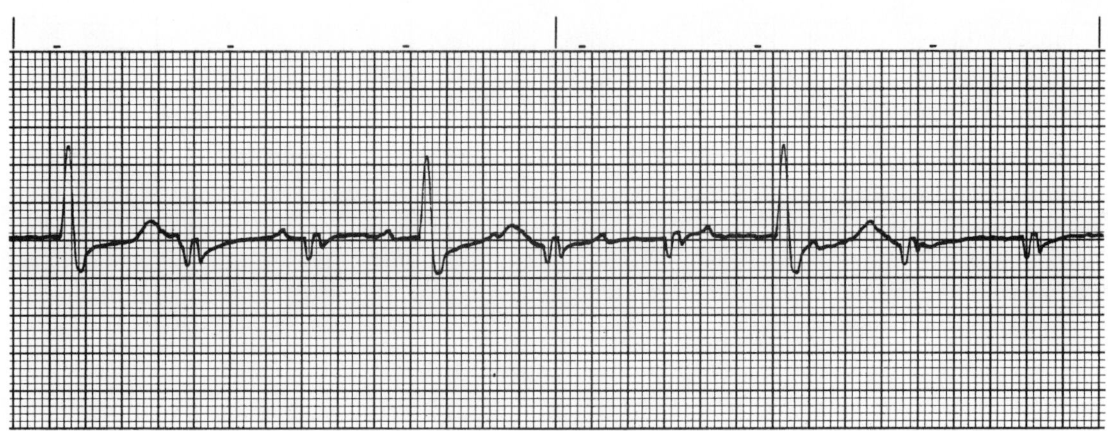

Practice Figure 9-99

Rate: ____________ Rhythm: ____________ P-R interval: ____________ QRS complex: ____________

Is there a P wave before every QRS complex? ____________________________

Is there a QRS complex after every P wave? ____________________________

Interpretation: ____________________________

____

Practice Figure 9-100

Rate: ____________ Rhythm: ____________ P-R interval: ____________ QRS complex: ____________

Is there a P wave before every QRS complex? ____________________________

Is there a QRS complex after every P wave? ____________________________

Interpretation: ____________________________

____

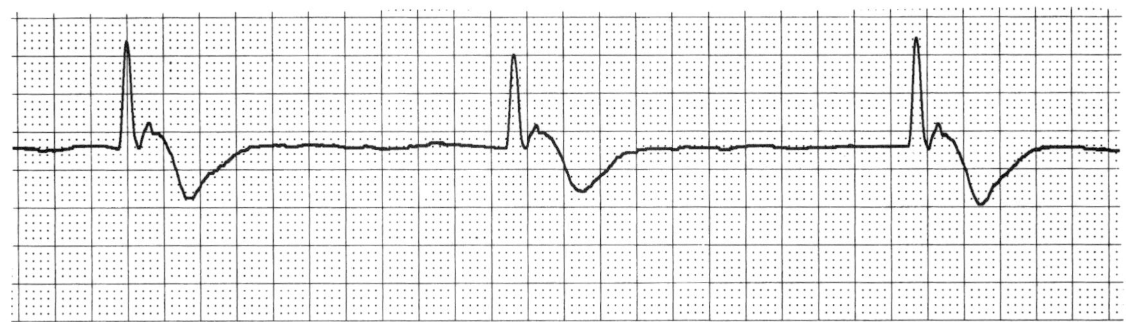

Practice Figure 9-101

Rate: ____________ Rhythm: ____________ P-R interval: ____________ QRS complex: ____________

Is there a P wave before every QRS complex? ____________

Is there a QRS complex after every P wave? ____________

Interpretation: ____________

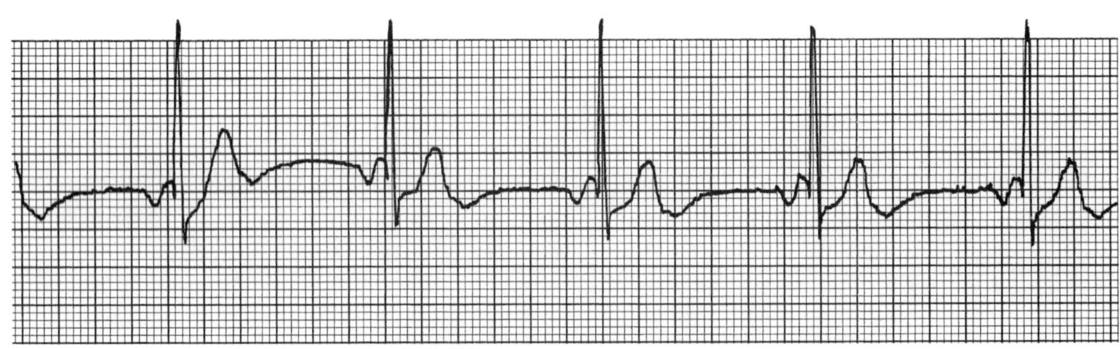

Practice Figure 9-102

Rate: ____________ Rhythm: ____________ P-R interval: ____________ QRS complex: ____________

Is there a P wave before every QRS complex? ____________

Is there a QRS complex after every P wave? ____________

Interpretation: ____________

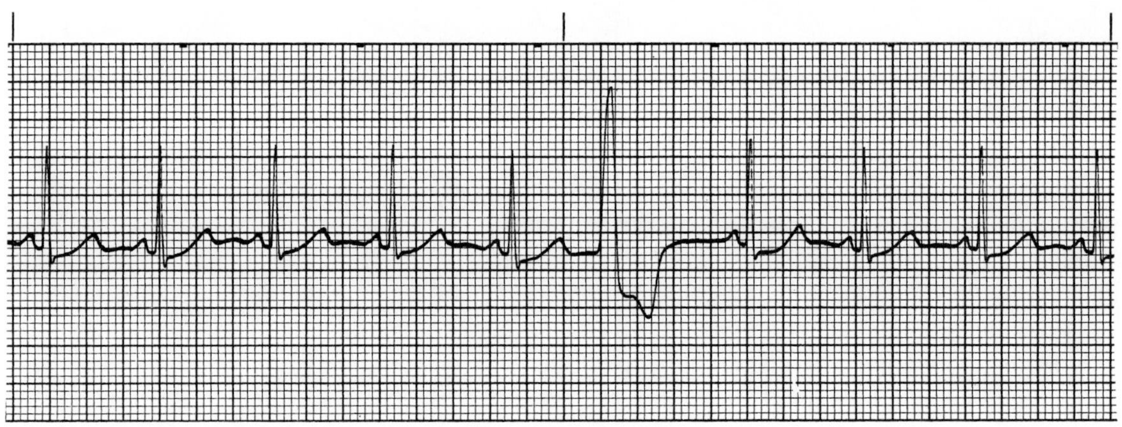

Practice Figure 9-103

Rate: ____________ Rhythm: ____________ P-R interval: ____________ QRS complex: ____________

Is there a P wave before every QRS complex? ____________

Is there a QRS complex after every P wave? ____________

Interpretation: ____________

____

Practice Figure 9-104

Rate: ____________ Rhythm: ____________ P-R interval: ____________ QRS complex: ____________

Is there a P wave before every QRS complex? ____________

Is there a QRS complex after every P wave? ____________

Interpretation: ____________

____

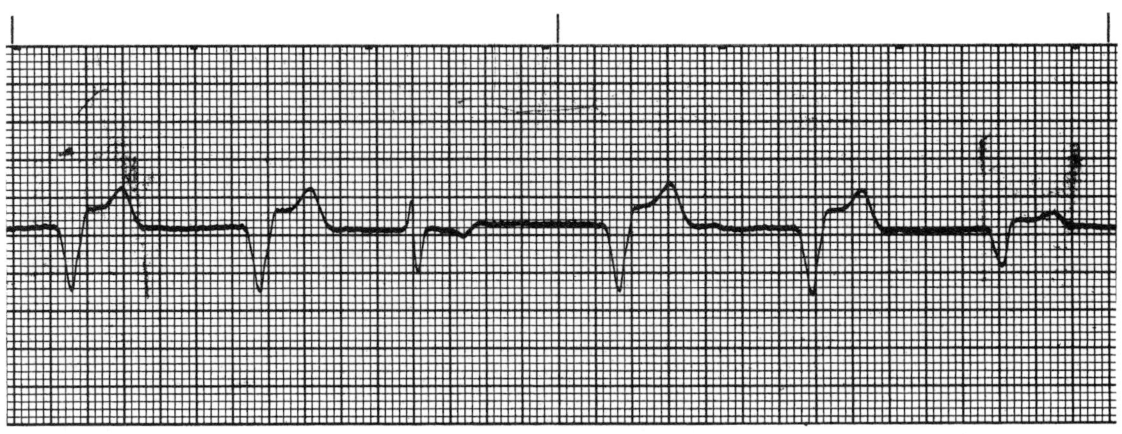

Practice Figure 9-105

Rate: ____________ Rhythm: ____________ P-R interval: ____________ QRS complex: ____________

Is there a P wave before every QRS complex? ____________

Is there a QRS complex after every P wave? ____________

Interpretation: ____________

____

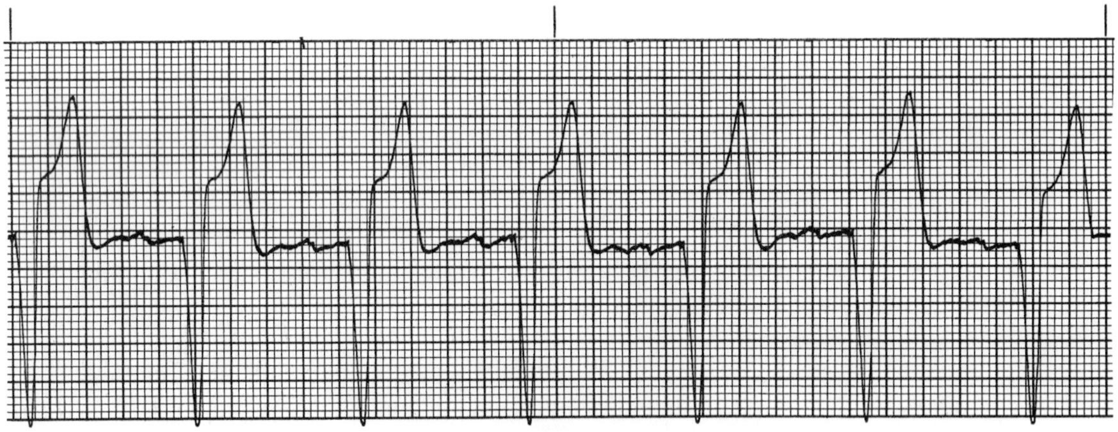

Practice Figure 9-106

Rate: ____________ Rhythm: ____________ P-R interval: ____________ QRS complex: ____________

Is there a P wave before every QRS complex? ____________

Is there a QRS complex after every P wave? ____________

Interpretation: ____________

____

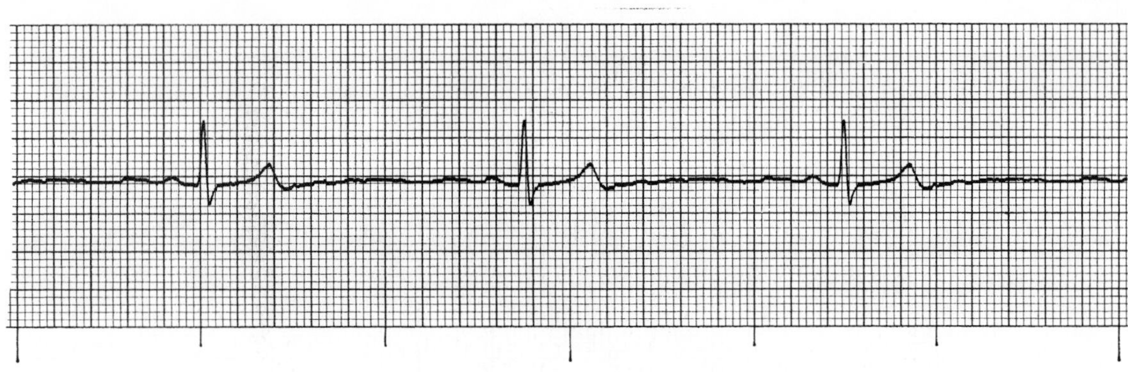

Practice Figure 9-107

Rate: ____________ Rhythm: ____________ P-R interval: ____________ QRS complex: ____________

Is there a P wave before every QRS complex? ____________

Is there a QRS complex after every P wave? ____________

Interpretation: ____________

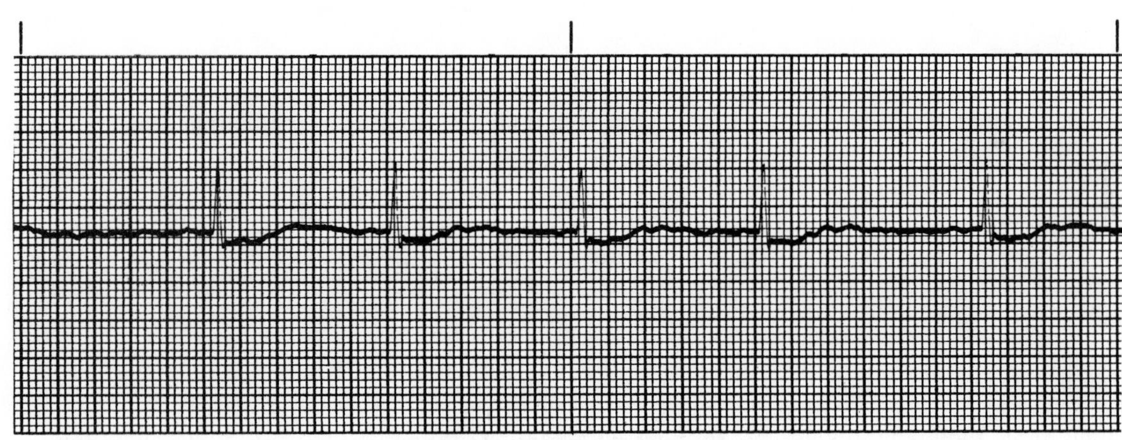

Practice Figure 9-108

Rate: ____________ Rhythm: ____________ P-R interval: ____________ QRS complex: ____________

Is there a P wave before every QRS complex? ____________

Is there a QRS complex after every P wave? ____________

Interpretation: ____________

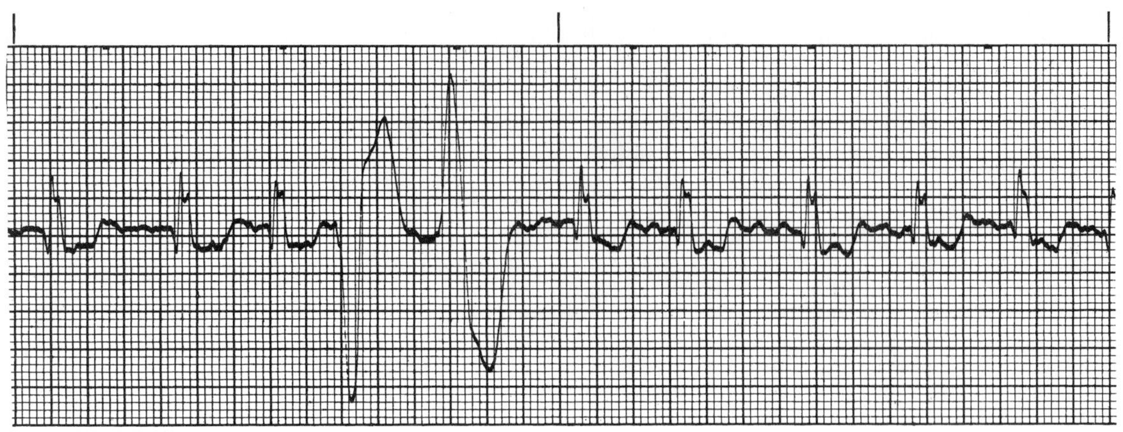

Practice Figure 9-109

Rate: ____________ Rhythm: ____________ P-R interval: ____________ QRS complex: ____________

Is there a P wave before every QRS complex? ______________________________

Is there a QRS complex after every P wave? ______________________________

Interpretation: ______________________________

____

Practice Figure 9-110

Rate: ____________ Rhythm: ____________ P-R interval: ____________ QRS complex: ____________

Is there a P wave before every QRS complex? ______________________________

Is there a QRS complex after every P wave? ______________________________

Interpretation: ______________________________

____

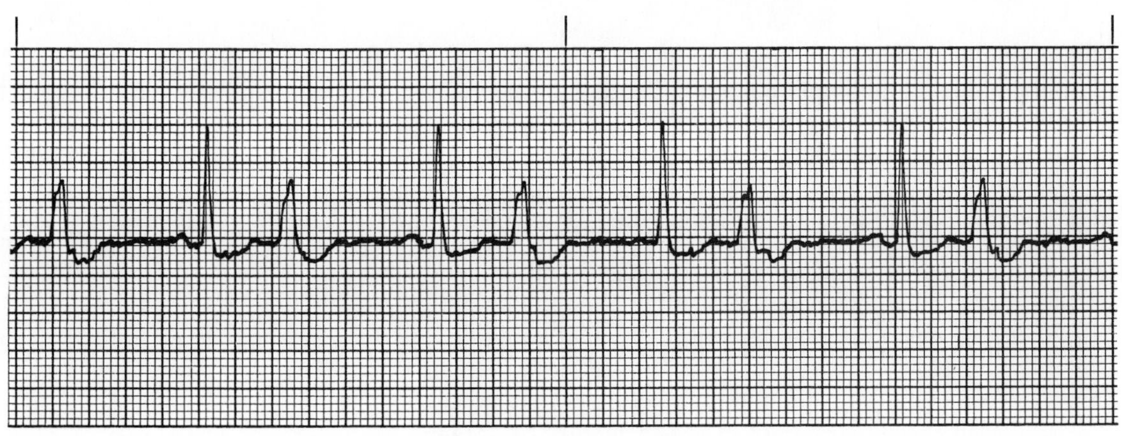

Practice Figure 9-111

Rate: ____________ Rhythm: ____________ P-R interval: ____________ QRS complex: ____________

Is there a P wave before every QRS complex? ____

Is there a QRS complex after every P wave? ____

Interpretation: ____

____

Practice Figure 9-112

Rate: ____________ Rhythm: ____________ P-R interval: ____________ QRS complex: ____________

Is there a P wave before every QRS complex? ____

Is there a QRS complex after every P wave? ____

Interpretation: ____

____

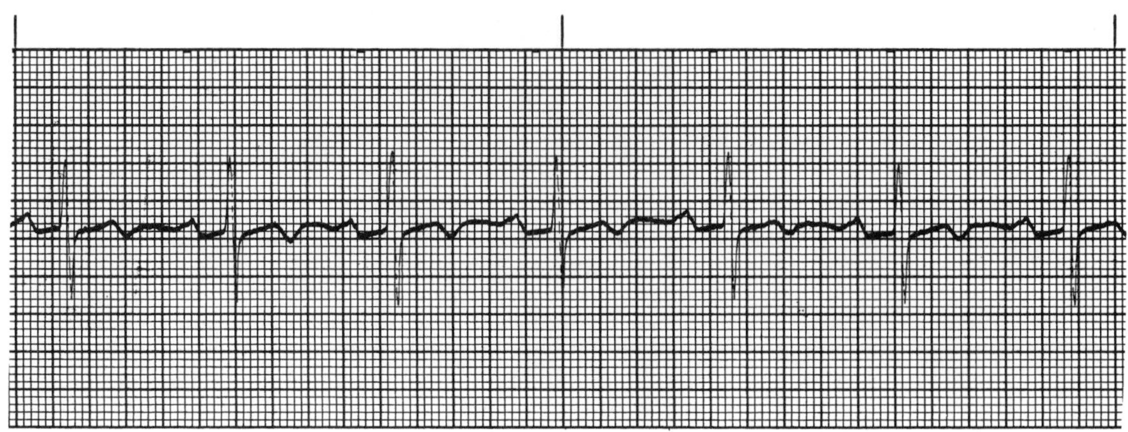

Practice Figure 9-113

Rate: ____________ Rhythm: ____________ P-R interval: ____________ QRS complex: ____________

Is there a P wave before every QRS complex? ____________

Is there a QRS complex after every P wave? ____________

Interpretation: ____________

____

ECG HR 30

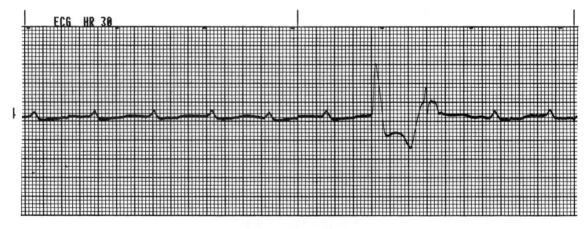

Practice Figure 9-114

Rate: ____________ Rhythm: ____________ P-R interval: ____________ QRS complex: ____________

Is there a P wave before every QRS complex? ____________

Is there a QRS complex after every P wave? ____________

Interpretation: ____________

____

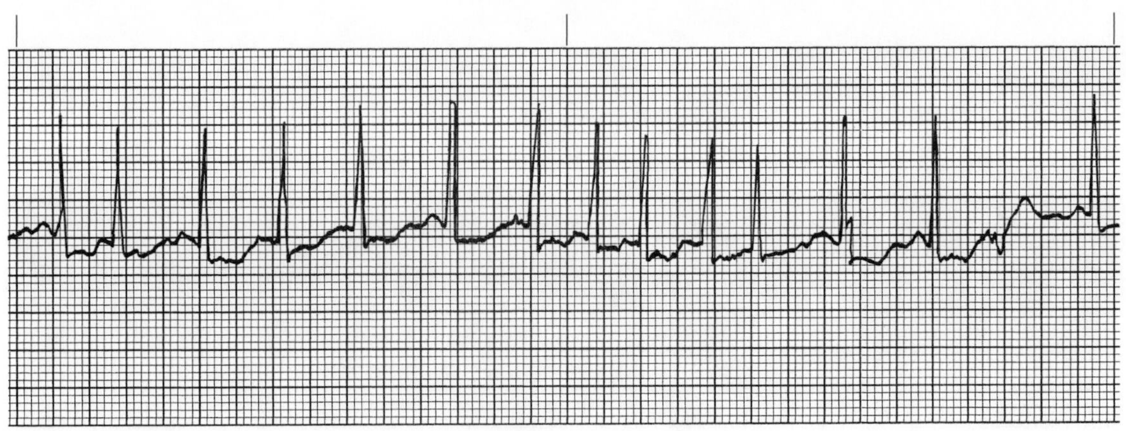

Practice Figure 9-115

Rate: ____________ Rhythm: ____________ P-R interval: ____________ QRS complex: ____________

Is there a P wave before every QRS complex? ____________

Is there a QRS complex after every P wave? ____________

Interpretation: ____________

____

Practice Figure 9-116

Rate: ____________ Rhythm: ____________ P-R interval: ____________ QRS complex: ____________

Is there a P wave before every QRS complex? ____________

Is there a QRS complex after every P wave? ____________

Interpretation: ____________

____

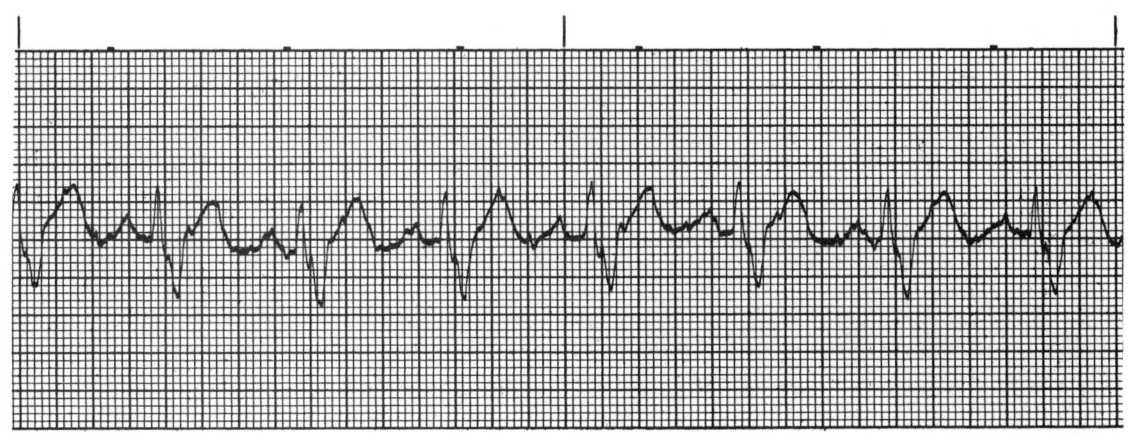

Practice Figure 9-117

Rate: ____________ Rhythm: ____________ P-R interval: ____________ QRS complex: ____________

Is there a P wave before every QRS complex? ____

Is there a QRS complex after every P wave? ____

Interpretation: ____

____

Practice Figure 9-118

Rate: ____________ Rhythm: ____________ P-R interval: ____________ QRS complex: ____________

Is there a P wave before every QRS complex? ____

Is there a QRS complex after every P wave? ____

Interpretation: ____

____

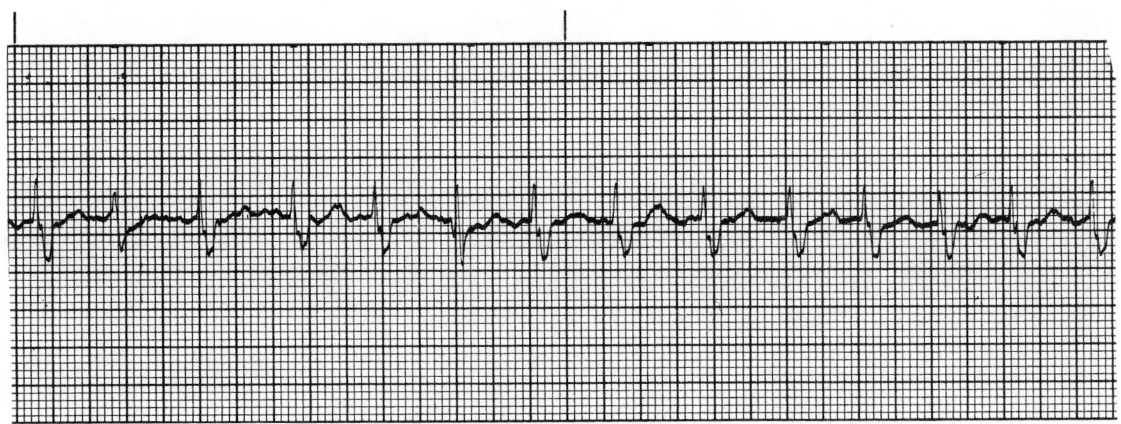

Practice Figure 9-119

Rate: ____________ Rhythm: ____________ P-R interval: ____________ QRS complex: ____________

Is there a P wave before every QRS complex? ____________

Is there a QRS complex after every P wave? ____________

Interpretation: ____________

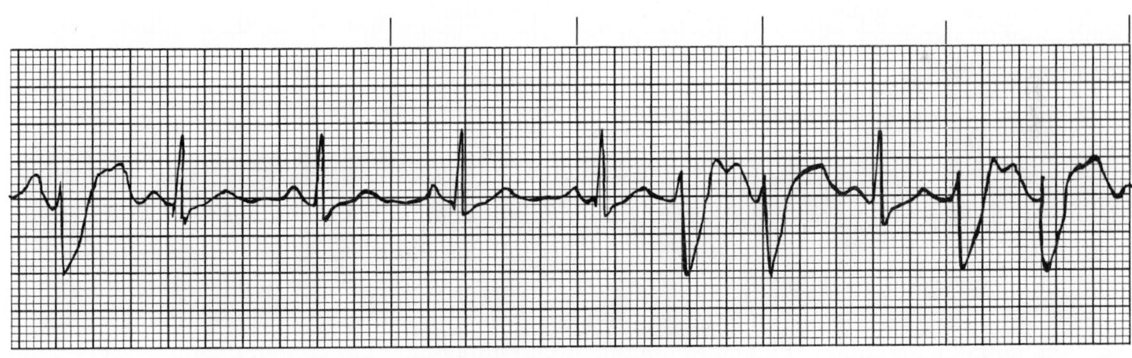

Practice Figure 9-120

Rate: ____________ Rhythm: ____________ P-R interval: ____________ QRS complex: ____________

Is there a P wave before every QRS complex? ____________

Is there a QRS complex after every P wave? ____________

Interpretation: ____________

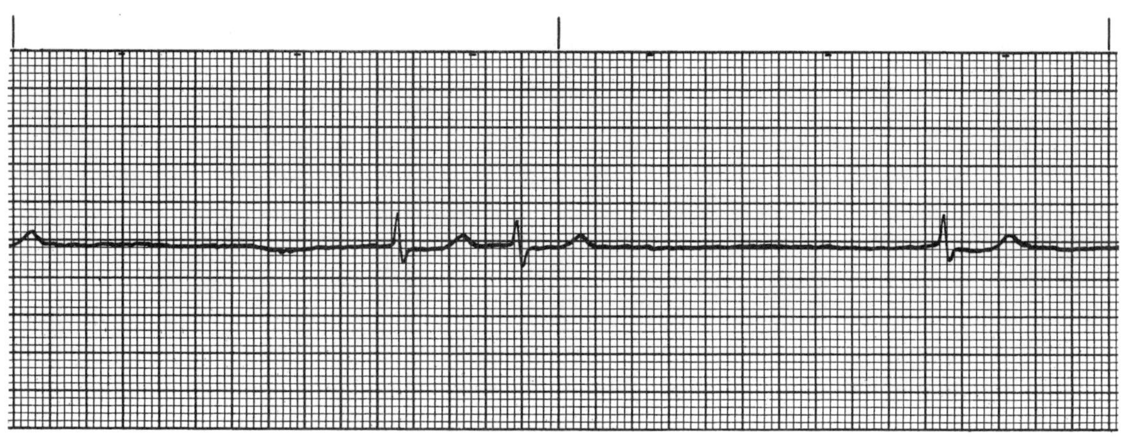

Practice Figure 9-121

Rate: ____________ Rhythm: ____________ P-R interval: ____________ QRS complex: ____________

Is there a P wave before every QRS complex? ____________

Is there a QRS complex after every P wave? ____________

Interpretation: ____________

Practice Figure 9-122

Rate: ____________ Rhythm: ____________ P-R interval: ____________ QRS complex: ____________

Is there a P wave before every QRS complex? ____________

Is there a QRS complex after every P wave? ____________

Interpretation: ____________

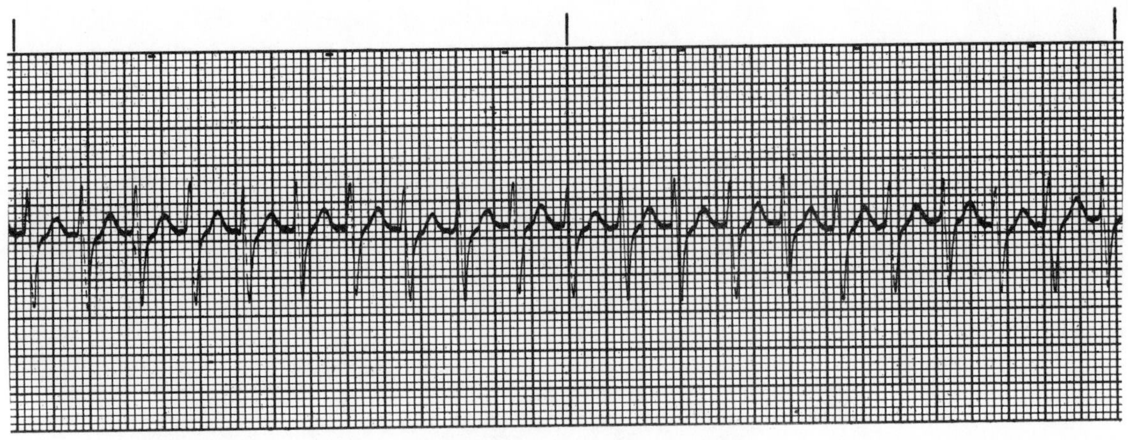

Practice Figure 9-123

Rate: ____________ Rhythm: ____________ P-R interval: ____________ QRS complex: ____________

Is there a P wave before every QRS complex? ____________

Is there a QRS complex after every P wave? ____________

Interpretation: ____________

____

Practice Figure 9-124

Rate: ____________ Rhythm: ____________ P-R interval: ____________ QRS complex: ____________

Is there a P wave before every QRS complex? ____________

Is there a QRS complex after every P wave? ____________

Interpretation: ____________

____

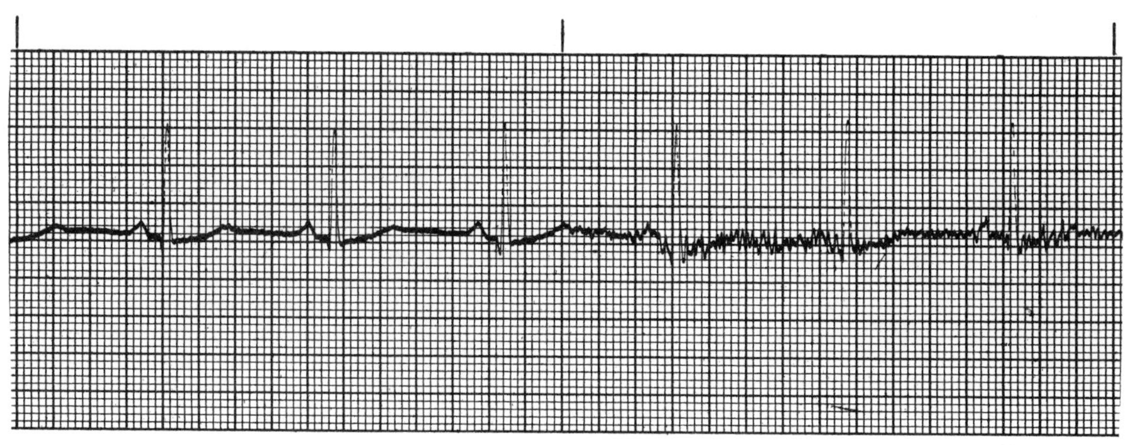

Practice Figure 9-125

Rate: ____________ Rhythm: ____________ P-R interval: ____________ QRS complex: ____________

Is there a P wave before every QRS complex? ____________

Is there a QRS complex after every P wave? ____________

Interpretation: ____________

____

Practice Figure 9-126

Rate: ____________ Rhythm: ____________ P-R interval: ____________ QRS complex: ____________

Is there a P wave before every QRS complex? ____________

Is there a QRS complex after every P wave? ____________

Interpretation: ____________

____

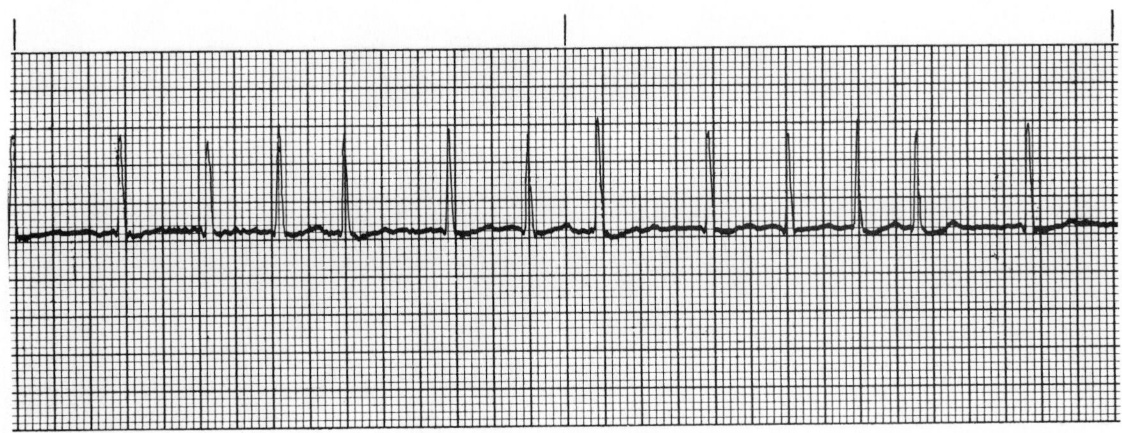

Practice Figure 9-127

Rate: __________ Rhythm: __________ P-R interval: __________ QRS complex: __________

Is there a P wave before every QRS complex? __________

Is there a QRS complex after every P wave? __________

Interpretation: __________

Practice Figure 9-128

Rate: __________ Rhythm: __________ P-R interval: __________ QRS complex: __________

Is there a P wave before every QRS complex? __________

Is there a QRS complex after every P wave? __________

Interpretation: __________

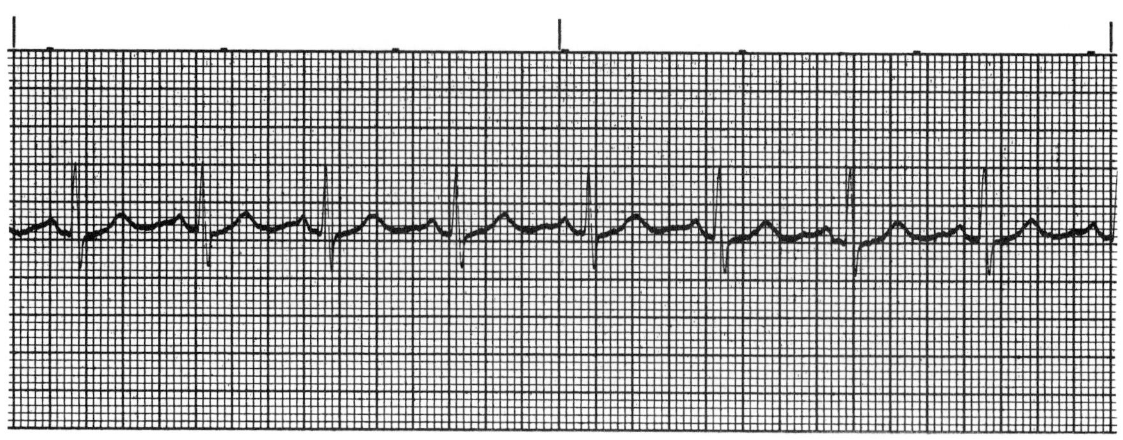

Practice Figure 9-129

Rate: ____________ Rhythm: ____________ P-R interval: ____________ QRS complex: ____________

Is there a P wave before every QRS complex? ____________

Is there a QRS complex after every P wave? ____________

Interpretation: ____________

____

Practice Figure 9-130

Rate: ____________ Rhythm: ____________ P-R interval: ____________ QRS complex: ____________

Is there a P wave before every QRS complex? ____________

Is there a QRS complex after every P wave? ____________

Interpretation: ____________

____

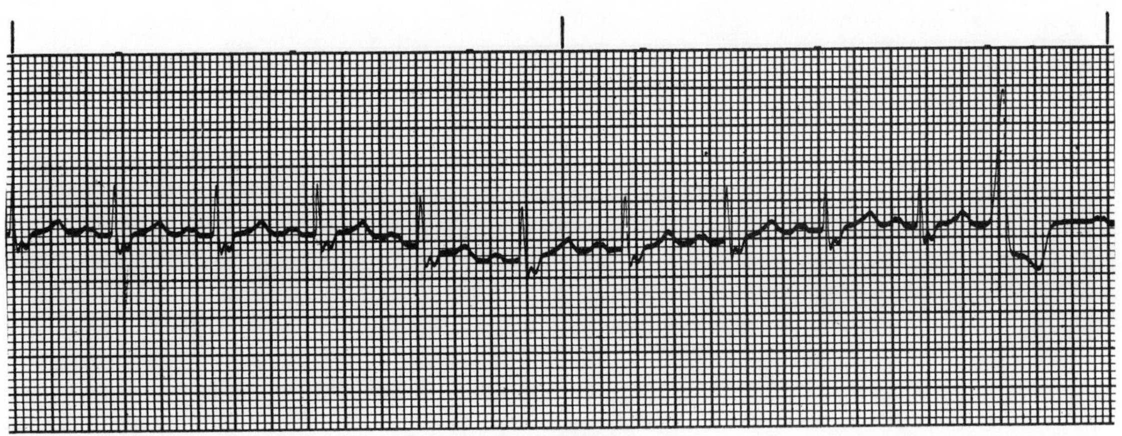

Practice Figure 9-131

Rate: ____________ Rhythm: ____________ P-R interval: ____________ QRS complex: ____________

Is there a P wave before every QRS complex? ____________

Is there a QRS complex after every P wave? ____________

Interpretation: ____________

Practice Figure 9-132

Rate: ____________ Rhythm: ____________ P-R interval: ____________ QRS complex: ____________

Is there a P wave before every QRS complex? ____________

Is there a QRS complex after every P wave? ____________

Interpretation: ____________

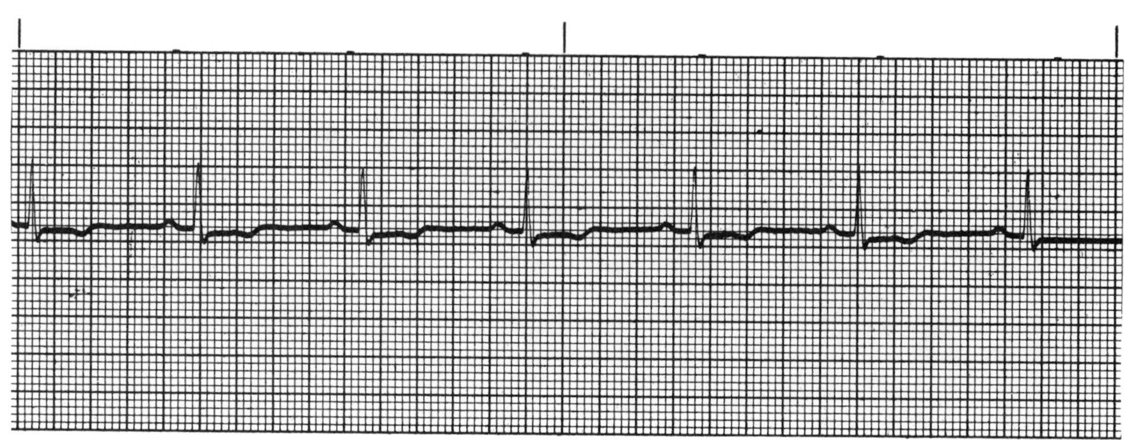

Practice Figure 9-133

Rate: ____________ Rhythm: ____________ P-R interval: ____________ QRS complex: ____________

Is there a P wave before every QRS complex? ____________

Is there a QRS complex after every P wave? ____________

Interpretation: ____________

____

Practice Figure 9-134

Rate: ____________ Rhythm: ____________ P-R interval: ____________ QRS complex: ____________

Is there a P wave before every QRS complex? ____________

Is there a QRS complex after every P wave? ____________

Interpretation: ____________

____

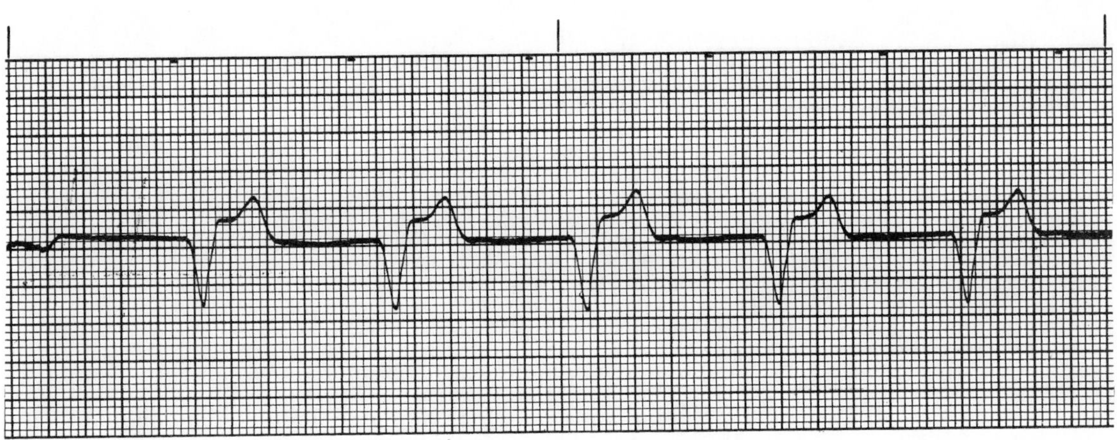

Practice Figure 9-135

Rate: ____________ Rhythm: ____________ P-R interval: ____________ QRS complex: ____________

Is there a P wave before every QRS complex? ____________

Is there a QRS complex after every P wave? ____________

Interpretation: ____________

____

Practice Figure 9-136

Rate: ____________ Rhythm: ____________ P-R interval: ____________ QRS complex: ____________

Is there a P wave before every QRS complex? ____________

Is there a QRS complex after every P wave? ____________

Interpretation: ____________

____

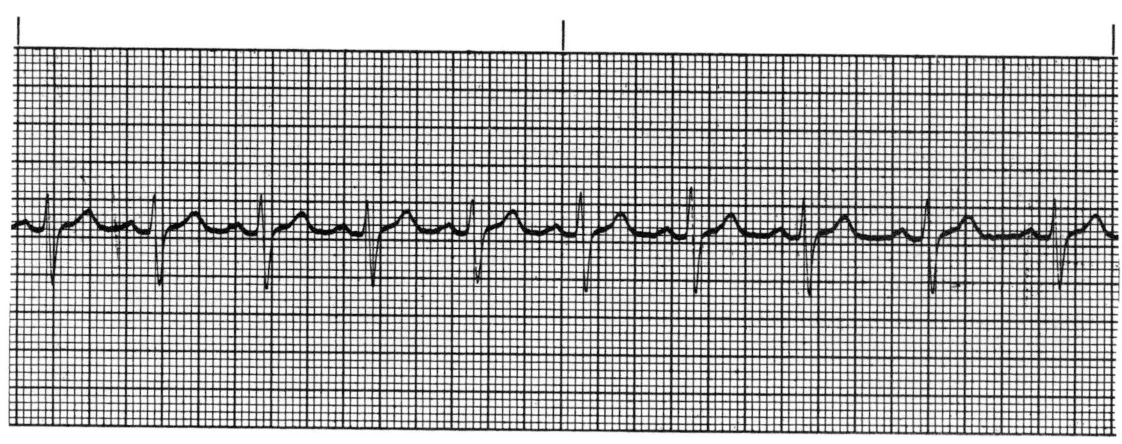

Practice Figure 9-137

Rate: ____________ Rhythm: ____________ P-R interval: ____________ QRS complex: ____________

Is there a P wave before every QRS complex? ____________

Is there a QRS complex after every P wave? ____________

Interpretation: ____________

____

Practice Figure 9-138

Rate: ____________ Rhythm: ____________ P-R interval: ____________ QRS complex: ____________

Is there a P wave before every QRS complex? ____________

Is there a QRS complex after every P wave? ____________

Interpretation: ____________

____

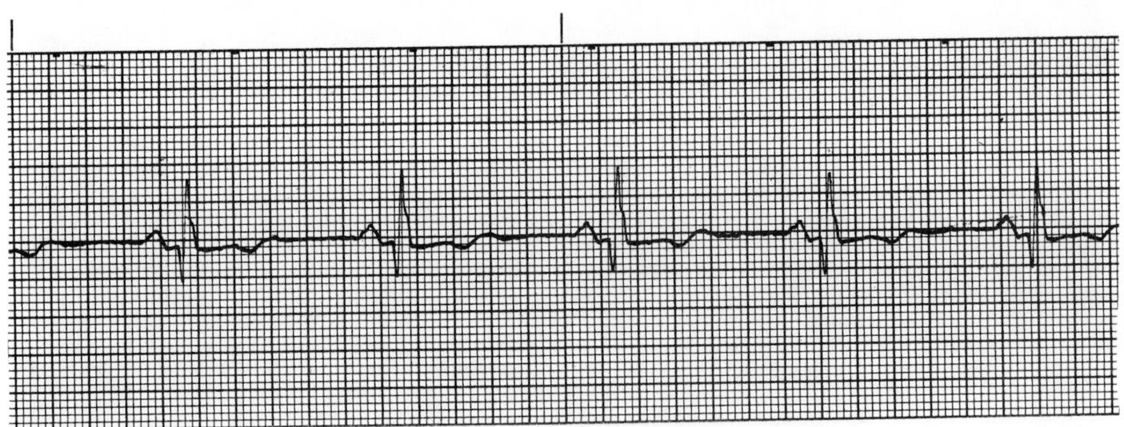

Practice Figure 9-139

Rate: ____________ Rhythm: ____________ P-R interval: ____________ QRS complex: ____________

Is there a P wave before every QRS complex? ____________

Is there a QRS complex after every P wave? ____________

Interpretation: ____________

____

Practice Figure 9-140

Rate: ____________ Rhythm: ____________ P-R interval: ____________ QRS complex: ____________

Is there a P wave before every QRS complex? ____________

Is there a QRS complex after every P wave? ____________

Interpretation: ____________

____

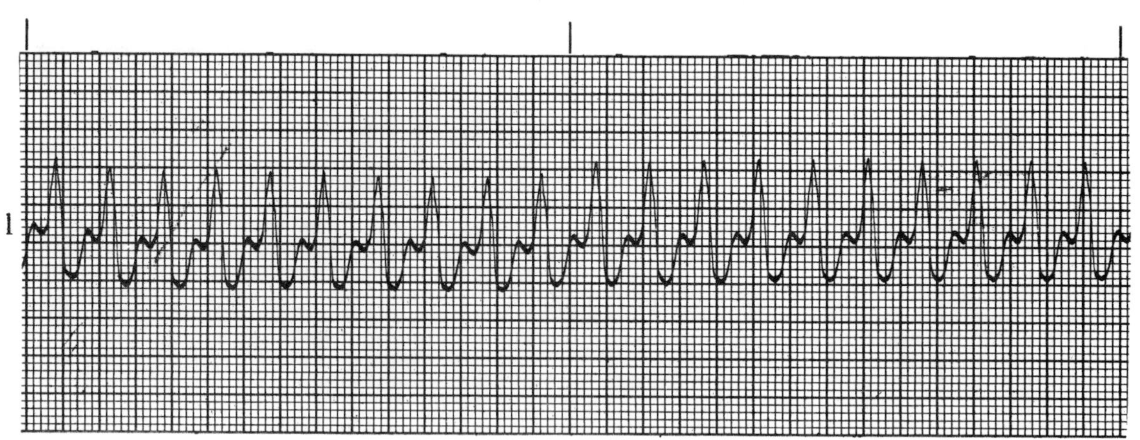

Practice Figure 9-141

Rate: ____________ Rhythm: ____________ P-R interval: ____________ QRS complex: ____________

Is there a P wave before every QRS complex? ____________

Is there a QRS complex after every P wave? ____________

Interpretation: ____________

____

Practice Figure 9-142

Rate: ____________ Rhythm: ____________ P-R interval: ____________ QRS complex: ____________

Is there a P wave before every QRS complex? ____________

Is there a QRS complex after every P wave? ____________

Interpretation: ____________

____

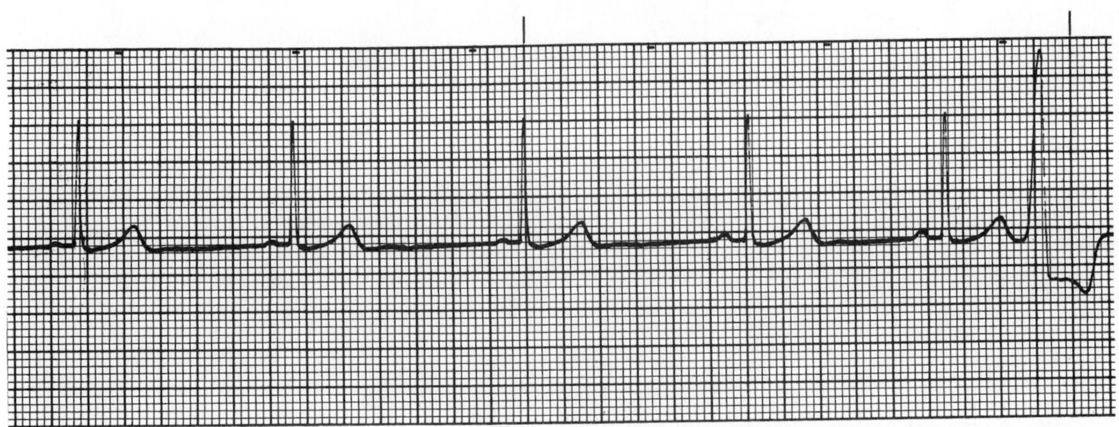

Practice Figure 9-143

Rate: ____________ Rhythm: ____________ P-R interval: ____________ QRS complex: ____________

Is there a P wave before every QRS complex? ____________

Is there a QRS complex after every P wave? ____________

Interpretation: ____________

____

Practice Figure 9-144

Rate: ____________ Rhythm: ____________ P-R interval: ____________ QRS complex: ____________

Is there a P wave before every QRS complex? ____________

Is there a QRS complex after every P wave? ____________

Interpretation: ____________

____

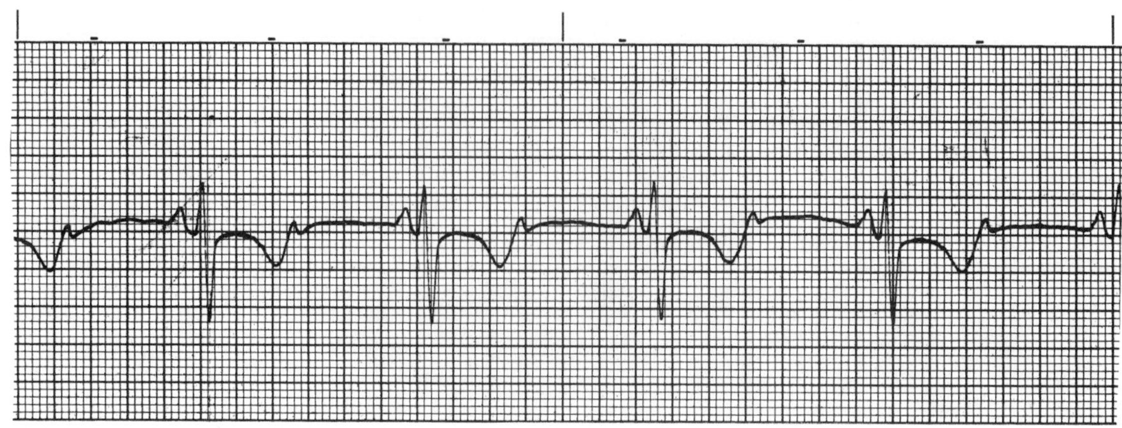

Practice Figure 9-145

Rate: ____________ Rhythm: ____________ P-R interval: ____________ QRS complex: ____________

Is there a P wave before every QRS complex? ____

Is there a QRS complex after every P wave? ____

Interpretation: ____

____

Practice Figure 9-146

Rate: ____________ Rhythm: ____________ P-R interval: ____________ QRS complex: ____________

Is there a P wave before every QRS complex? ____

Is there a QRS complex after every P wave? ____

Interpretation: ____

____

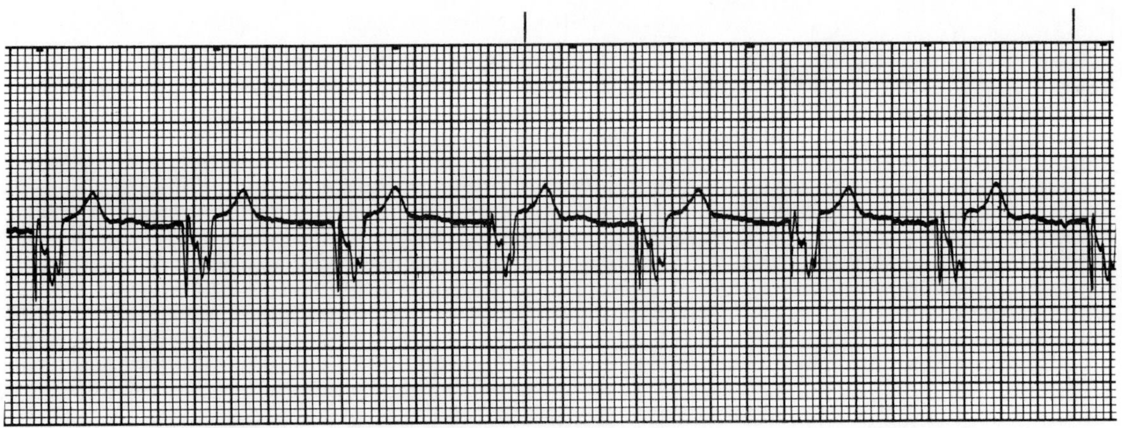

Practice Figure 9-147

Rate: ____________ Rhythm: ____________ P-R interval: ____________ QRS complex: ____________

Is there a P wave before every QRS complex? ____________

Is there a QRS complex after every P wave? ____________

Interpretation: ____________

____

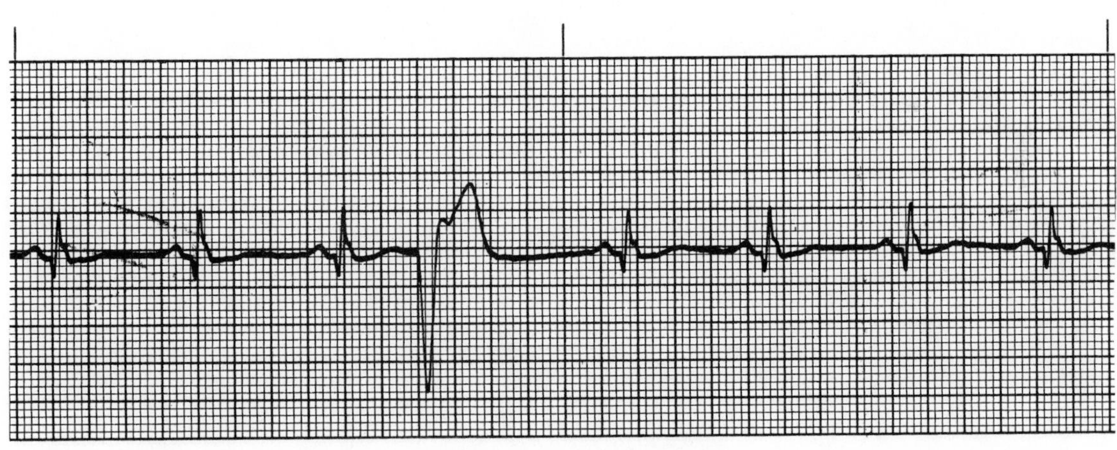

Practice Figure 9-148

Rate: ____________ Rhythm: ____________ P-R interval: ____________ QRS complex: ____________

Is there a P wave before every QRS complex? ____________

Is there a QRS complex after every P wave? ____________

Interpretation: ____________

____

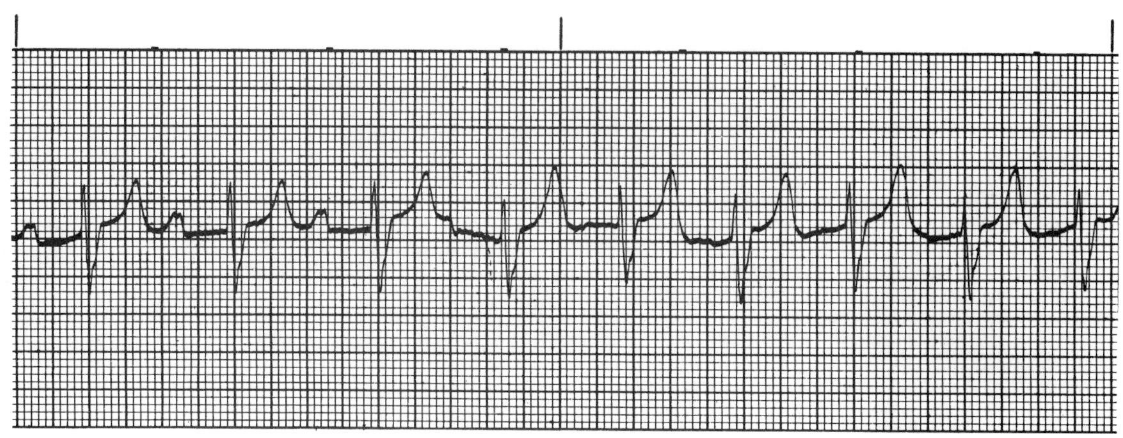

Practice Figure 9-149

Rate: ____________ Rhythm: ____________ P-R interval: ____________ QRS complex: ____________

Is there a P wave before every QRS complex? ____________

Is there a QRS complex after every P wave? ____________

Interpretation: ____________

____

Practice Figure 9-150

Rate: ____________ Rhythm: ____________ P-R interval: ____________ QRS complex: ____________

Is there a P wave before every QRS complex? ____________

Is there a QRS complex after every P wave? ____________

Interpretation: ____________

____

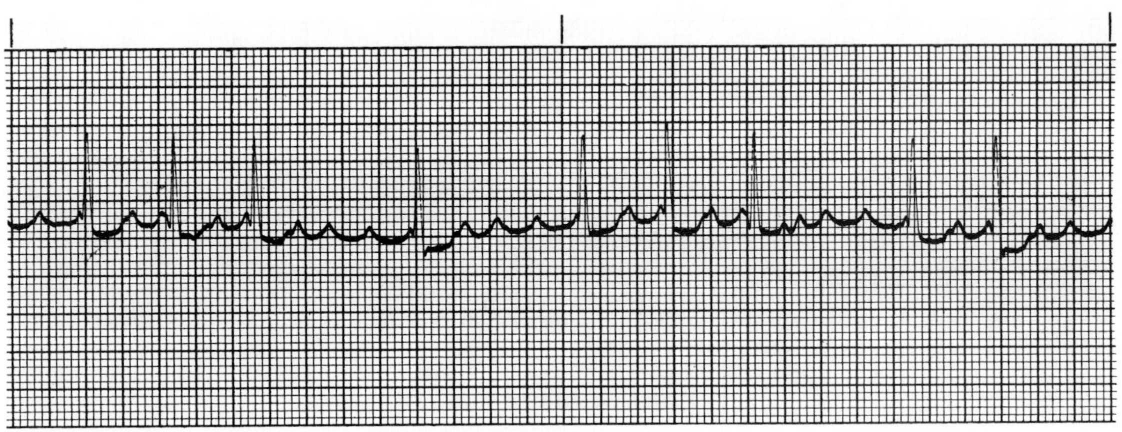

Practice Figure 9-151

Rate: ____________ Rhythm: ____________ P-R interval: ____________ QRS complex: ____________

Is there a P wave before every QRS complex? ____________

Is there a QRS complex after every P wave? ____________

Interpretation: ____________

____

Practice Figure 9-152

Rate: ____________ Rhythm: ____________ P-R interval: ____________ QRS complex: ____________

Is there a P wave before every QRS complex? ____________

Is there a QRS complex after every P wave? ____________

Interpretation: ____________

____

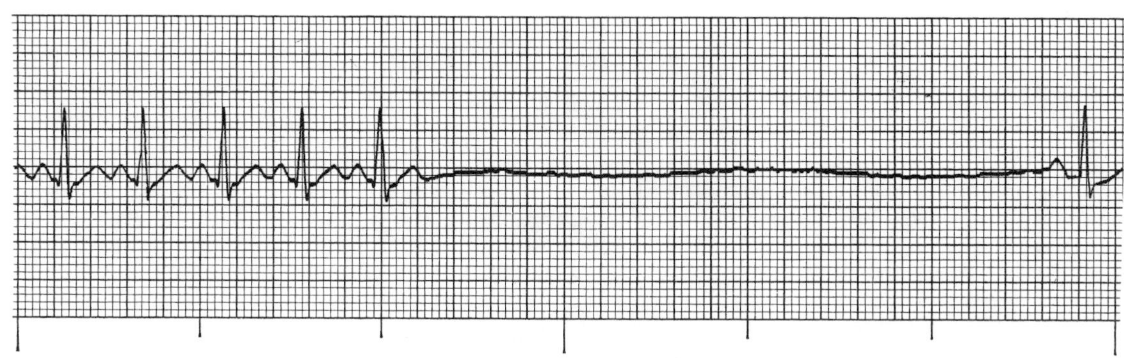

Practice Figure 9-153

Rate: ____________ Rhythm: ____________ P-R interval: ____________ QRS complex: ____________

Is there a P wave before every QRS complex? ____________

Is there a QRS complex after every P wave? ____________

Interpretation: ____________

____

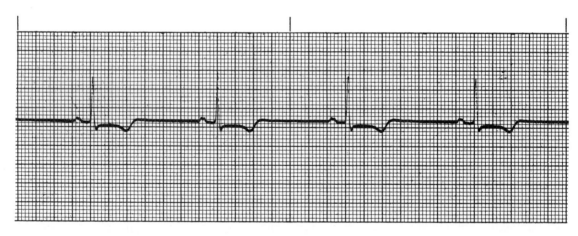

Practice Figure 9-154

Rate: ____________ Rhythm: ____________ P-R interval: ____________ QRS complex: ____________

Is there a P wave before every QRS complex? ____________

Is there a QRS complex after every P wave? ____________

Interpretation: ____________

____

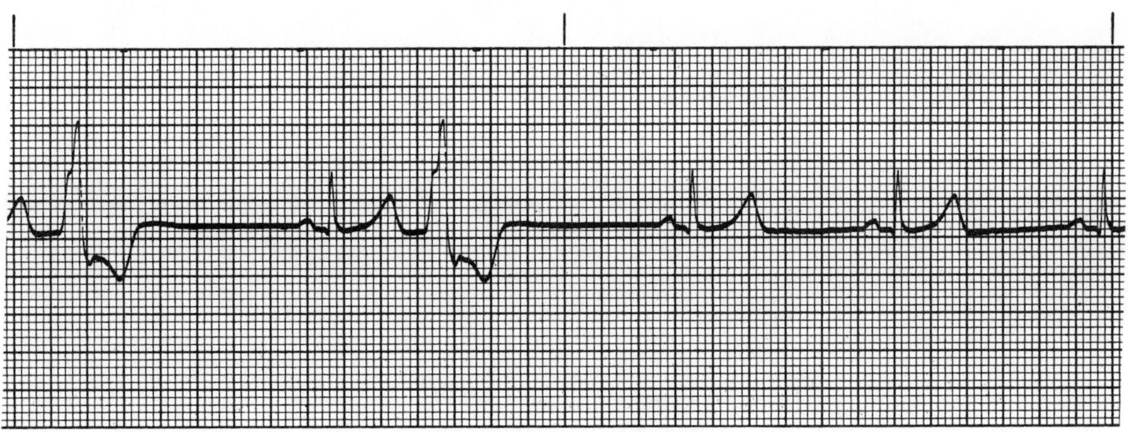

Practice Figure 9-155

Rate: ____________ Rhythm: ____________ P-R interval: ____________ QRS complex: ____________

Is there a P wave before every QRS complex? ________________________________

Is there a QRS complex after every P wave? ________________________________

Interpretation: ____

____

Practice Figure 9-156

Rate: ____________ Rhythm: ____________ P-R interval: ____________ QRS complex: ____________

Is there a P wave before every QRS complex? ________________________________

Is there a QRS complex after every P wave? ________________________________

Interpretation: ____

____

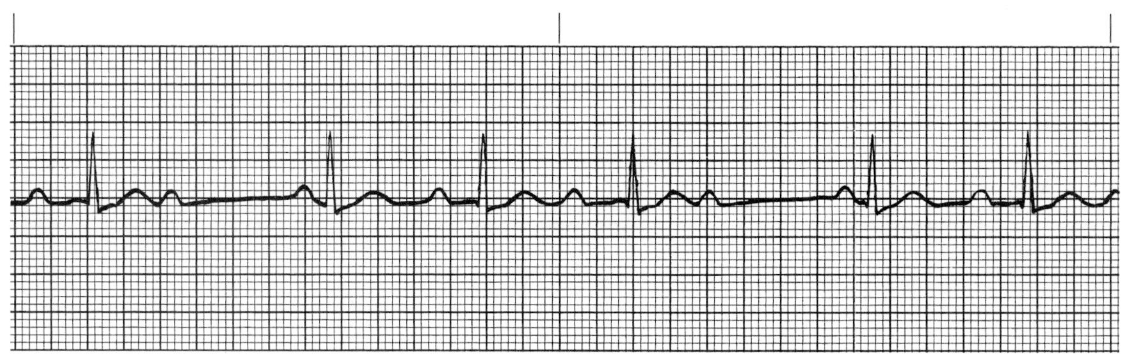

Practice Figure 9-157

Rate: ________ Rhythm: ________ P-R interval: ________ QRS complex: ________

Is there a P wave before every QRS complex? ________

Is there a QRS complex after every P wave? ________

Interpretation: ________

____

Practice Figure 9-158

Rate: ________ Rhythm: ________ P-R interval: ________ QRS complex: ________

Is there a P wave before every QRS complex? ________

Is there a QRS complex after every P wave? ________

Interpretation: ________

____

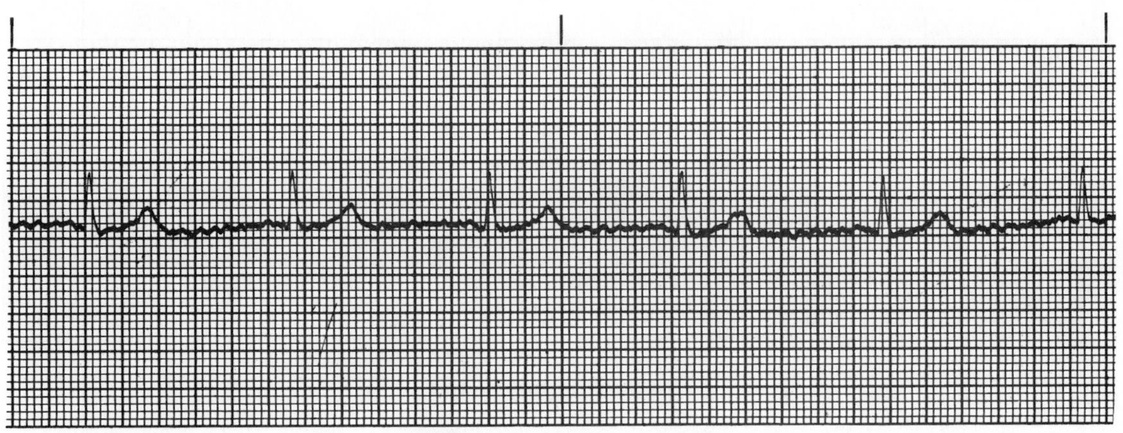

Practice Figure 9-159

Rate: ____________ Rhythm: ____________ P-R interval: ____________ QRS complex: ____________

Is there a P wave before every QRS complex? ____

Is there a QRS complex after every P wave? ____

Interpretation: ____

____

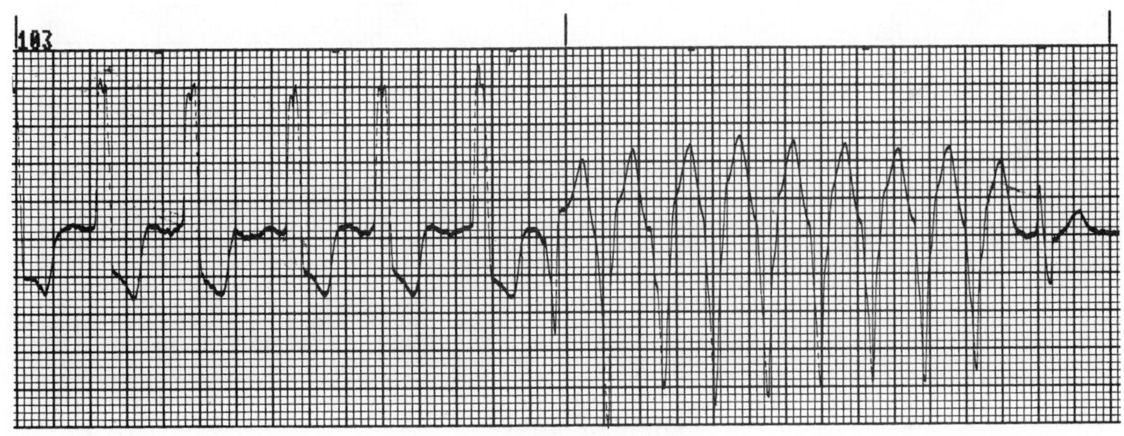

Practice Figure 9-160

Rate: ____________ Rhythm: ____________ P-R interval: ____________ QRS complex: ____________

Is there a P wave before every QRS complex? ____

Is there a QRS complex after every P wave? ____

Interpretation: ____

____

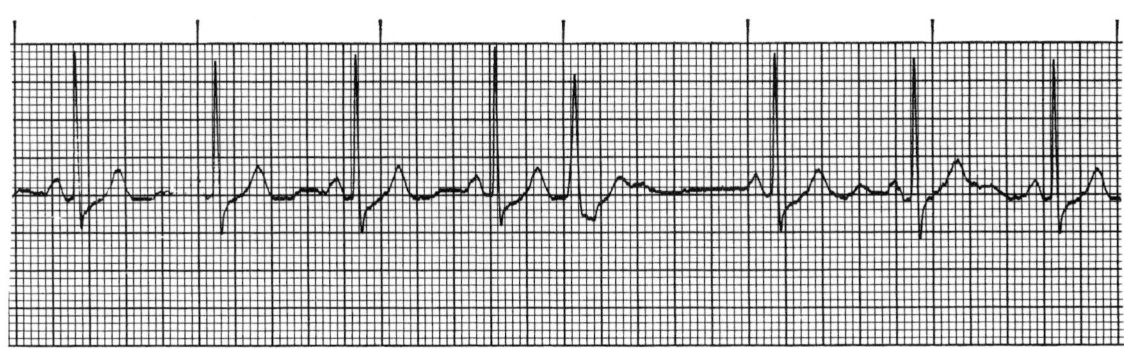

Practice Figure 9-161

Rate: ____________ Rhythm: ____________ P-R interval: ____________ QRS complex: ____________

Is there a P wave before every QRS complex? ____________

Is there a QRS complex after every P wave? ____________

Interpretation: ____________

Practice Figure 9-162

Rate: ____________ Rhythm: ____________ P-R interval: ____________ QRS complex: ____________

Is there a P wave before every QRS complex? ____________

Is there a QRS complex after every P wave? ____________

Interpretation: ____________

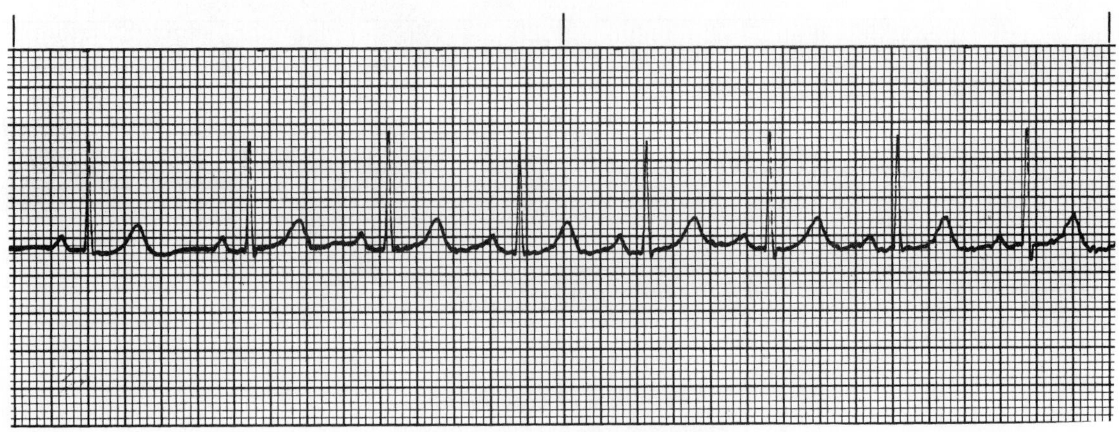

Practice Figure 9-163

Rate: ____________ Rhythm: ____________ P-R interval: ____________ QRS complex: ____________

Is there a P wave before every QRS complex? ____________

Is there a QRS complex after every P wave? ____________

Interpretation: ____________

____

Practice Figure 9-164

Rate: ____________ Rhythm: ____________ P-R interval: ____________ QRS complex: ____________

Is there a P wave before every QRS complex? ____________

Is there a QRS complex after every P wave? ____________

Interpretation: ____________

____

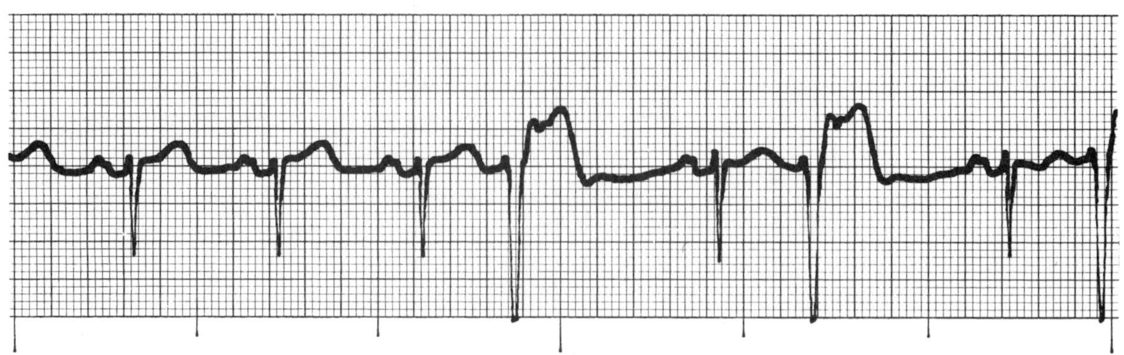

Practice Figure 9-165

Rate: ____________ Rhythm: ____________ P-R interval: ____________ QRS complex: ____________

Is there a P wave before every QRS complex? ____________

Is there a QRS complex after every P wave? ____________

Interpretation: ____________

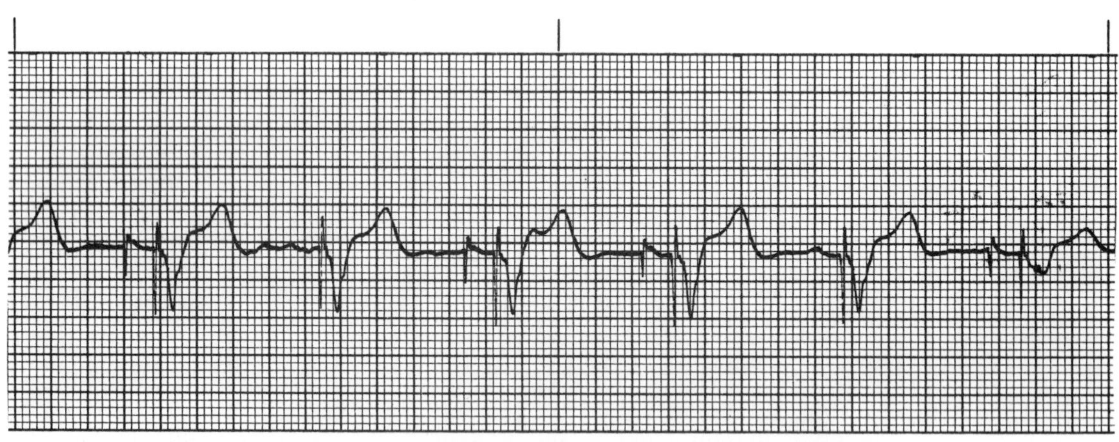

Practice Figure 9-166

Rate: ____________ Rhythm: ____________ P-R interval: ____________ QRS complex: ____________

Is there a P wave before every QRS complex? ____________

Is there a QRS complex after every P wave? ____________

Interpretation: ____________

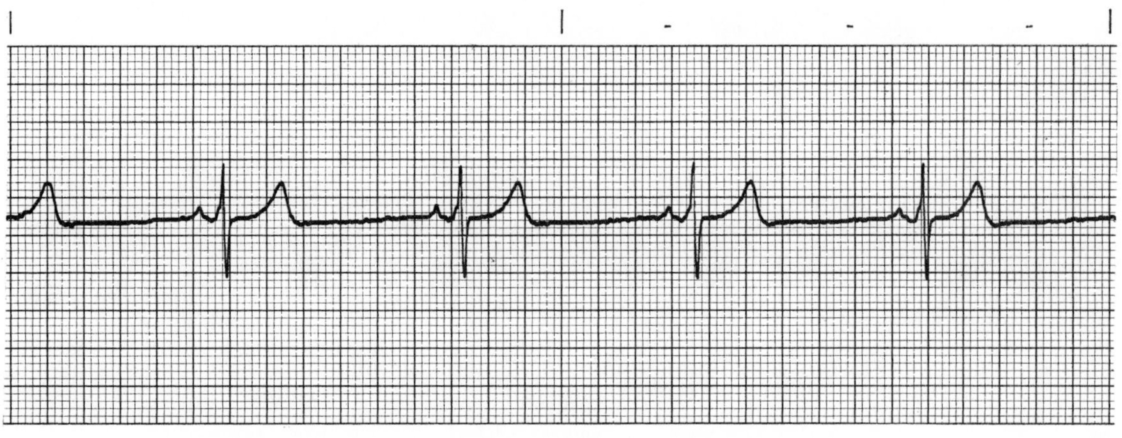

Practice Figure 9-167

Rate: __________ Rhythm: __________ P-R interval: __________ QRS complex: __________

Is there a P wave before every QRS complex? __________

Is there a QRS complex after every P wave? __________

Interpretation: __________

Practice Figure 9-168

Rate: __________ Rhythm: __________ P-R interval: __________ QRS complex: __________

Is there a P wave before every QRS complex? __________

Is there a QRS complex after every P wave? __________

Interpretation: __________

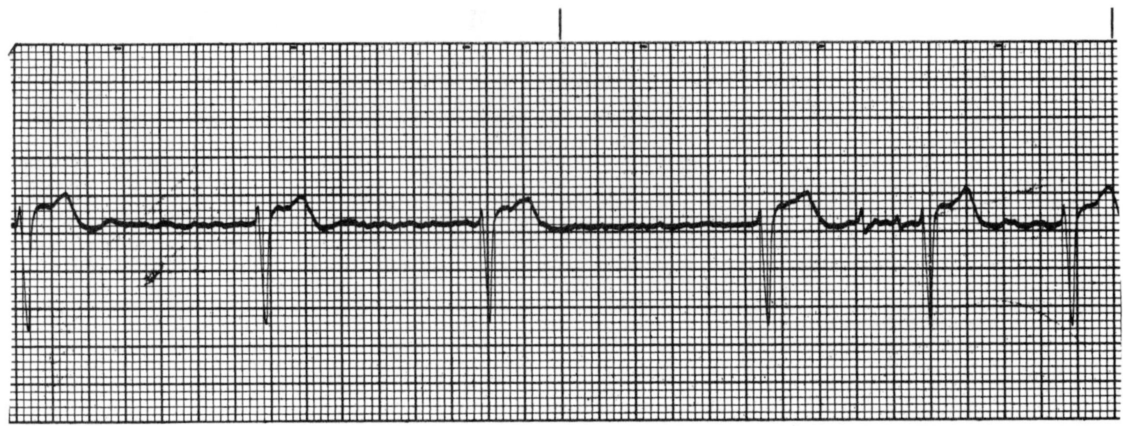

Practice Figure 9-169

Rate: ____________ Rhythm: ____________ P-R interval: ____________ QRS complex: ____________

Is there a P wave before every QRS complex? ____________

Is there a QRS complex after every P wave? ____________

Interpretation: ____________

Practice Figure 9-170

Rate: ____________ Rhythm: ____________ P-R interval: ____________ QRS complex: ____________

Is there a P wave before every QRS complex? ____________

Is there a QRS complex after every P wave? ____________

Interpretation: ____________

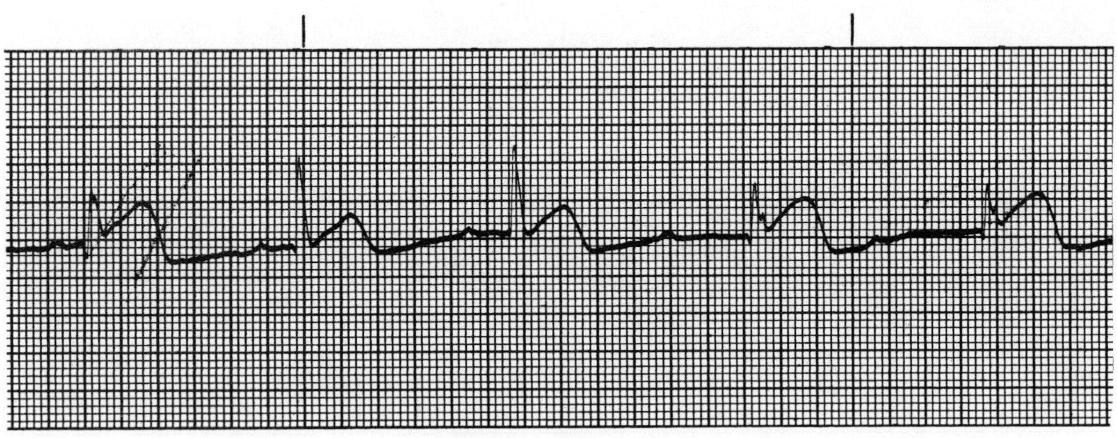

Practice Figure 9-171

Rate: ____________ Rhythm: ____________ P-R interval: ____________ QRS complex: ____________

Is there a P wave before every QRS complex? ____________

Is there a QRS complex after every P wave? ____________

Interpretation: ____________

____

Practice Figure 9-172

Rate: ____________ Rhythm: ____________ P-R interval: ____________ QRS complex: ____________

Is there a P wave before every QRS complex? ____________

Is there a QRS complex after every P wave? ____________

Interpretation: ____________

____

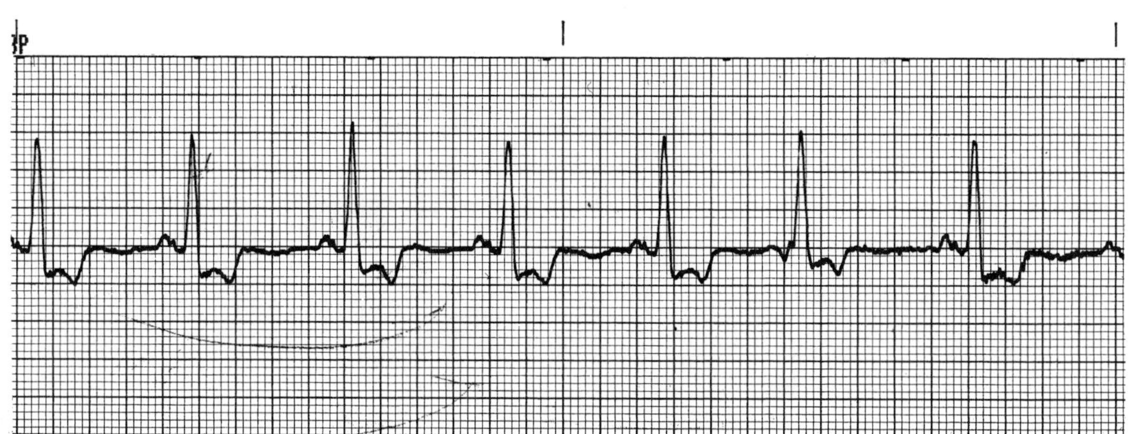

Practice Figure 9-173

Rate: ____________ Rhythm: ____________ P-R interval: ____________ QRS complex: ____________

Is there a P wave before every QRS complex? ____

Is there a QRS complex after every P wave? ____

Interpretation: ____

____

Practice Figure 9-174

Rate: ____________ Rhythm: ____________ P-R interval: ____________ QRS complex: ____________

Is there a P wave before every QRS complex? ____

Is there a QRS complex after every P wave? ____

Interpretation: ____

____

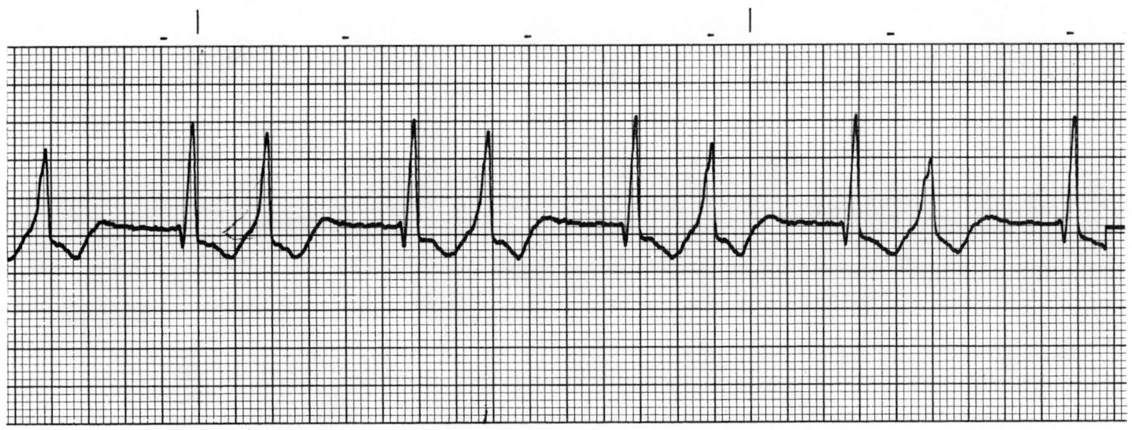

Practice Figure 9-175

Rate: ____________ Rhythm: ____________ P-R interval: ____________ QRS complex: ____________

Is there a P wave before every QRS complex? ______________________________

Is there a QRS complex after every P wave? ______________________________

Interpretation: ______________________________

____

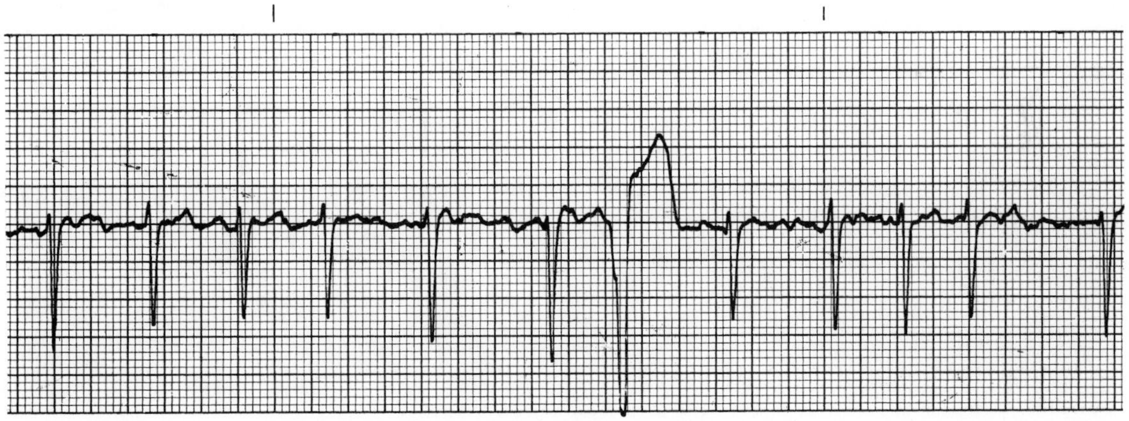

Practice Figure 9-176

Rate: ____________ Rhythm: ____________ P-R interval: ____________ QRS complex: ____________

Is there a P wave before every QRS complex? ______________________________

Is there a QRS complex after every P wave? ______________________________

Interpretation: ______________________________

____

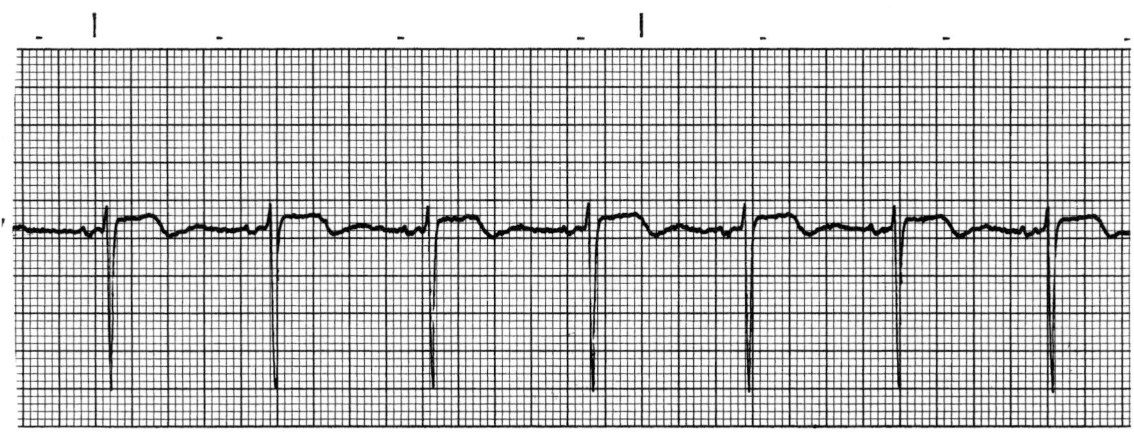

Practice Figure 9-177

Rate: ____________ Rhythm: ____________ P-R interval: ____________ QRS complex: ____________

Is there a P wave before every QRS complex? ____

Is there a QRS complex after every P wave? ____

Interpretation: ____

____

Practice Figure 9-178

Rate: ____________ Rhythm: ____________ P-R interval: ____________ QRS complex: ____________

Is there a P wave before every QRS complex? ____

Is there a QRS complex after every P wave? ____

Interpretation: ____

____

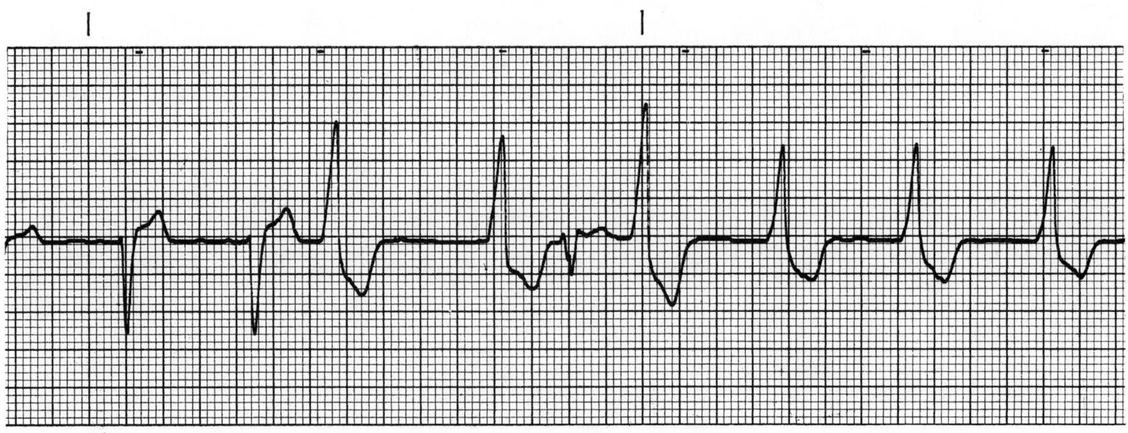

Practice Figure 9-179

Rate: ____________ Rhythm: ____________ P-R interval: ____________ QRS complex: ____________

Is there a P wave before every QRS complex? ____________

Is there a QRS complex after every P wave? ____________

Interpretation: ____________

____

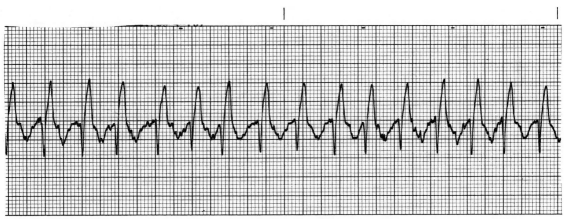

Practice Figure 9-180

Rate: ____________ Rhythm: ____________ P-R interval: ____________ QRS complex: ____________

Is there a P wave before every QRS complex? ____________

Is there a QRS complex after every P wave? ____________

Interpretation: ____________

____

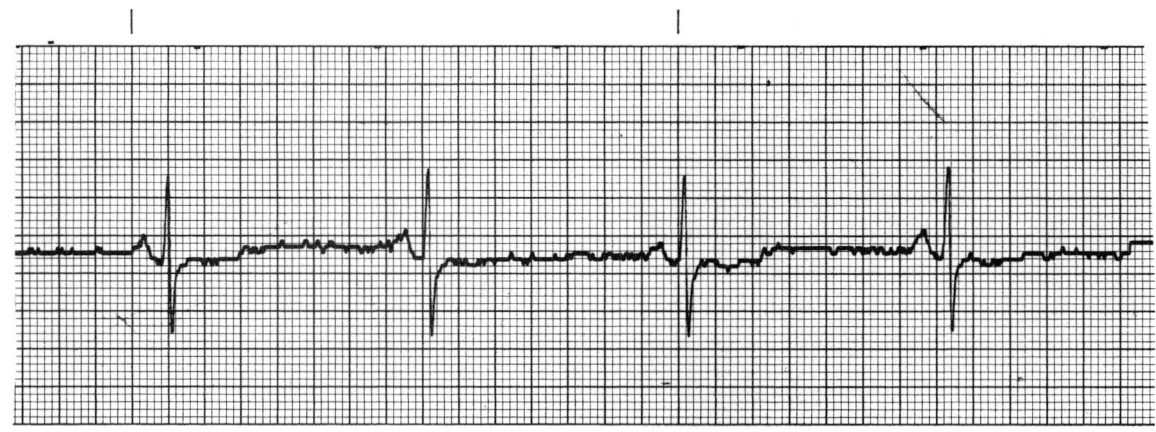

Practice Figure 9-181

Rate: ____________ Rhythm: ____________ P-R interval: ____________ QRS complex: ____________

Is there a P wave before every QRS complex? ____________

Is there a QRS complex after every P wave? ____________

Interpretation: ____________

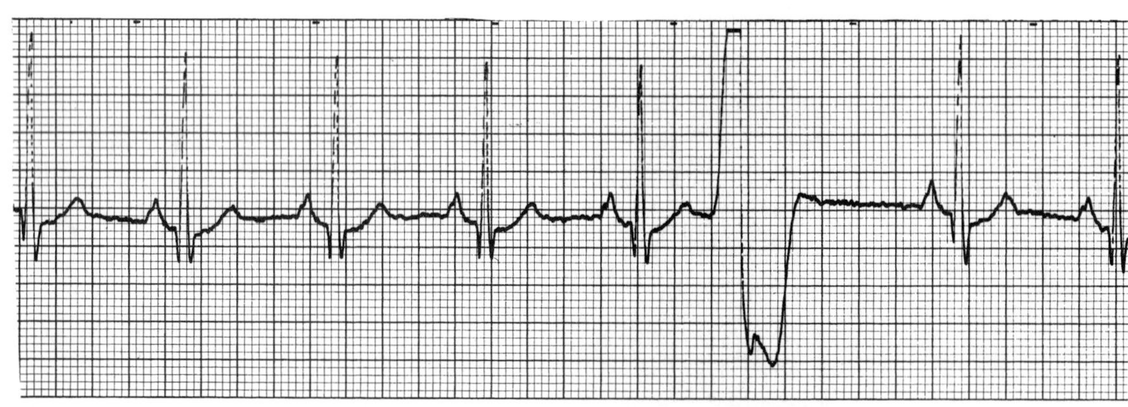

Practice Figure 9-182

Rate: ____________ Rhythm: ____________ P-R interval: ____________ QRS complex: ____________

Is there a P wave before every QRS complex? ____________

Is there a QRS complex after every P wave? ____________

Interpretation: ____________

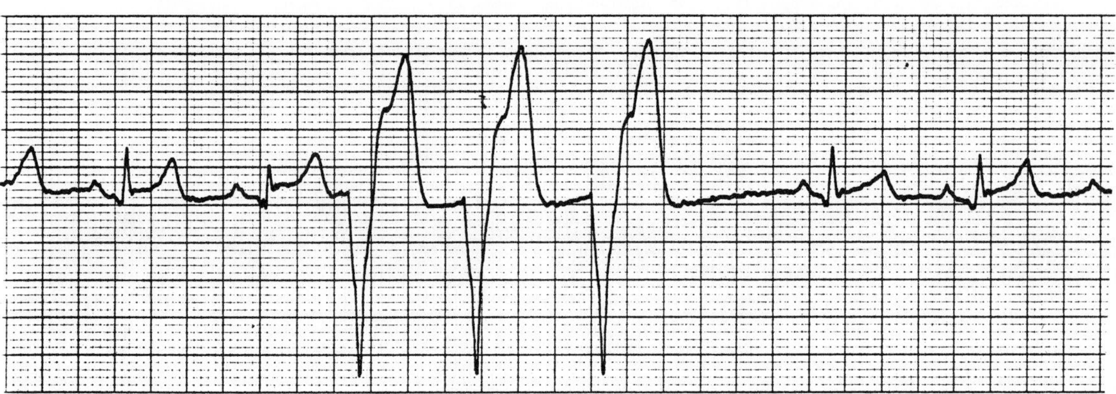

Practice Figure 9-183

Rate: ____________ Rhythm: ____________ P-R interval: ____________ QRS complex: ____________

Is there a P wave before every QRS complex? ____________

Is there a QRS complex after every P wave? ____________

Interpretation: ____________

____

Practice Figure 9-184

Rate: ____________ Rhythm: ____________ P-R interval: ____________ QRS complex: ____________

Is there a P wave before every QRS complex? ____________

Is there a QRS complex after every P wave? ____________

Interpretation: ____________

____

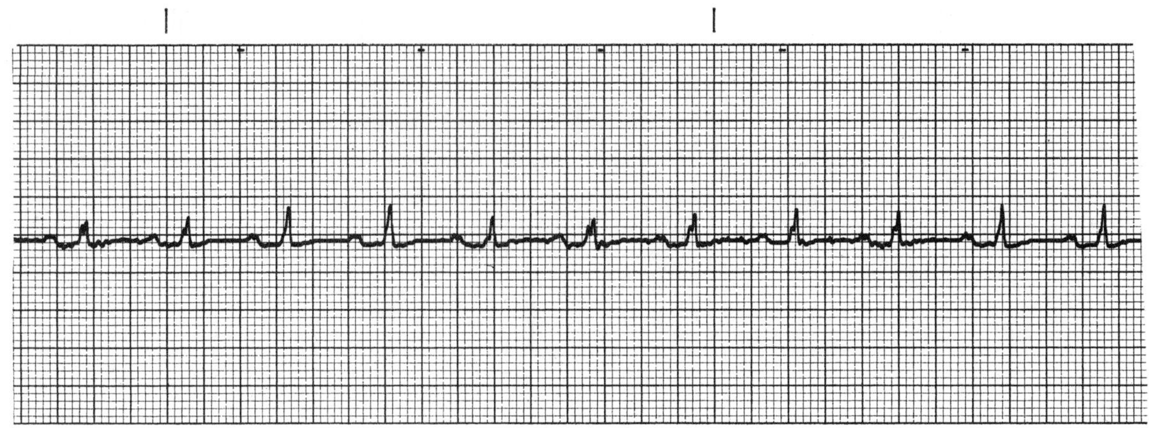

Practice Figure 9-185

Rate: ____________ Rhythm: ____________ P-R interval: ____________ QRS complex: ____________

Is there a P wave before every QRS complex? ____________

Is there a QRS complex after every P wave? ____________

Interpretation: ____________

Practice Figure 9-186

Rate: ____________ Rhythm: ____________ P-R interval: ____________ QRS complex: ____________

Is there a P wave before every QRS complex? ____________

Is there a QRS complex after every P wave? ____________

Interpretation: ____________

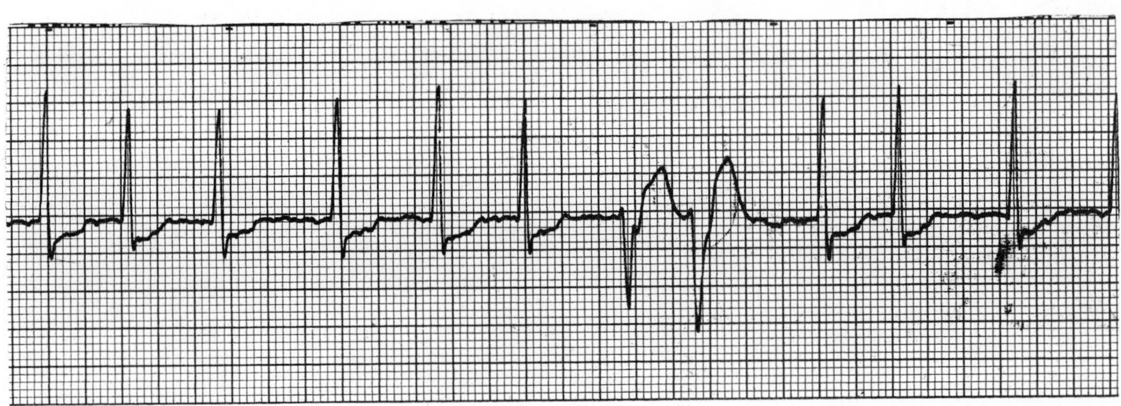

Practice Figure 9-187

Rate: ________ Rhythm: ________ P-R interval: ________ QRS complex: ________

Is there a P wave before every QRS complex? ________

Is there a QRS complex after every P wave? ________

Interpretation: ________

Practice Figure 9-188

Rate: ________ Rhythm: ________ P-R interval: ________ QRS complex: ________

Is there a P wave before every QRS complex? ________

Is there a QRS complex after every P wave? ________

Interpretation: ________

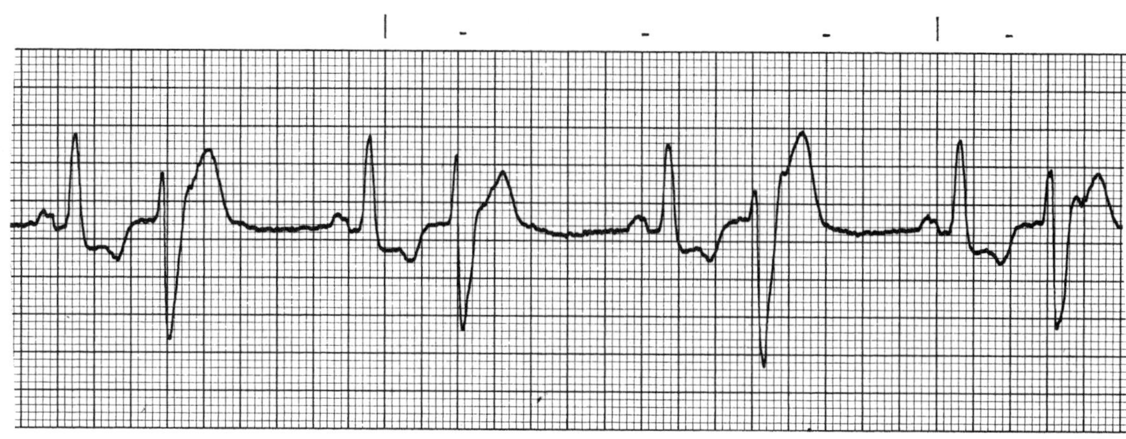

Practice Figure 9-189

Rate: ____________ Rhythm: ____________ P-R interval: ____________ QRS complex: ____________

Is there a P wave before every QRS complex? ____________

Is there a QRS complex after every P wave? ____________

Interpretation: ____________

Practice Figure 9-190

Rate: ____________ Rhythm: ____________ P-R interval: ____________ QRS complex: ____________

Is there a P wave before every QRS complex? ____________

Is there a QRS complex after every P wave? ____________

Interpretation: ____________

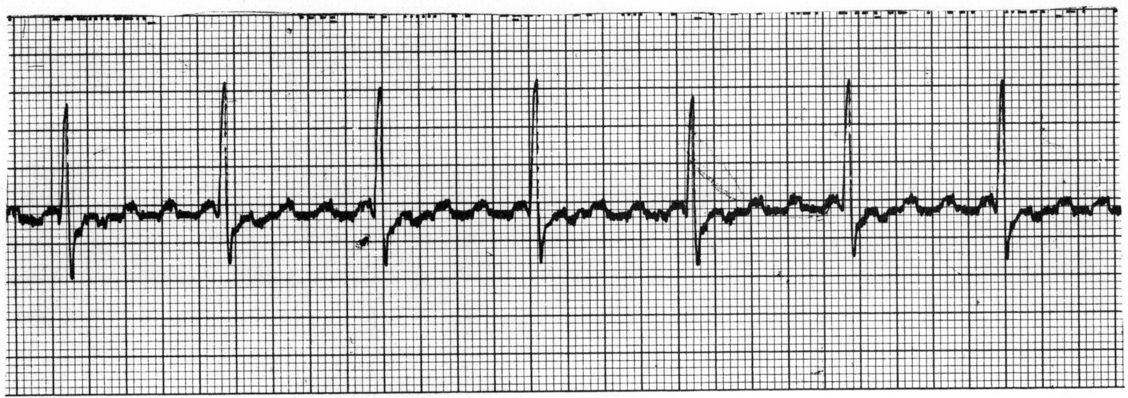

Practice Figure 9-191

Rate: ___________ Rhythm: ___________ P-R interval: ___________ QRS complex: ___________

Is there a P wave before every QRS complex? ___________

Is there a QRS complex after every P wave? ___________

Interpretation: ___________

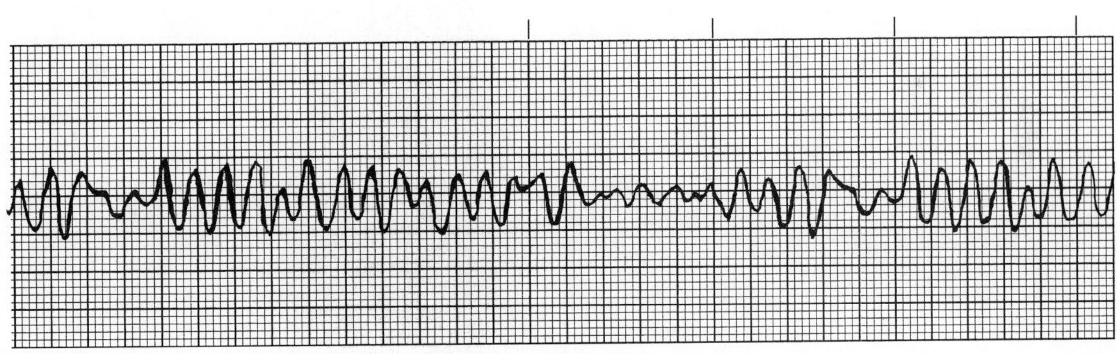

Practice Figure 9-192

Rate: ___________ Rhythm: ___________ P-R interval: ___________ QRS complex: ___________

Is there a P wave before every QRS complex? ___________

Is there a QRS complex after every P wave? ___________

Interpretation: ___________

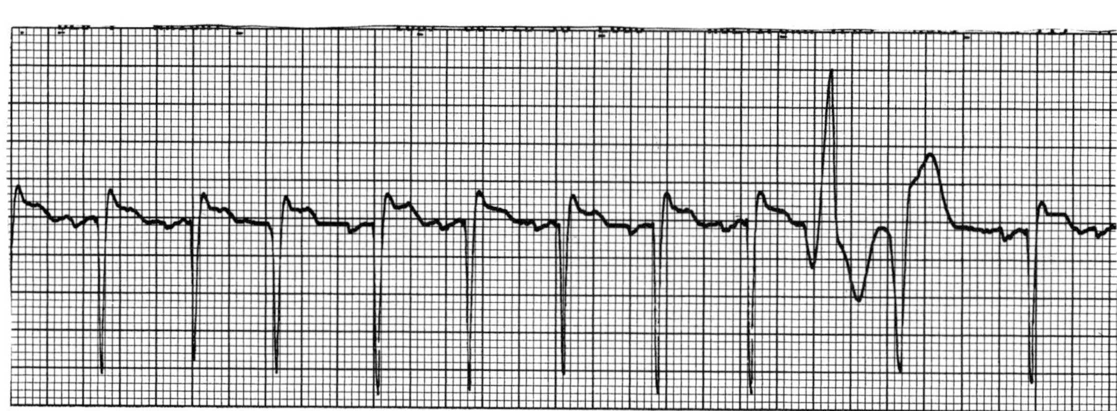

Practice Figure 9-193

Rate: ____________ Rhythm: ____________ P-R interval: ____________ QRS complex: ____________

Is there a P wave before every QRS complex? ____________

Is there a QRS complex after every P wave? ____________

Interpretation: ____________

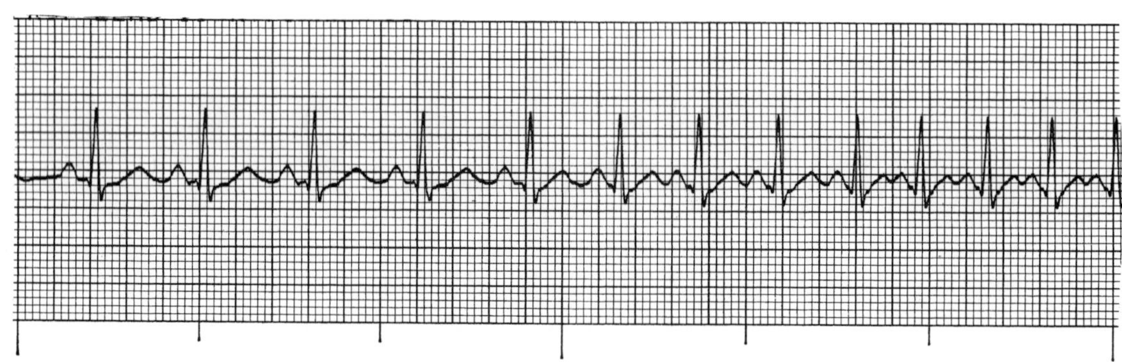

Practice Figure 9-194

Rate: ____________ Rhythm: ____________ P-R interval: ____________ QRS complex: ____________

Is there a P wave before every QRS complex? ____________

Is there a QRS complex after every P wave? ____________

Interpretation: ____________

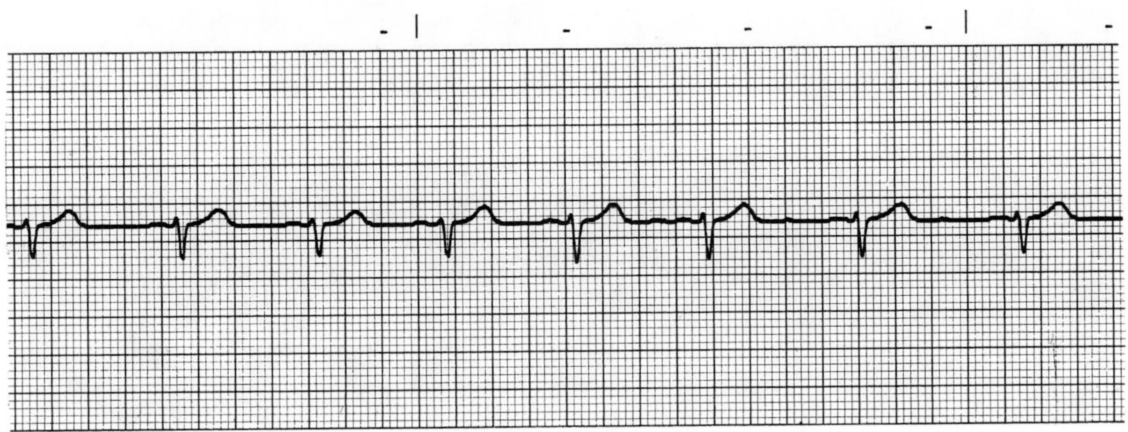

Practice Figure 9-195

Rate: ____________ Rhythm: ____________ P-R interval: ____________ QRS complex: ____________

Is there a P wave before every QRS complex? ________________________________

Is there a QRS complex after every P wave? ________________________________

Interpretation: ____

____

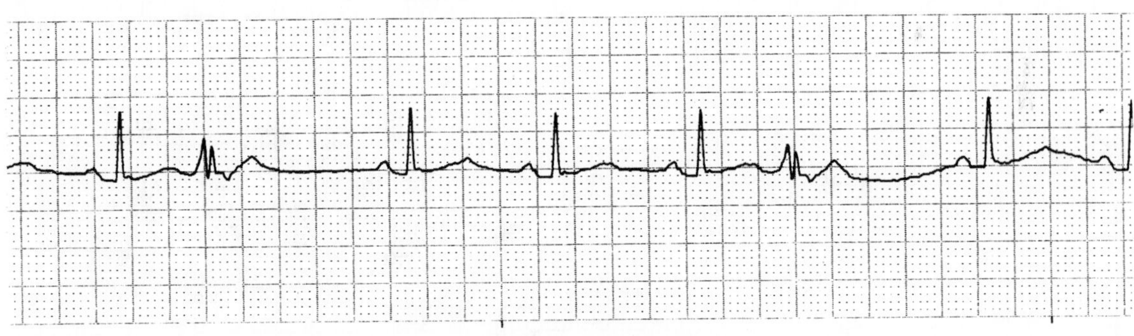

Practice Figure 9-196

Rate: ____________ Rhythm: ____________ P-R interval: ____________ QRS complex: ____________

Is there a P wave before every QRS complex? ________________________________

Is there a QRS complex after every P wave? ________________________________

Interpretation: ____

____

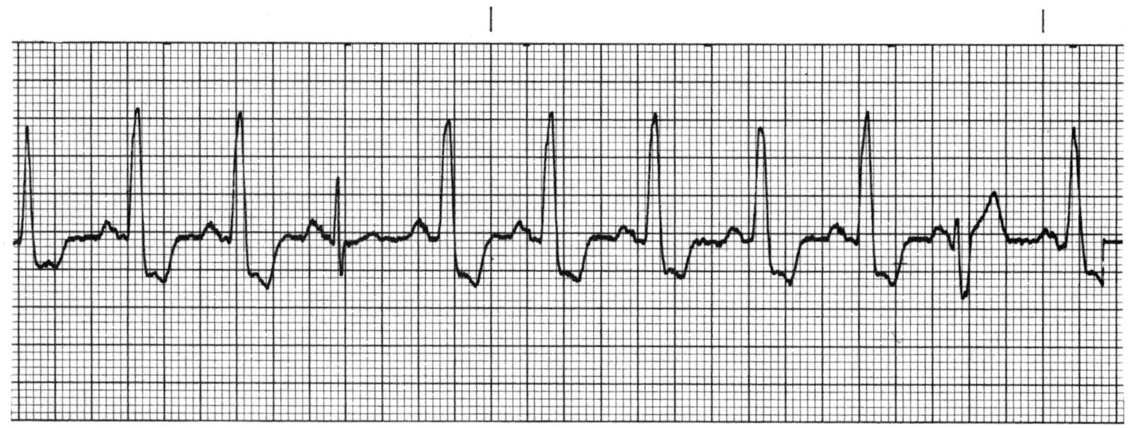

Practice Figure 9-197

Rate: ____________ Rhythm: ____________ P-R interval: ____________ QRS complex: ____________

Is there a P wave before every QRS complex? ____________

Is there a QRS complex after every P wave? ____________

Interpretation: ____________

____

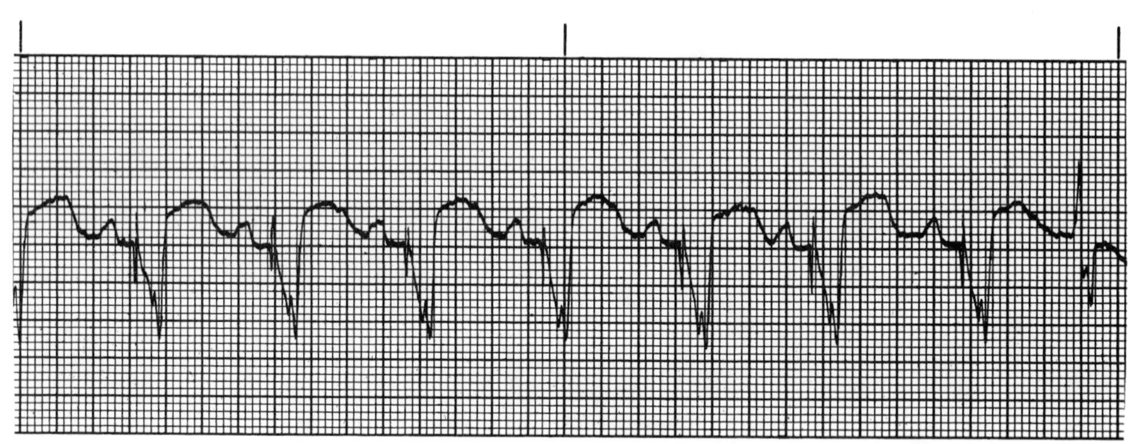

Practice Figure 9-198

Rate: ____________ Rhythm: ____________ P-R interval: ____________ QRS complex: ____________

Is there a P wave before every QRS complex? ____________

Is there a QRS complex after every P wave? ____________

Interpretation: ____________

____

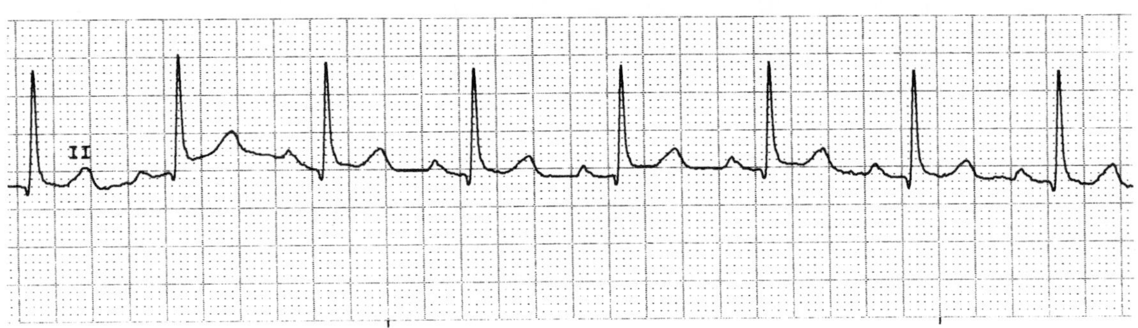

Practice Figure 9-199

Rate: ____________ Rhythm: ____________ P-R interval: ____________ QRS complex: ____________

Is there a P wave before every QRS complex? ____________

Is there a QRS complex after every P wave? ____________

Interpretation: ____________

____

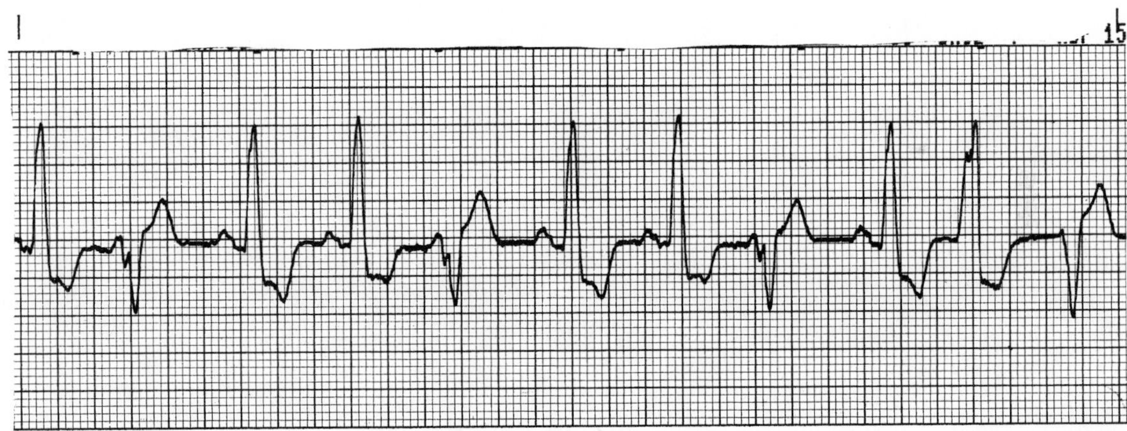

Practice Figure 9-200

Rate: ____________ Rhythm: ____________ P-R interval: ____________ QRS complex: ____________

Is there a P wave before every QRS complex? ____________

Is there a QRS complex after every P wave? ____________

Interpretation: ____________

____

10

Case Scenarios

CASE 1

Scenario: (Actual EMS Call)

A 68-year-old male comes into the emergency department, complaining of feeling light-headed and dizzy and having slight chest pressure. He had an episode of syncope lasting 30 to 60 seconds. His medical history includes hypertension, anemia, and COPD. He smoked two packs of cigarettes per day for the past 50 years. He also has consumed a considerable amount of coffee over the past few months because of stress in his home life. Vital signs are BP, 112/60; P, 80 and irregular; and R, 20. He is alert, oriented ×4, and his skin is pink, warm, and dry. Lung sounds are decreased but clear. On the monitor you see the following rhythm:

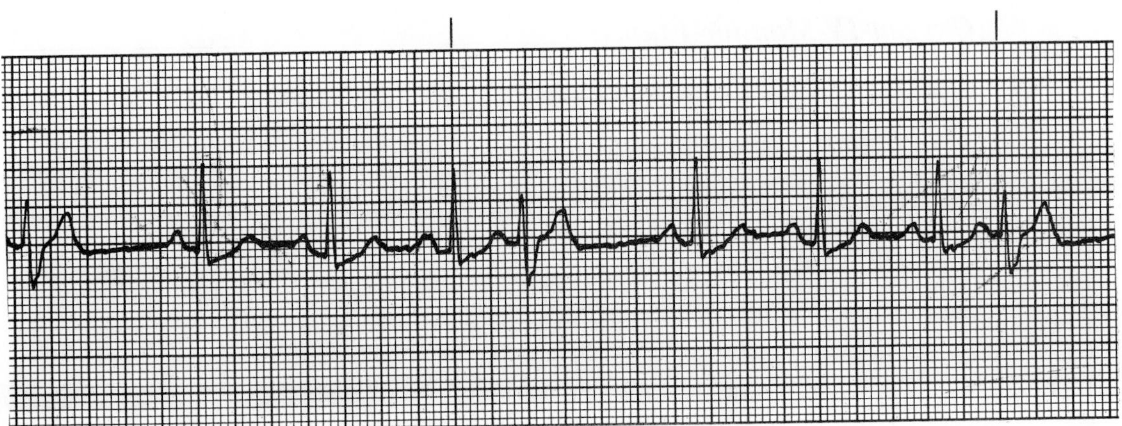

Identify the Rhythm

What is the rate? ____________ What is the rhythm (regular or irregular)? ____________

Is there a P wave before every QRS complex? ____________ Is there a QRS complex after every P wave? ____________

What is the P-R interval? ____________ QRS complex duration? ____________

Interpretation:

____

____

Case 1 Self-Test

In the spaces below give your treatment for the Primary Survey and Secondary Survey, plus the continued care under Oxygen-IV-Monitor-Fluids and Vital Signs. How would you care for this patient, and what orders would you expect from the physician? At the bottom list your potential diagnosis or impression of the patient's problem.

Primary Survey	*Secondary Survey*
A.	A.
B.	B.
C.	C.
D.	D.

Oxygen-IV-Monitor-Fluids: ____

____

Vital Signs: ____

____

Your Impression: ____

____

CASE 2

Scenario (Actual EMS Call)

You are called to the local gas station for a patient with "abdominal pain." When you arrive, you find a 38-year-old female complaining of lower abdominal pain. She tells you it began early this morning. Also, she says she had some chest pain yesterday but awoke this morning to find the pain had moved to her lower abdomen, which has become worse over the last hour. There is nothing in her medical history. Vital signs are BP, 110/72; P, 115 and regular; R, 20; and an Sao_2 of 96%. She is alert and oriented ×4. Her skin is pink, warm, and dry. Lung sounds are clear. When she is connected to the monitor because of the chest pain yesterday, you note the following rhythm:

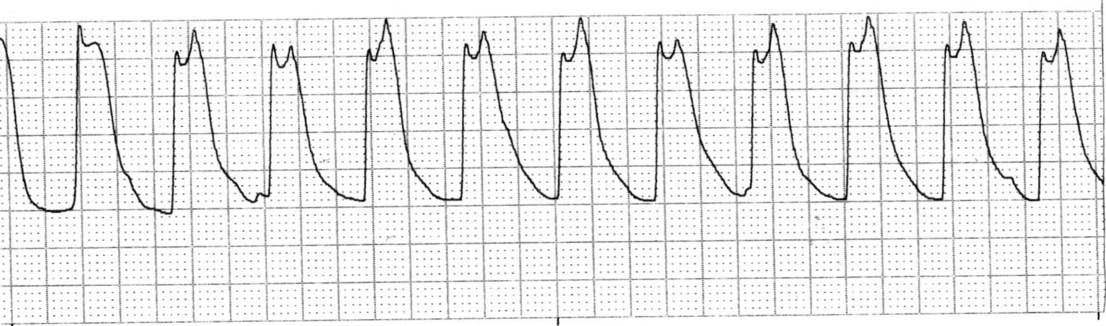

Identify the Rhythm

What is the rate? ____________ What is the rhythm (regular or irregular)? ____________

Is there a P wave before every QRS complex? ____________ Is there a QRS complex after every P wave? ____________

What is the P-R interval? ____________ QRS complex duration? ____________

Interpretation:

____

____

Case 2 Self-Test

In the spaces below give your treatment for the Primary Survey and Secondary Survey, plus the continued care under Oxygen-IV-Monitor-Fluids and Vital Signs. How would you care for this patient and what orders would you expect from the physician? At the bottom list your potential diagnosis or impression of the patient's problem.

Primary Survey

A.

B.

C.

D.

Secondary Survey

A.

B.

C.

D.

Oxygen-IV-Monitor-Fluids: ____

____

Vital Signs: ____

____

Your Impression: ____

____

CASE 3

Scenario

A 42-year-old female has had nausea, vomiting, fever, and a headache for the past 3 days. She appears very weak and pale. Her medical history includes diabetes mellitus and arthritis. Her medications include Glucotrol and ibuprofen. Fingerstick with a glucometer resulted in a blood glucose level of 108. Vital signs are BP, 110/56; P, 176 and regular; and R, 22. She is alert and oriented ×4. Her skin is pale, cool, and moist. Lung sounds are clear. You see the following on the monitor:

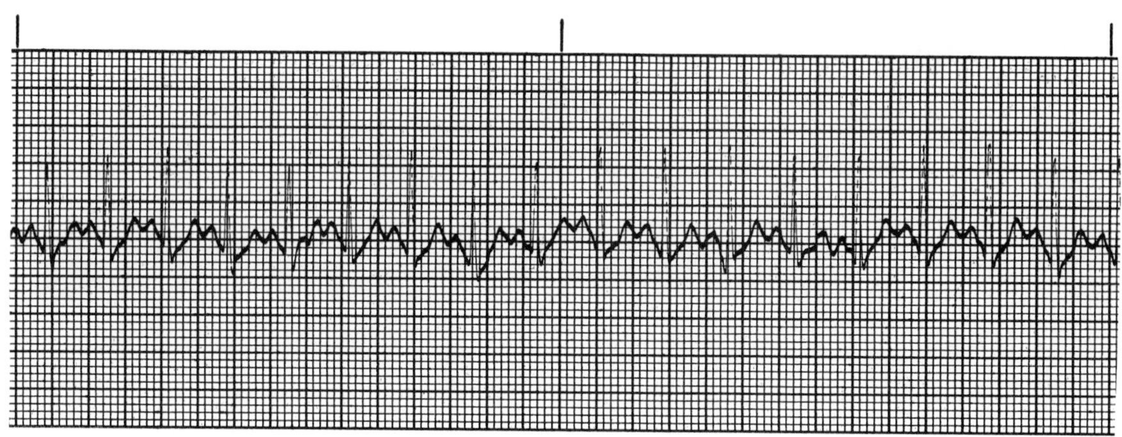

Identify the Rhythm

What is the rate? ____________ What is the rhythm (regular or irregular)? ____________

Is there a P wave before every QRS complex? ____________ Is there a QRS complex after every P wave? ____________

What is the P-R interval? ____________ QRS complex duration? ____________

Interpretation:

____

____

Case 3 Self-Test

In the spaces below give your treatment for the Primary Survey and Secondary Survey, plus the continued care under Oxygen-IV-Monitor-Fluids and Vital Signs. How would you care for this patient, and what orders would you expect from the physician? At the bottom list your potential diagnosis or impression of the patient's problem.

Primary Survey

A.

B.

C.

D.

Secondary Survey

A.

B.

C.

D.

Oxygen-IV-Monitor-Fluids: ______________________________

____

Vital Signs: ______________________________

____

Your Impression: ______________________________

____

CASE 4

Scenario

A 67-year-old male presents with confusion, nausea, and abdominal cramps, and appears apathetic. He tells you he has been feeling weak and dizzy for the past 3 to 5 days, but today his wife says he is very confused, which is not normal for him. He denies any chest pain and shortness of breath. He has a history of an MI 4 years ago and also has CHF, COPD, and high blood pressure. His medications include propranolol, furosemide, K-lor, and a Proventil inhaler. Vital signs are BP, 100/48; P, 45 beats per minute and regular; and R, 20. He is alert but oriented only to person and place. His skin is pink, cool, and dry, and his lung sounds are clear. You see the following on the monitor:

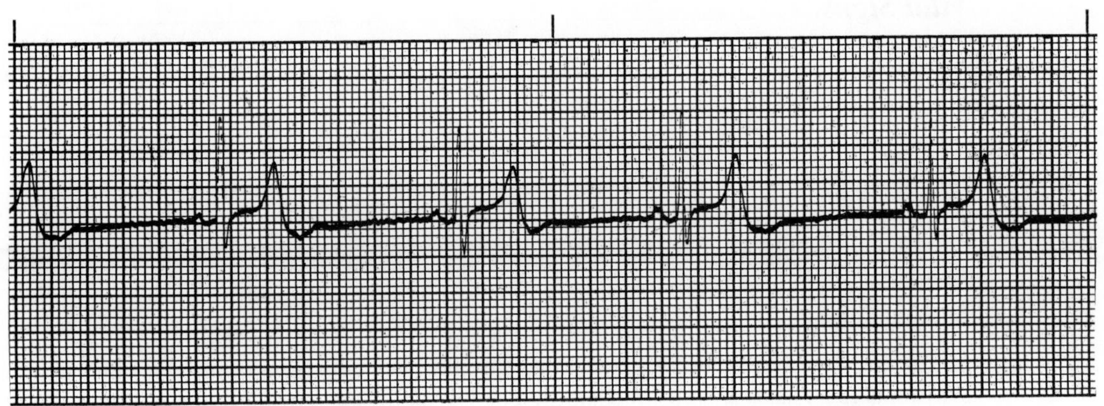

Identify the Rhythm

What is the rate? ____________ What is the rhythm (regular or irregular)? ____________

Is there a P wave before every QRS complex? ____________ Is there a QRS complex after every P wave? ____________

What is the P-R interval? ______________ QRS complex duration? ______________

Interpretation:

____

____

Case 4 Self-Test

In the spaces below give your treatment for the Primary Survey and Secondary Survey, plus the continued care under Oxygen-IV-Monitor-Fluids and Vital Signs. How would you care for this patient, and what orders would you expect from the physician? At the bottom list your potential diagnosis or impression of the patient's problem.

Primary Survey

A.

B.

C.

D.

Secondary Survey

A.

B.

C.

D.

Oxygen-IV-Monitor-Fluids: ______________________________

____

Vital Signs: ______________________________________

____

Your Impression: __________________________________

____

CASE 5

Scenario

You have a 71-year-old male who comes into the emergency department with complaints of flulike symptoms (e.g., nausea, chills, feeling tired and weak off and on) for the past 2 days. He also complains of slight chest pressure but believes this is due to a cold he has had for the past week. He denies any cough, and his lungs have decreased breath sounds but are clear. The patient is alert and oriented to person and place. His skin is pale, cool, and clammy with slight lip cyanosis noted. Vital signs are BP, 92/60; P, 46 to 50 and weak but regular; and R, 24. You see the following on the monitor:

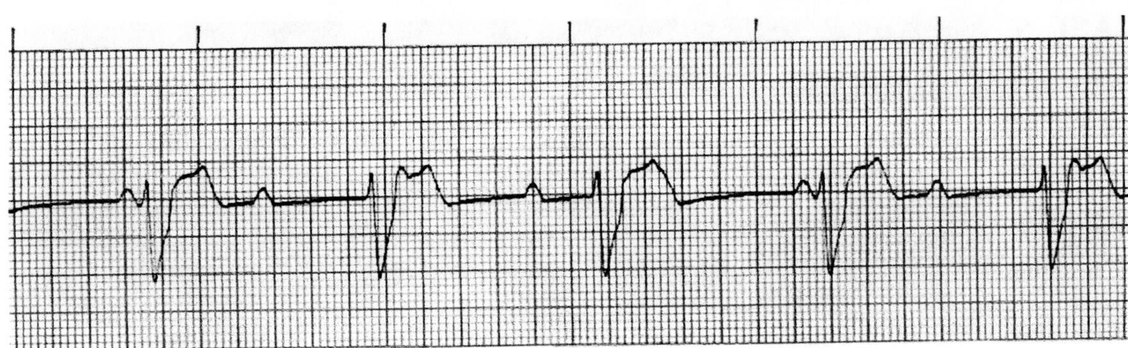

Identify the Rhythm

What is the rate? ____________ What is the rhythm (regular or irregular)? ____________

Is there a P wave before every QRS complex? ____________ Is there a QRS complex after every P wave? ____________

What is the P-R interval? ____________ QRS complex duration? ____________

Interpretation:

____

____

Case 5 Self-Test

In the spaces below give your treatment for the Primary Survey and Secondary Survey, plus the continued care under Oxygen-IV-Monitor-Fluids and Vital Signs. How would you care for this patient, and what orders would you expect from the physician? At the bottom list your potential diagnosis or impression of the patient's problem.

Primary Survey

A.

B.

C.

D.

Secondary Survey

A.

B.

C.

D.

Oxygen-IV-Monitor-Fluids: ____

____

Vital Signs: ____

____

Your Impression: ____

____

CASE 6

Scenario

A 35-year-old female had an episode of syncope while shopping. She is alert and oriented ×4 at present. She denies any recent illnesses. Her only complaint at present is feeling light-headed when she sits up. She is not complaining of chest pain, nausea, diaphoresis, shortness of breath, or weakness. Her skin is pink, warm, and dry. The Sao_2 = 96% on room air, and lung sounds are clear. Vital signs are BP, 118/74; pulse, rapid and weak; and R, 22. You see the following on the monitor:

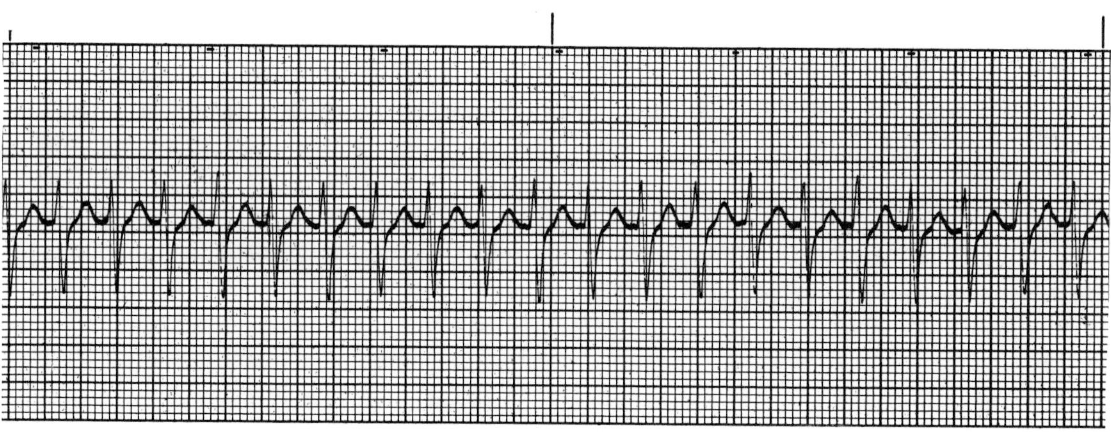

Identify the Rhythm

What is the rate? ____________ What is the rhythm (regular or irregular)? ____________

Is there a P wave before every QRS complex? ____________ Is there a QRS complex after every P wave? ____________

What is the P-R interval? ____________ QRS complex duration? ____________

Interpretation:

____

____

Case 6 Self-Test

In the spaces below give your treatment for the Primary Survey and Secondary Survey, plus the continued care under Oxygen-IV-Monitor-Fluids and Vital Signs. How would you care for this patient, and what orders would you expect from the physician? At the bottom list your potential diagnosis or impression of the patient's problem.

Primary Survey

A.

B.

C.

D.

Secondary Survey

A.

B.

C.

D.

Oxygen-IV-Monitor-Fluids: ____________________

____

Vital Signs: ____________________

____

Your Impression: ____________________

____

CASE 7

Scenario

A car pulls up in front of the emergency department with a 69-year-old male who is unconscious. Your initial primary survey reveals no respirations and no pulse. His wife tells you that he has a history of two MIs and bypass surgery 5 years ago. She says he had not been feeling well and complained of an upset stomach with nausea but no vomiting for the past 2 to 3 hours. You take a quick look with the paddles and see the following:

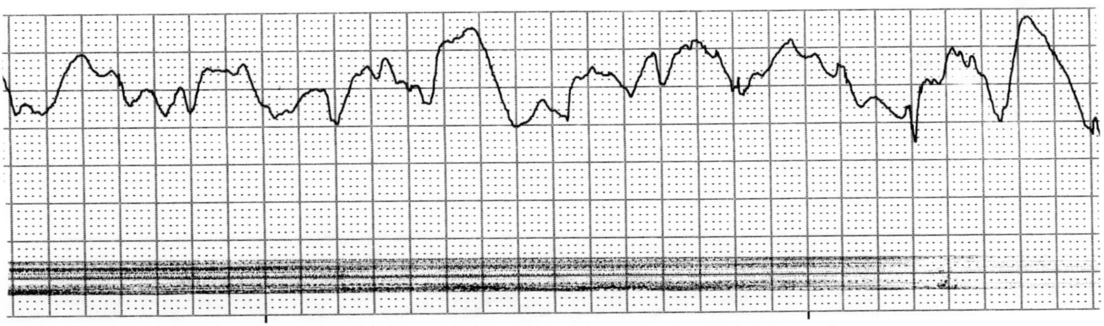

Identify the Rhythm

What is the rate? ____________ What is the rhythm (regular or irregular)? ____________

Is there a P wave before every QRS complex? ____________ Is there a QRS complex after every P wave? ____________

What is the P-R interval? ____________ QRS complex duration? ____________

Interpretation:

____

____

Case 7 Self-Test

In the spaces below give your treatment for the Primary Survey and Secondary Survey, plus the continued care under Oxygen-IV-Monitor-Fluids and Vital Signs. How would you care for this patient, and what orders would you expect from the physician? At the bottom list your potential diagnosis or impression of the patient's problem.

Primary Survey	***Secondary Survey***
A.	A.
B.	B.
C.	C.
D.	D.

Oxygen-IV-Monitor-Fluids: ____

____

Vital Signs: ____

____

Your Impression: ____

____

CASE 8

Scenario

A 71-year-old male is complaining of intermittent dizziness and tells you "it feels like my heart is skipping a beat." He denies any chest pain and other associated cardiac symptoms. His wife says he has a history of cardiac problems, but she is not sure what. He did have a pacemaker put in 6 years ago, but she is not sure why. She also tells you that he has diabetes but does not take insulin. His medications include furosemide, Lanoxin, and Glucophage. He is alert and oriented ×4. His skin is pink, warm, and dry. Vital signs are BP, 114/70; P, 50 and irregular; and R, 20. You see the following on the monitor:

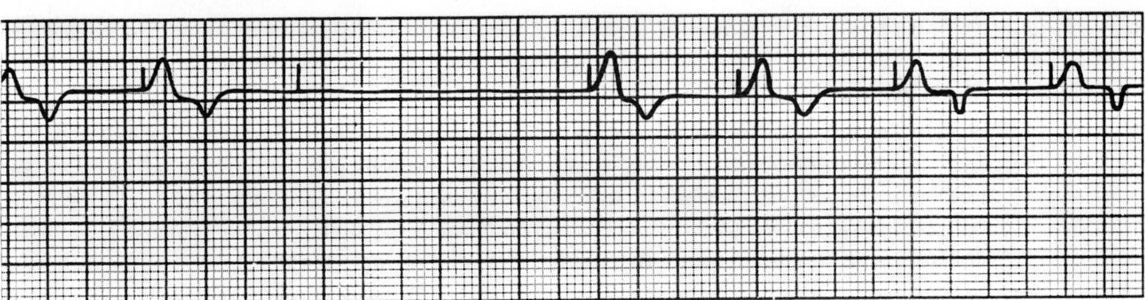

Identify the Rhythm

What is the rate? ____________ What is the rhythm (regular or irregular)? ____________

Is there a P wave before every QRS complex? ____________ Is there a QRS complex after every P wave? ____________

What is the P-R interval? ______________ QRS complex duration? ____________

Interpretation:

____

____

Case 8 Self-Test

In the spaces below give your treatment for the Primary Survey and Secondary Survey, plus the continued care under Oxygen-IV-Monitor-Fluids and Vital Signs. How would you care for this patient, and what orders would you expect from the physician? At the bottom list your potential diagnosis or impression of the patient's problem.

Primary Survey

A.

B.

C.

D.

Secondary Survey

A.

B.

C.

D.

Oxygen-IV-Monitor-Fluids: ______________________________

____

Vital Signs: ______________________________

____

Your Impression: ______________________________

____

CASE 9

Scenario

You are seeing a 38-year-old female who had an episode of syncope. At present she is alert and oriented ×4 but states she still feels weak and dizzy. She tells you her only medical history was a problem she had with her blood sugar, and now she takes insulin every day. Lungs are clear, and her skin is cool and slightly moist. The result of a fingerstick is a blood glucose level of 48. The Sao_2 is 98%. Vital signs are BP, 102/60; P, 90 and regular; and R, 22. You see the following on the monitor:

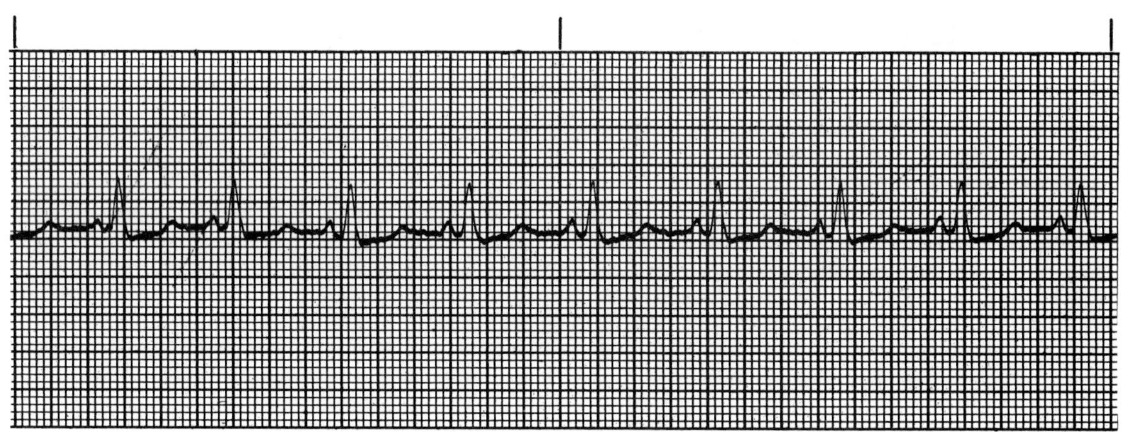

Identify the Rhythm

What is the rate? ____________ What is the rhythm (regular or irregular)? ____________

Is there a P wave before every QRS complex? ____________ Is there a QRS complex after every P wave? ____________

What is the P-R interval? ____________ QRS complex duration? ____________

Interpretation:

____

____

Case 9 Self-Test

In the spaces below give your treatment for the Primary Survey and Secondary Survey, plus the continued care under Oxygen-IV-Monitor-Fluids and Vital Signs. How would you care for this patient, and what orders would you expect from the physician? At the bottom list your potential diagnosis or impression of the patient's problem.

Primary Survey

A.

B.

C.

D.

Secondary Survey

A.

B.

C.

D.

Oxygen-IV-Monitor-Fluids: ______________________________

____

Vital Signs: ______________________________

____

Your Impression: ______________________________

____

CASE 10

Scenario

Your patient is a 61-year-old male who is complaining of weakness, slight chest pressure, and nausea and admits to an episode of syncope. He says he is just not feeling well. His medical history includes two MIs, COPD, and arthritis. Medications are nitroglycerin SL as needed, Proventil as needed, and one baby aspirin a day. He is alert and oriented ×4. Skin is pink, warm, and dry, and lung sounds are clear. Sao_2 = 94%. Vital signs are BP, 126/84; P, 55 and regular; and R, 22. You see the following on the monitor:

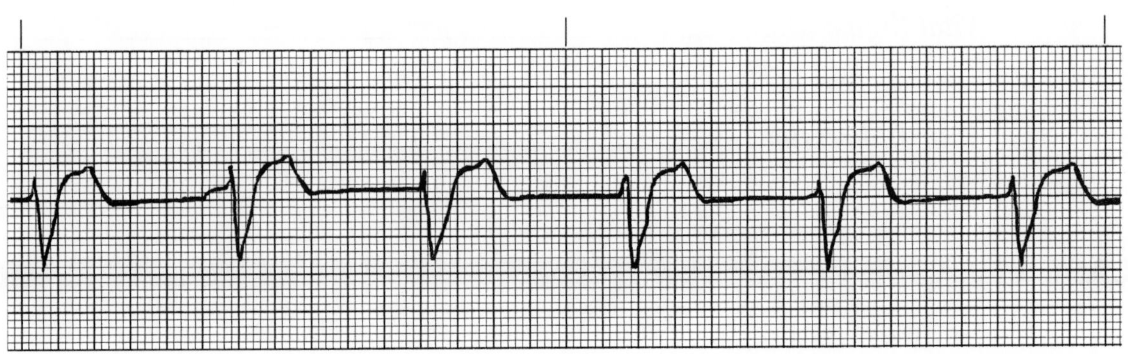

Identify the Rhythm

What is the rate? ____________ What is the rhythm (regular or irregular)? ____________

Is there a P wave before every QRS complex? ____________ Is there a QRS complex after every P wave? ____________

What is the P-R interval? ____________ QRS complex duration? ____________

Interpretation:

____

____

Case 10 Self-Test

In the spaces below give your treatment for the Primary Survey and Secondary Survey, plus the continued care under Oxygen-IV-Monitor-Fluids and Vital Signs. How would you care for this patient, and what orders would you expect from the physician? At the bottom list your potential diagnosis or impression of the patient's problem.

Primary Survey	*Secondary Survey*
A.	A.
B.	B.
C.	C.
D.	D.

Oxygen-IV-Monitor-Fluids: ____

____

Vital Signs: ____

____

Your Impression: ____

____

CASE 11

Scenario

A 25-year-old female was working in a lumberyard when she was struck in the chest with lumber being loaded by a forklift. When you get to her, she is unresponsive. She is not breathing, and there is no pulse. You do notice a large bruise on the center of her chest. CPR was immediately initiated but with difficulty because of several fractured ribs. You see the following on the monitor:

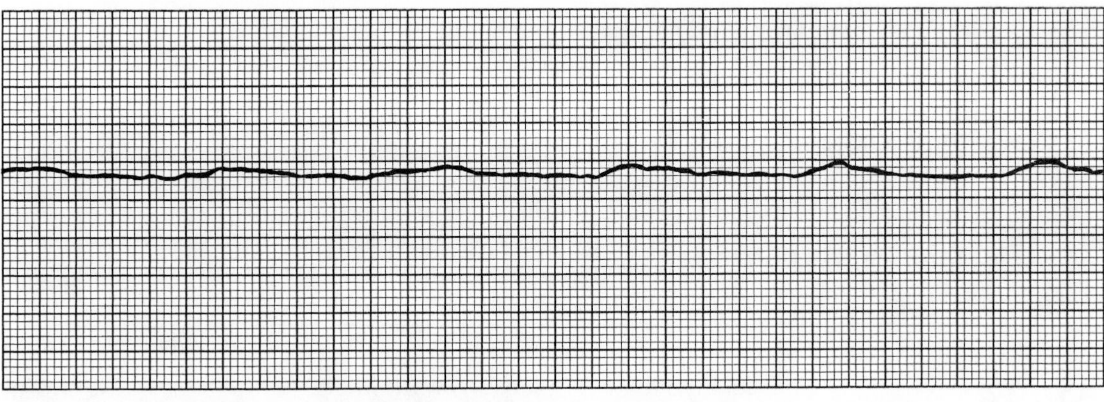

Identify the Rhythm

What is the rate? ____________ What is the rhythm (regular or irregular)? ____________

Is there a P wave before every QRS complex? ____________ Is there a QRS complex after every P wave? ____________

What is the P-R interval? ______________ QRS complex duration? ______________

Interpretation:

____

____

Case 11 Self-Test

In the spaces below give your treatment for the Primary Survey and Secondary Survey, plus the continued care under Oxygen-IV-Monitor-Fluids and Vital Signs. How would you care for this patient, and what orders would you expect from the physician? At the bottom list your potential diagnosis or impression of the patient's problem.

Primary Survey

A.

B.

C.

D.

Secondary Survey

A.

B.

C.

D.

Oxygen-IV-Monitor-Fluids: ______________________________

____

Vital Signs: ______________________________

____

Your Impression: ______________________________

____

CASE 12

Scenario

You have a 72-year-old female who has been ill for the past 4 days with flu symptoms. She has nausea, vomiting, and diarrhea and is complaining at present of some shortness of breath. There is nothing in her medical history, and she is not taking any medications. She is alert and oriented ×4, and her skin is pale, cool, and dry with signs of dehydration noted (poor skin turgor and dry mucous membranes). Vital signs are BP, 90/60; P, 56 and regular; and R, 26. Her lungs have decreased breath sounds, and the Sao_2 = 91%. On the monitor you see the following:

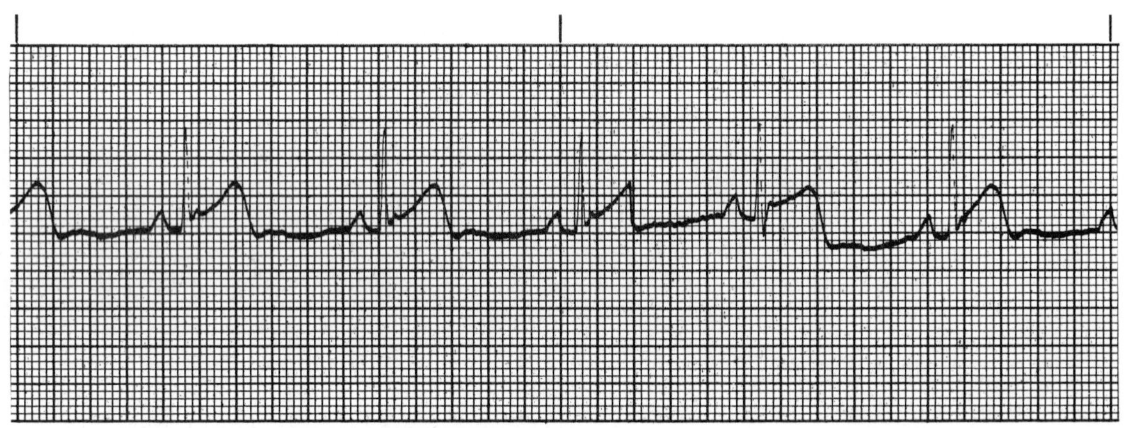

Identify the Rhythm

What is the rate? __________ What is the rhythm (regular or irregular)? __________

Is there a P wave before every QRS complex? __________ Is there a QRS complex after every P wave? __________

What is the P-R interval? __________ QRS complex duration? __________

Interpretation:

____

____

Case 12 Self-Test

In the spaces below give your treatment for the Primary Survey and Secondary Survey, plus the continued care under Oxygen-IV-Monitor-Fluids and Vital Signs. How would you care for this patient, and what orders would you expect from the physician? At the bottom list your potential diagnosis or impression of the patient's problem.

Primary Survey

A.

B.

C.

D.

Secondary Survey

A.

B.

C.

D.

Oxygen-IV-Monitor-Fluids: ______________________________

____

Vital Signs: ______________________________

____

Your Impression: ______________________________

____

CASE 13

Scenario

Your patient is a 68-year-old female complaining of severe shortness of breath. She is sitting, leaning forward on the edge of the bed. She is very diaphoretic and appears extremely anxious and apprehensive. She is unable to tell you her medical history or medications she is taking. Lung sounds reveal crackles and wheezes throughout all lung fields. Skin is pale, cool, and moist. She is alert but not oriented. Vital signs BP, 190/106; P, 140; and R, 36 and labored. Her Sao_2 = 84%. On the monitor you see the following:

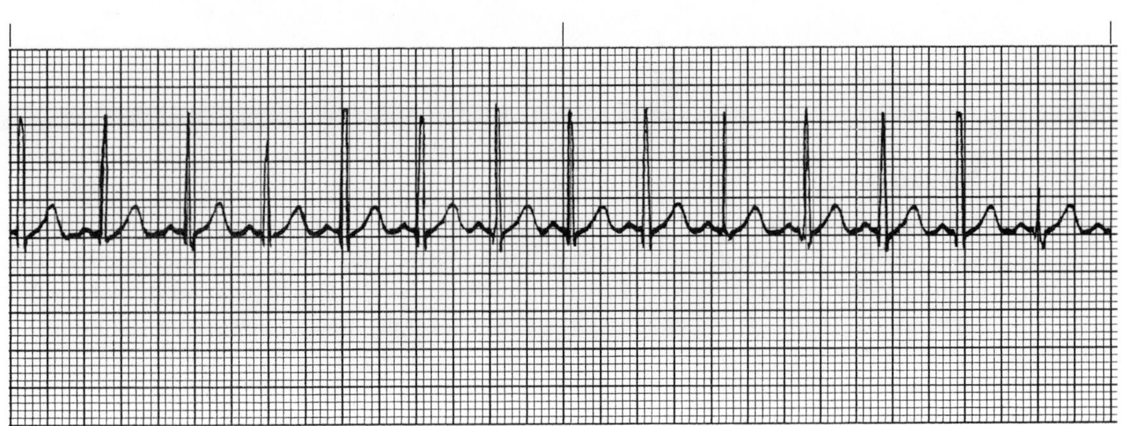

Identify the Rhythm

What is the rate? ____________ What is the rhythm (regular or irregular)? ____________

Is there a P wave before every QRS complex? ____________ Is there a QRS complex after every P wave? ____________

What is the P-R interval? ____________ QRS complex duration? ____________

Interpretation:

____

____

Case 13 Self-Test

In the spaces below give your treatment for the Primary Survey and Secondary Survey, plus the continued care under Oxygen-IV-Monitor-Fluids and Vital Signs. How would you care for this patient, and what orders would you expect from the physician? At the bottom list your potential diagnosis or impression of the patient's problem.

Primary Survey	*Secondary Survey*
A.	A.
B.	B.
C.	C.
D.	D.

Oxygen-IV-Monitor-Fluids: ____

____

Vital Signs: ____

____

Your Impression: ____

____

CASE 14

Scenario

You see a 41-year-old female who is complaining of feeling weak and dizzy and says she has a funny feeling in her chest. She really cannot describe it to you. She is alert and oriented ×4, has nothing in her medical history, and takes no medications. Her skin is pink, warm, and dry. Vital signs are BP, 108/68; P, 204 and regular; and R, 22. On the monitor you see the following:

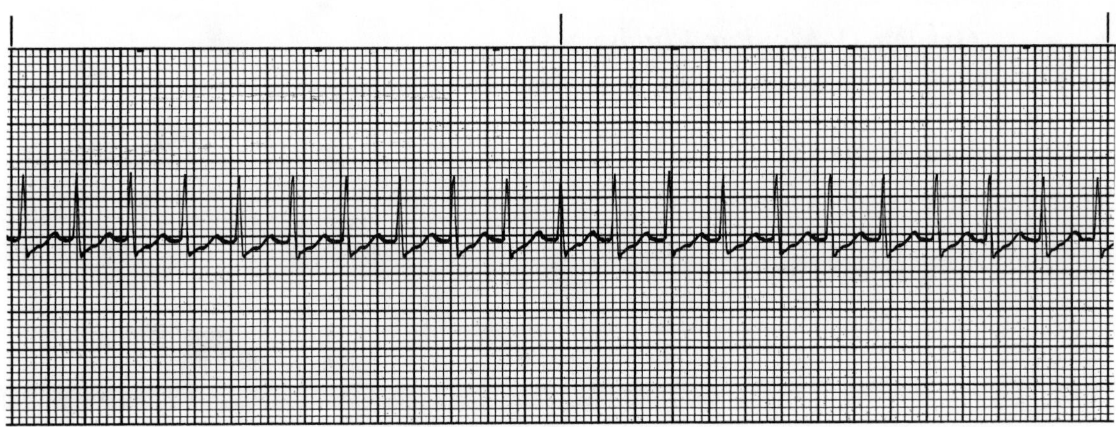

Identify the Rhythm

What is the rate? ______________ What is the rhythm (regular or irregular)? ______________

Is there a P wave before every QRS complex? ______________ Is there a QRS complex after every P wave? ______________

What is the P-R interval? ________________ QRS complex duration? ________________

Interpretation:

____

____

Case 14 Self-Test

In the spaces below give your treatment for the Primary Survey and Secondary Survey, plus the continued care under Oxygen-IV-Monitor-Fluids and Vital Signs. How would you care for this patient, and what orders would you expect from the physician? At the bottom list your potential diagnosis or impression of the patient's problem.

Primary Survey

A.

B.

C.

D.

Secondary Survey

A.

B.

C.

D.

Oxygen-IV-Monitor-Fluids: ______________________________

____

Vital Signs: ______________________________

____

Your Impression: ______________________________

____

CASE 15

Scenario

You have a 49-year-old male who is complaining of fever for the past week. Today he had chest discomfort accompanied with fatigue, a slight cough, and some difficulty in breathing. There is nothing in his medical history, but he tells you he has been tired for the past 3 months. He is not taking medications. He is alert and oriented ×4. His skin is pink, warm, and dry. Lung sounds reveal scattered wheezes and a few crackles. Vital signs are BP, 114/78; P, 47; R, 24; and a temperature of 101° F. You see the following on the monitor:

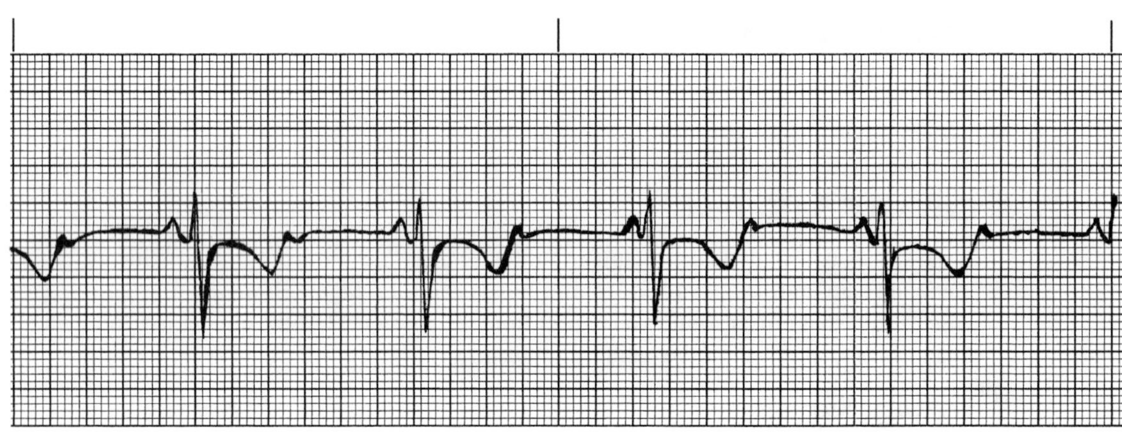

Identify the Rhythm

What is the rate? ____________ What is the rhythm (regular or irregular)? ____________

Is there a P wave before every QRS complex? ____________ Is there a QRS complex after every P wave? ____________

What is the P-R interval? ____________ QRS complex duration? ____________

Interpretation:

____

____

Case 15 Self-Test

In the spaces below give your treatment for the Primary Survey and Secondary Survey, plus the continued care under Oxygen-IV-Monitor-Fluids and Vital Signs. How would you care for this patient, and what orders would you expect from the physician? At the bottom list your potential diagnosis or impression of the patient's problem.

Primary Survey	*Secondary Survey*
A.	A.
B.	B.
C.	C.
D.	D.

Oxygen-IV-Monitor-Fluids: ______________________________

____

Vital Signs: ______________________________

____

Your Impression: ______________________________

____

CASE 16

Scenario

A 39-year-old male complains of chest pain. He rates the pain as a 10 on a scale of 1 to 10 and says it is radiating to his left arm and to the back of his neck. He states he is having dizziness and weakness but denies nausea or difficulty breathing. He did have one episode of syncope but did not tell anyone. There is nothing in his medical history, and he is not taking any medications. He is alert and oriented ×4. Skin is pink, warm, and dry. Vital signs are BP, 132/88; P, 71 and regular; and R, 20. You see the following on the monitor:

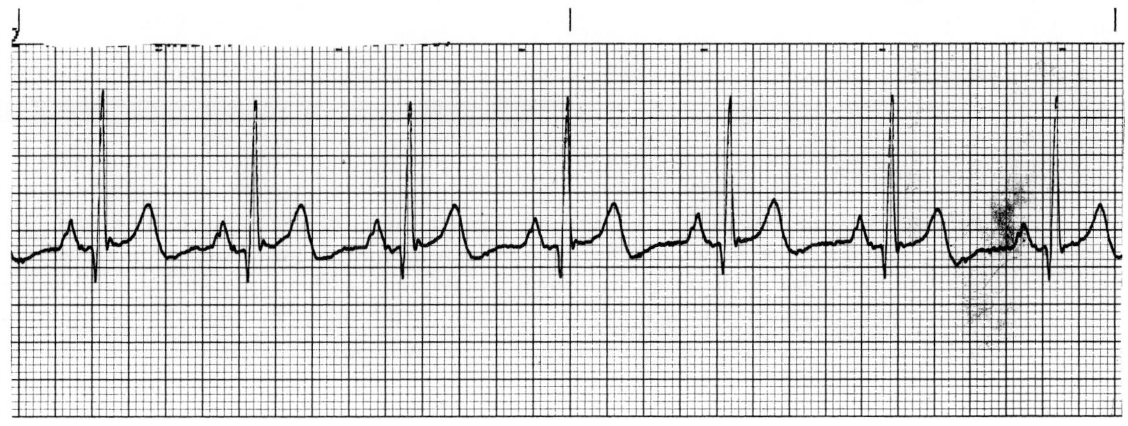

Identify the Rhythm

What is the rate? ____________ What is the rhythm (regular or irregular)? ____________

Is there a P wave before every QRS complex? ____________ Is there a QRS complex after every P wave? ____________

What is the P-R interval? ______________ QRS complex duration? ______________

Interpretation:

____

____

Case 16 Self-Test

In the spaces below give your treatment for the Primary Survey and Secondary Survey, plus the continued care under Oxygen-IV-Monitor-Fluids and Vital Signs. How would you care for this patient, and what orders would you expect from the physician? At the bottom list your potential diagnosis or impression of the patient's problem.

Primary Survey

A.

B.

C.

D.

Secondary Survey

A.

B.

C.

D.

Oxygen-IV-Monitor-Fluids: ______________________________________

____

Vital Signs: ____

____

Your Impression: ____

____

CASE 17

Scenario

Your patient is a 31-year-old male who was involved in a one-car motor vehicle crash. The patient was the driver and was not wearing a seat belt. There is major damage to the vehicle. When rescue arrives on the scene, the patient is unresponsive. There are multiple abrasions and lacerations on his body. A large bruise is noted over the left side of the chest. The patient is not breathing, and you cannot feel a pulse. CPR is begun, and you see the following on the monitor:

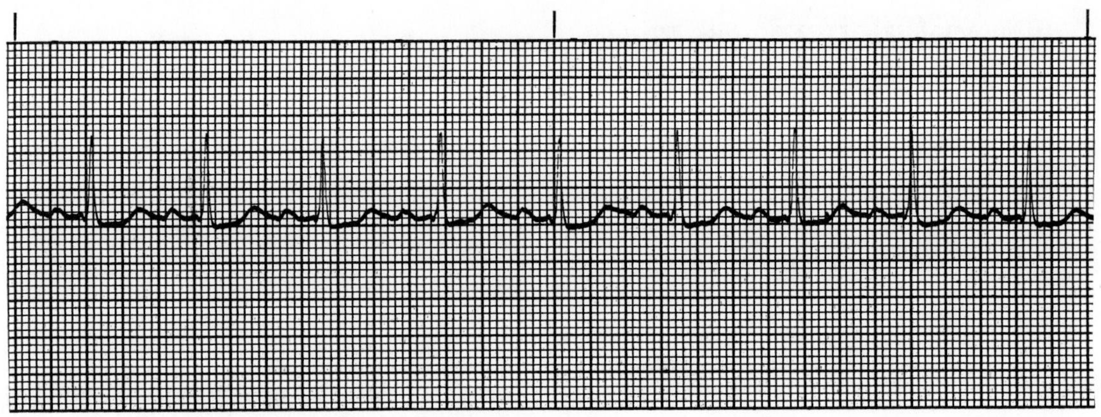

Identify the Rhythm

What is the rate? ____________ What is the rhythm (regular or irregular)? ____________

Is there a P wave before every QRS complex? ____________ Is there a QRS complex after every P wave? ____________

What is the P-R interval? ____________ QRS complex duration? ____________

Interpretation:

____

____

Case 17 Self-Test

In the spaces below give your treatment for the Primary Survey and Secondary Survey, plus the continued care under Oxygen-IV-Monitor-Fluids and Vital Signs. How would you care for this patient, and what orders would you expect from the physician? At the bottom list your potential diagnosis or impression of the patient's problem.

Primary Survey

A.

B.

C.

D.

Secondary Survey

A.

B.

C.

D.

Oxygen-IV-Monitor-Fluids: ______________________________

____

Vital Signs: ______________________________

____

Your Impression: ______________________________

____

CASE 18

Scenario

A 38-year-old female has had cold symptoms, cough, and fever for the past 5 days. She has a productive cough with yellow sputum and sometimes rust-colored sputum. She also tells you she has been having some chest discomfort for the past 24 hours. There is nothing in her medical history, and she is not taking any medications. She is alert and oriented ×4, and her skin is pink, warm, and moist. Vital signs are BP, 122/74; P, 124; R, 24; and Sao_2 = 93%, and her temperature is 102.8° F. You see the following on the monitor:

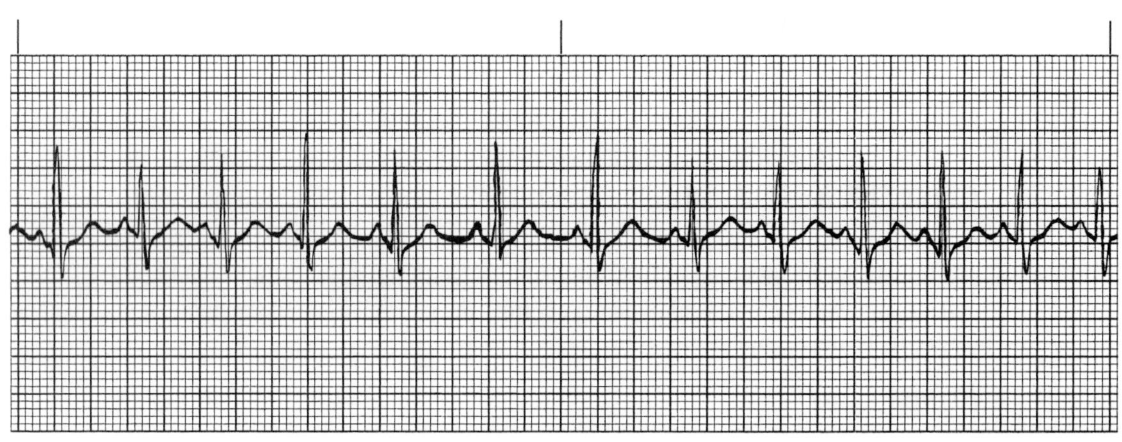

Identify the Rhythm

What is the rate? __________ What is the rhythm (regular or irregular)? __________

Is there a P wave before every QRS complex? __________ Is there a QRS complex after every P wave? __________

What is the P-R interval? __________ QRS complex duration? __________

Interpretation:

____

____

Case 18 Self-Test

In the spaces below give your treatment for the Primary Survey and Secondary Survey, plus the continued care under Oxygen-IV-Monitor-Fluids and Vital Signs. How would you care for this patient, and what orders would you expect from the physician? At the bottom list your potential diagnosis or impression of the patient's problem.

Primary Survey

A.

B.

C.

D.

Secondary Survey

A.

B.

C.

D.

Oxygen-IV-Monitor-Fluids: ______________________________

____

Vital Signs: ______________________________

____

Your Impression: ______________________________

____

CASE 19

Scenario

A 79-year-old male is complaining of nausea, vomiting, diarrhea, and yellow vision at times. His family tells you that he has been confused for the past few weeks. He is alert but not oriented to time. His skin is pale, warm, and dry. Vital signs are BP, 122/68; P, 45; and R, 20. He does have a history of cardiac problems but no other medical problems. The only medication he is taking is digoxin, 0.25 mg once a day, and nitroglycerin SL, 0.4 mg, as needed. You see the following on the monitor:

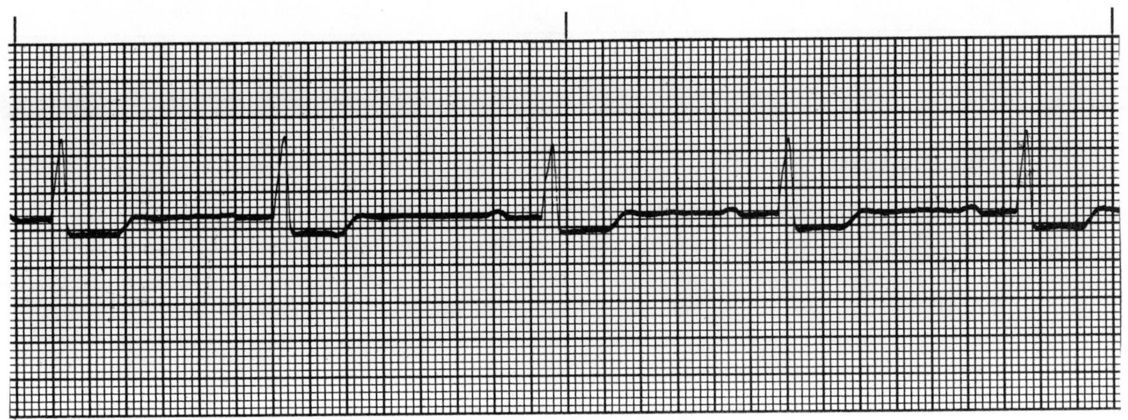

Identify the Rhythm

What is the rate? ____________ What is the rhythm (regular or irregular)? ____________

Is there a P wave before every QRS complex? ____________ Is there a QRS complex after every P wave? ____________

What is the P-R interval? ____________ QRS complex duration? ____________

Interpretation:

____

____

Case 19 Self-Test

In the spaces below give your treatment for the Primary Survey and Secondary Survey, plus the continued care under Oxygen-IV-Monitor-Fluids and Vital Signs. How would you care for this patient, and what orders would you expect from the physician? At the bottom list your potential diagnosis or impression of the patient's problem.

Primary Survey

A.

B.

C.

D.

Secondary Survey

A.

B.

C.

D.

Oxygen-IV-Monitor-Fluids: ____

____

Vital Signs: ____

____

Your Impression: ____

____

CASE 20

Scenario

A 63-year-old male is complaining of intermittent episodes of syncope for the past 2 to 3 days. He just had open heart surgery 2 weeks ago without any complications. At this time he denies any chest pain but says he has been light-headed and has passed out about four times in the past 24 hours. His medical history includes cardiac problems, with the open heart surgery and arthritis. He is alert and oriented ×4 at present. Vital signs are BP, 90/62; P, 60 and regular; and R, 22. You see the following on the monitor:

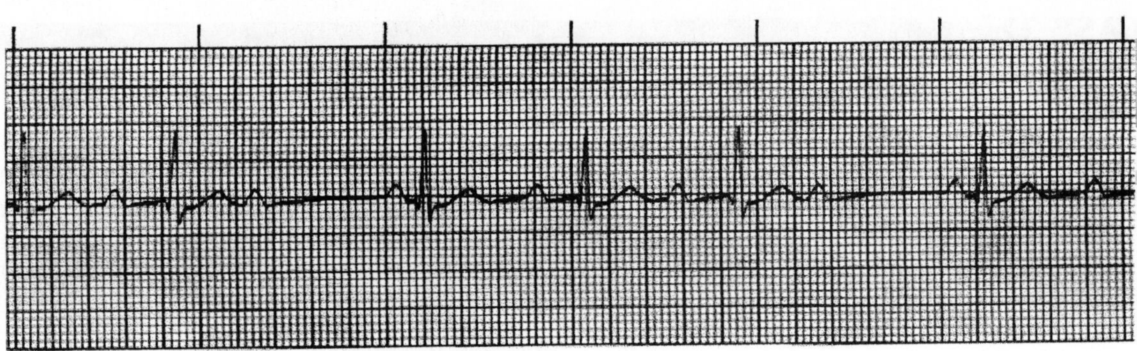

Identify the Rhythm

What is the rate? ____________ What is the rhythm (regular or irregular)? ____________

Is there a P wave before every QRS complex? ____________ Is there a QRS complex after every P wave? ____________

What is the P-R interval? ______________ QRS complex duration? ______________

Interpretation:

____

____

Case 20 Self-Test

In the spaces below give your treatment for the Primary Survey and Secondary Survey, plus the continued care under Oxygen-IV-Monitor-Fluids and Vital Signs. How would you care for this patient, and what orders would you expect from the physician? At the bottom list your potential diagnosis or impression of the patient's problem.

Primary Survey

A.

B.

C.

D.

Secondary Survey

A.

B.

C.

D.

Oxygen-IV-Monitor-Fluids: ______________________________________

____

Vital Signs: ____

____

Your Impression: ____

____

CASE 21

Scenario

A 39-year-old male is brought into the emergency department with dizziness and blurred vision for the past 12 hours. He denies any chest pain, difficulty in breathing, headache, or recent head trauma. He tells you that he has no medical history. After further questioning, his wife tells you he is an alcoholic and has been for years. He is alert and oriented to person and place. His skin is pale, cool, and dry. Lung sounds are clear. Vital signs are BP, 102/62; P, 40 to 60 and very irregular; and R, 22. You see the following on the monitor:

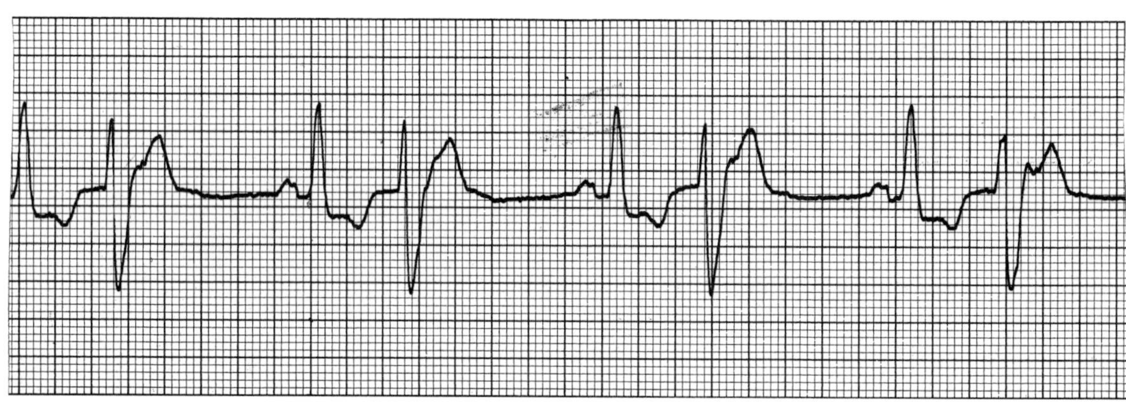

Identify the Rhythm

What is the rate? ____________ What is the rhythm (regular or irregular)? ____________

Is there a P wave before every QRS complex? ____________ Is there a QRS complex after every P wave? ____________

What is the P-R interval? ____________ QRS complex duration? ____________

Interpretation:

____

____

Case 21 Self-Test

In the spaces below give your treatment for the Primary Survey and Secondary Survey, plus the continued care under Oxygen-IV-Monitor-Fluids and Vital Signs. How would you care for this patient, and what orders would you expect from the physician? At the bottom list your potential diagnosis or impression of the patient's problem.

Primary Survey

A.

B.

C.

D.

Secondary Survey

A.

B.

C.

D.

Oxygen-IV-Monitor-Fluids: ____________________

____

Vital Signs: ____________________

____

Your Impression: ____________________

____

CASE 22

Scenario

A 51-year-old male walks into your emergency department complaining of chest pain. He states it began 3 hours ago and radiates to the left shoulder. He is also complaining of dizziness, but denies nausea, shortness of breath, or weakness. He does not have a medical history and is not taking any medications. He is allergic to sulfa. He tells you the pain began as 6 on a 1 to 10 scale. He smokes half a pack of cigarettes per day and has a very stressful job. Vital signs are BP, 116/78; P, 55; and R, 20. His Sao_2 = 100%, and lung sounds are decreased but clear. You see the following on the monitor:

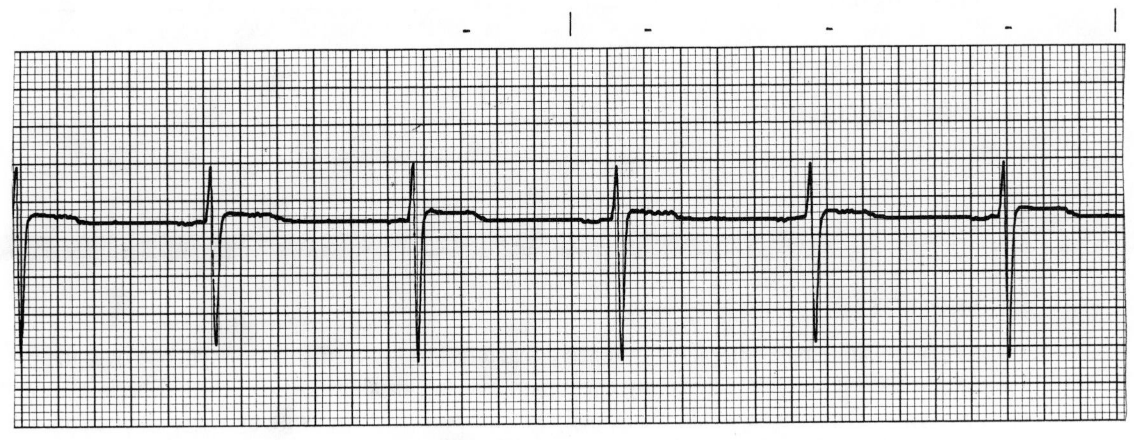

Identify the Rhythm

What is the rate? ____________ What is the rhythm (regular or irregular)? ____________

Is there a P wave before every QRS complex? ____________ Is there a QRS complex after every P wave? ____________

What is the P-R interval? ____________ QRS complex duration? ____________

Interpretation:

____

____

Case 22 Self-Test

In the spaces below give your treatment for the Primary Survey and Secondary Survey, plus the continued care under Oxygen-IV-Monitor-Fluids and Vital Signs. How would you care for this patient, and what orders would you expect from the physician? At the bottom list your potential diagnosis or impression of the patient's problem.

Primary Survey

A.

B.

C.

D.

Secondary Survey

A.

B.

C.

D.

Oxygen-IV-Monitor-Fluids: ____

____

Vital Signs: ____

____

Your Impression: ____

____

CASE 23

Scenario

A 31-year-old female complains of dizziness and has had two episodes of syncope over the past 6 hours. At present she denies any chest pain, nausea, or shortness of breath. She is alert and oriented ×4, but feeling weak, dizzy, and says she feels like she is going to pass out again. Her skin is pale, cool, and moist. Vital signs are BP, 88/52; P, weak, very rapid but regular; R, 24; and Sao_2 = 92%. You see the following on the monitor:

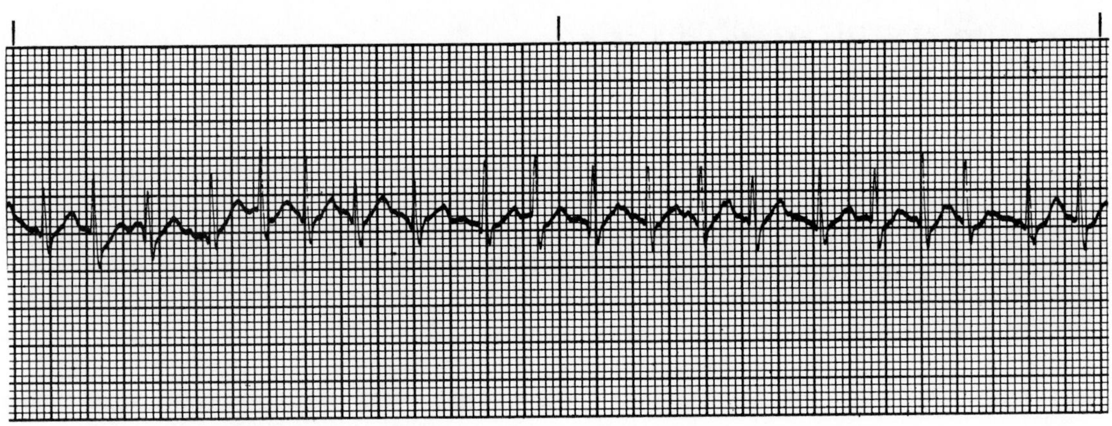

Identify the Rhythm

What is the rate? ____________ What is the rhythm (regular or irregular)? ____________

Is there a P wave before every QRS complex? ____________ Is there a QRS complex after every P wave? ____________

What is the P-R interval? ____________ QRS complex duration? ____________

Interpretation:

____

____

Case 23 Self-Test

In the spaces below give your treatment for the Primary Survey and Secondary Survey, plus the continued care under Oxygen-IV-Monitor-Fluids and Vital Signs. How would you care for this patient, and what orders would you expect from the physician? At the bottom list your potential diagnosis or impression of the patient's problem.

Primary Survey

A.

B.

C.

D.

Secondary Survey

A.

B.

C.

D.

Oxygen-IV-Monitor-Fluids: ______________________________

____

Vital Signs: ______________________________

____

Your Impression: ______________________________

____

CASE 24

Scenario

A 58-year-old female calls the ambulance because of three syncopal episodes today. She denies any recent trauma and chest pain. She tells you she has had a fluid problem, CHF for the past year, and is taking K-lor and furosemide. However, she has had the flu for the past week and is not sure if she took her medications or how much she may have taken. She is alert and oriented ×4 at present. Vital signs are BP, 106/60; P, 64 and irregular; and R, 20, and temperature is 100.6.° F. Her skin is pink, warm, and slightly moist. Lungs sounds are clear, and Sao_2 = 94%. You see the following on the monitor:

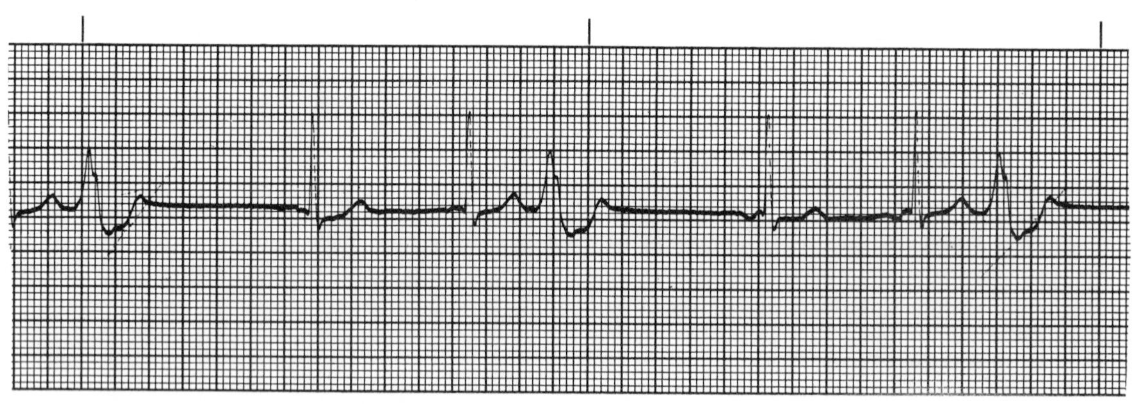

Identify the Rhythm

What is the rate? ____________ What is the rhythm (regular or irregular)? ____________

Is there a P wave before every QRS complex? ____________ Is there a QRS complex after every P wave? ____________

What is the P-R interval? ____________ QRS complex duration? ____________

Interpretation:

____

____

Case 24 Self-Test

In the spaces below give your treatment for the Primary Survey and Secondary Survey, plus the continued care under Oxygen-IV-Monitor-Fluids and Vital Signs. How would you care for this patient, and what orders would you expect from the physician? At the bottom list your potential diagnosis or impression of the patient's problem.

Primary Survey	***Secondary Survey***
A.	A.
B.	B.
C.	C.
D.	D.

Oxygen-IV-Monitor-Fluids: ____________________

____

Vital Signs: ____________________

____

Your Impression: ____________________

____

CASE 25

Scenario

A 63-year-old male comes to the emergency department complaining of midsternal chest pain that is radiating to the left shoulder and arm. He also complains of nausea, vomiting ×1, weakness, dizziness, and a feeling of impending doom. He is slightly short of breath and very diaphoretic. He rates the pain as 7 on a scale of 1 to 10 and describes it as a heaviness in his chest. His medical history includes angina and CHF. Medications include nitroglycerin SL, as needed, and bumetanide. He has no allergies. He is alert and oriented ×4; skin is pale, cool, and moist. Lung sounds reveal crackles at the bases, and his Sao_2 = 94%. Vital signs are BP, 100/56; P, 50 and irregular; and R, 24. You see the following on the monitor:

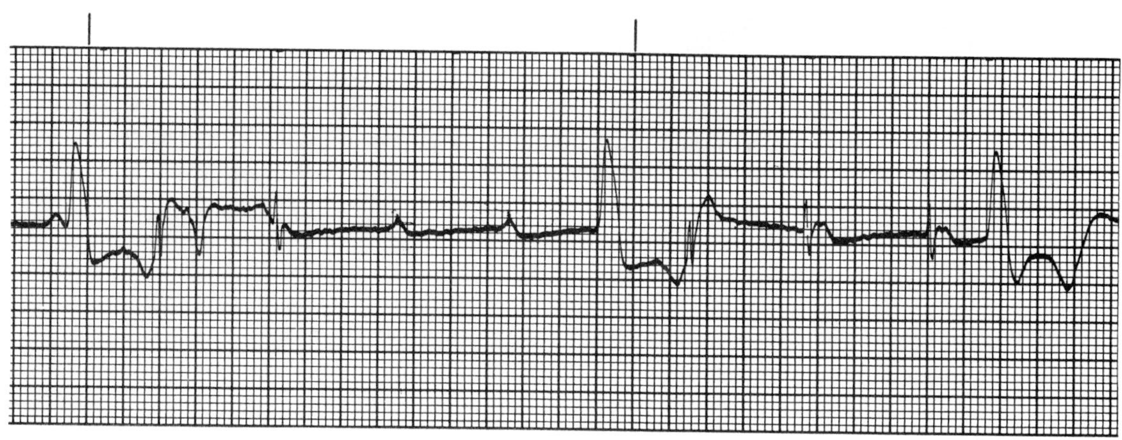

Identify the Rhythm

What is the rate? ______________ What is the rhythm (regular or irregular)? ______________

Is there a P wave before every QRS complex? ______________ Is there a QRS complex after every P wave? ______________

What is the P-R interval? ______________ QRS complex duration? ______________

Interpretation:

____

____

Case 25 Self-Test

In the spaces below give your treatment for the Primary Survey and Secondary Survey, plus the continued care under Oxygen-IV-Monitor-Fluids and Vital Signs. How would you care for this patient, and what orders would you expect from the physician? At the bottom list your potential diagnosis or impression of the patient's problem.

Primary Survey

A.

B.

C.

D.

Secondary Survey

A.

B.

C.

D.

Oxygen-IV-Monitor-Fluids: ____________________

____

Vital Signs: ____________________

____

Your Impression: ____________________

____

CASE 26

Scenario (Actual EMS Call)

You are called for a 57-year-old male who was outside shoveling snow off the sidewalk by his house, when ice on the edge of the roof broke loose and fell. You find him on the ground, unresponsive. He is not breathing and has no pulse. CPR was initiated by rescue unit. You see the following on the monitor:

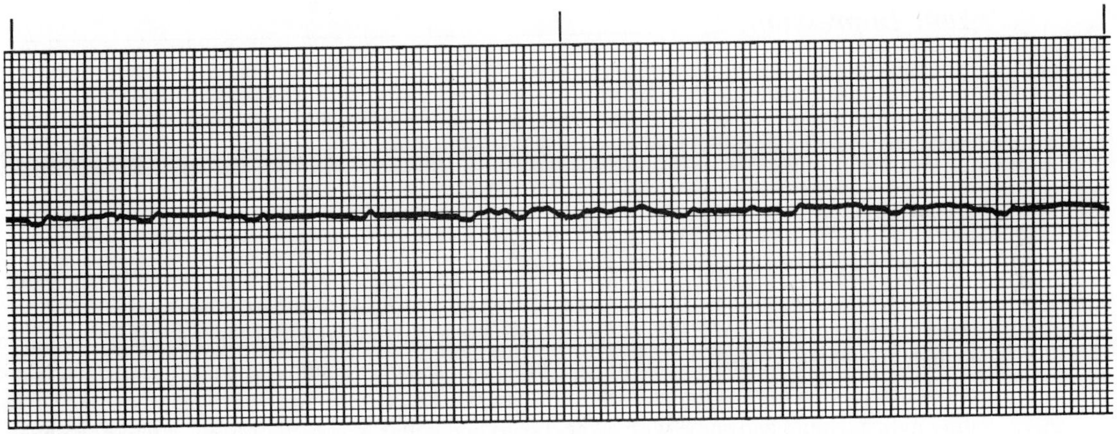

Identify the Rhythm

What is the rate? __________ What is the rhythm (regular or irregular)? __________

Is there a P wave before every QRS complex? __________ Is there a QRS complex after every P wave? __________

What is the P-R interval? __________ QRS complex duration? __________

Interpretation:

____

____

Case 26 Self-Test

In the spaces below give your treatment for the Primary Survey and Secondary Survey, plus the continued care under Oxygen-IV-Monitor-Fluids and Vital Signs. How would you care for this patient, and what orders would you expect from the physician? At the bottom list your potential diagnosis or impression of the patient's problem.

Primary Survey

A.

B.

C.

D.

Secondary Survey

A.

B.

C.

D.

Oxygen-IV-Monitor-Fluids: ______________________________

____

Vital Signs: ______________________________

____

Your Impression: ______________________________

____

CASE 27

Scenario

You are called for an 86-year-old female who fell out of bed. She is awake, but rambling, making no sense when you arrive. You note a deformity on her left hip with external rotation of the left foot. She has a history of Parkinson's disease, arthritis, and cardiac problems. Her medications include ibuprofen, captopril, and nitroglycerin SL, as needed, and she has a pacemaker. Neuro checks are within normal limits. Vital signs are BP, 150/108; P, 102 and regular; and R, 22. You immobilize the hip and spine with a backboard and collar. You begin transport when she begins having difficulty breathing. An IV line is established. You see the following on the monitor:

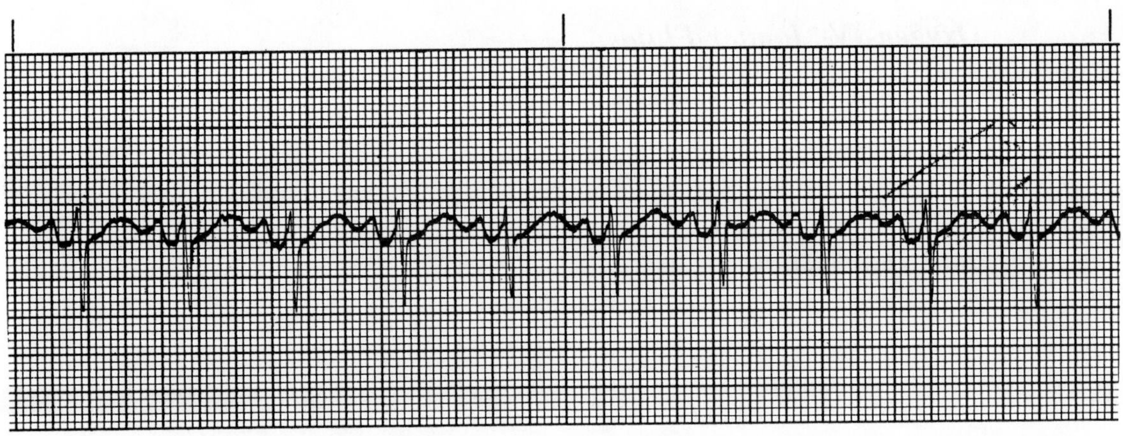

Identify the Rhythm

What is the rate? ____________ What is the rhythm (regular or irregular)? ____________

Is there a P wave before every QRS complex? ____________ Is there a QRS complex after every P wave? ____________

What is the P-R interval? ____________ QRS complex duration? ____________

Interpretation:

____

____

Case 27 Self-Test

In the spaces below give your treatment for the Primary Survey and Secondary Survey, plus the continued care under Oxygen-IV-Monitor-Fluids and Vital Signs. How would you care for this patient, and what orders would you expect from the physician? At the bottom list your potential diagnosis or impression of the patient's problem.

Primary Survey

A.

B.

C.

D.

Secondary Survey

A.

B.

C.

D.

Oxygen-IV-Monitor-Fluids: ______________________________

____

Vital Signs: ______________________________

____

Your Impression: ______________________________

____

CASE 28

Scenario (Actual EMS Call)

You are called for a 50-year-old male complaining of dizziness and weakness. He is literally unable to get up from the living room chair. He tells you that he has had a sinus infection for the past week and was given long-acting Sudafed 3 days ago. There is nothing in his medical history, and he is not taking other medications. He is lethargic and not oriented to time. Skin is pale, cool, and moist. Vital signs are BP, 89/58; P, too weak to obtain; R, 20; and Sao_2 = 97%. You see the following on the monitor:

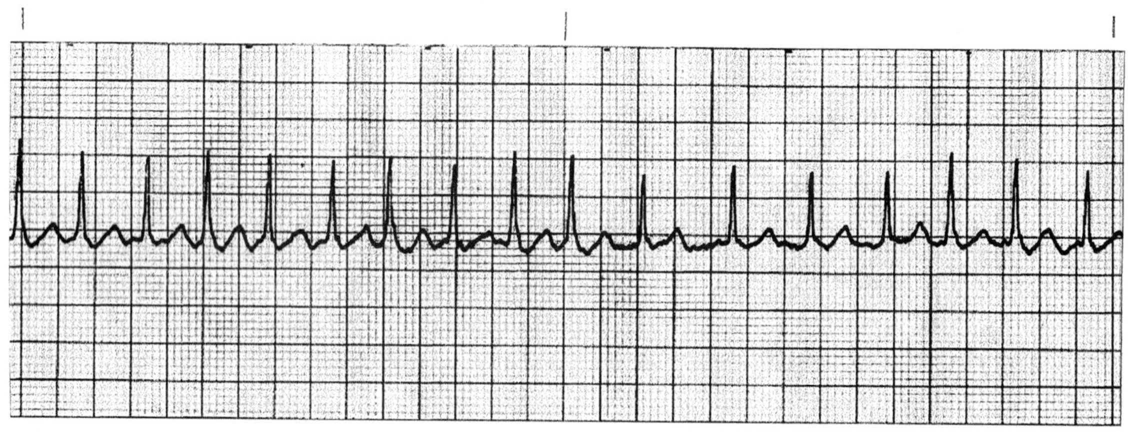

Identify the Rhythm

What is the rate? ____________ What is the rhythm (regular or irregular)? ____________

Is there a P wave before every QRS complex? ____________ Is there a QRS complex after every P wave? ____________

What is the P-R interval? ____________ QRS complex duration? ____________

Interpretation:

____

____

Case 28 Self-Test

In the spaces below give your treatment for the Primary Survey and Secondary Survey, plus the continued care under Oxygen-IV-Monitor-Fluids and Vital Signs. How would you care for this patient, and what orders would you expect from the physician? At the bottom list your potential diagnosis or impression of the patient's problem.

Primary Survey

A.

B.

C.

D.

Secondary Survey

A.

B.

C.

D.

Oxygen-IV-Monitor-Fluids: ______________________________

____

Vital Signs: ______________________________

____

Your Impression: ______________________________

____

CASE 29

Scenario (Actual EMS Call)

A 24-year-old female collapses while jogging 5 miles on a hot summer day. When you evaluate her, she is complaining of abdominal and leg cramps. She tells you she had some water but ran out 3 miles back. She is alert and oriented ×4. Her skin is pale, cool, and moist. She has no medical history and is not taking any medications. Vital signs are BP, 104/48; P, 104; and R, 20. You see the following on the monitor:

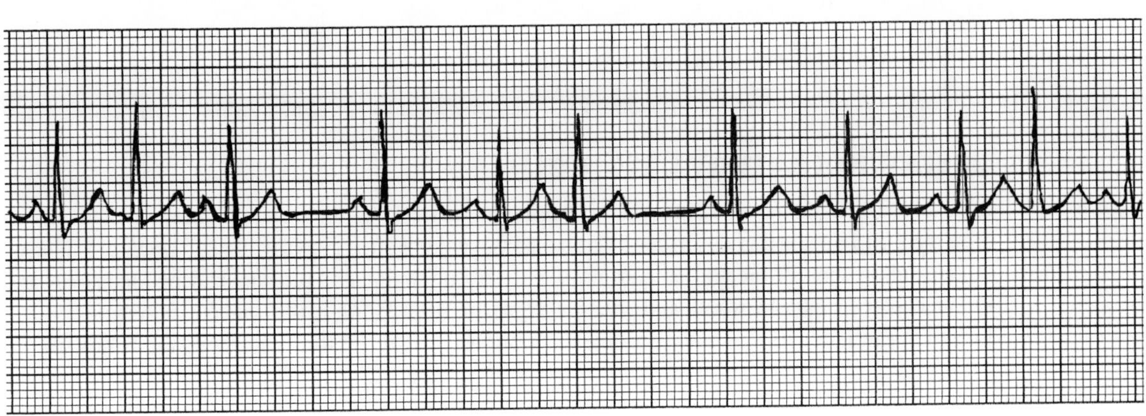

Identify the Rhythm

What is the rate? ______________ What is the rhythm (regular or irregular)? ______________

Is there a P wave before every QRS complex? ______________ Is there a QRS complex after every P wave? ______________

What is the P-R interval? ______________ QRS complex duration? ______________

Interpretation:

____

____

Case 29 Self-Test

In the spaces below give your treatment for the Primary Survey and Secondary Survey, plus the continued care under Oxygen-IV-Monitor-Fluids and Vital Signs. How would you care for this patient, and what orders would you expect from the physician? At the bottom list your potential diagnosis or impression of the patient's problem.

Primary Survey

A.

B.

C.

D.

Secondary Survey

A.

B.

C.

D.

Oxygen-IV-Monitor-Fluids: ______________________________

____

Vital Signs: ______________________________

____

Your Impression: ______________________________

____

CASE 30

Scenario (Actual EMS Call)

A 71-year-old male has had chest pain radiating to his neck for the past hour. He rates the pain as 5 on the 1 to 10 scale and describes it "like a heavy weight sitting on my chest." He denies nausea but is slightly short of breath. He does have a history of angina and prostate cancer. He is alert and oriented ×4. Skin is pale, warm, and dry. Vital signs are BP, 128/90; P, 180; and R, 18. As you connect him to the monitor he suddenly becomes unresponsive. The rhythm you see is the following:

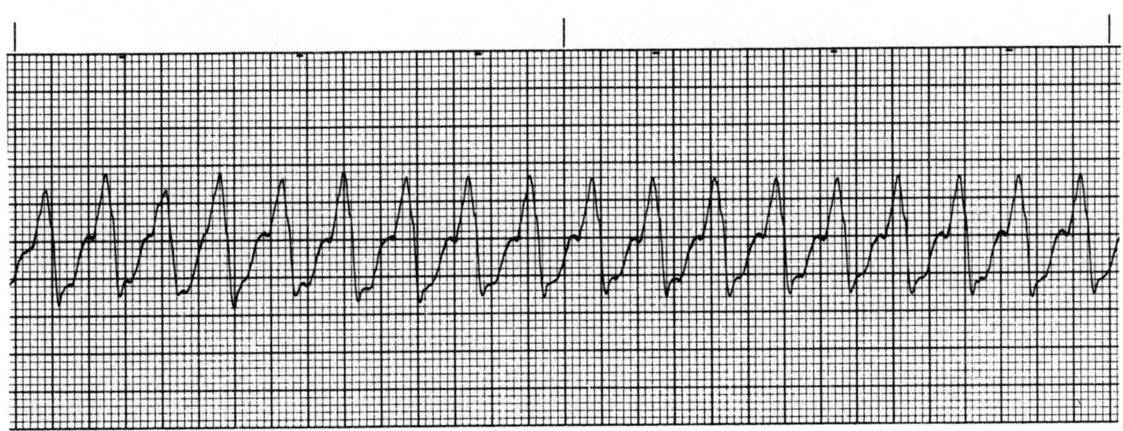

Identify the Rhythm

What is the rate? ____________ What is the rhythm (regular or irregular)? ____________

Is there a P wave before every QRS complex? ____________ Is there a QRS complex after every P wave? ____________

What is the P-R interval? ____________ QRS complex duration? ____________

Interpretation:

____

____

Case 30 Self-Test

In the spaces below give your treatment for the Primary Survey and Secondary Survey, plus the continued care under Oxygen-IV-Monitor-Fluids and Vital Signs. How would you care for this patient, and what orders would you expect from the physician? At the bottom list your potential diagnosis or impression of the patient's problem.

Primary Survey

A.

B.

C.

D.

Secondary Survey

A.

B.

C.

D.

Oxygen-IV-Monitor-Fluids: ______________________________

____

Vital Signs: ______________________________

____

Your Impression: ______________________________

____

CASE 31

Scenario

An 89-year-old female has difficulty breathing. She tells you it started 3 days ago and became worse today. She is also complaining of nonradiating chest pain on the right side. You note 3+ pedal edema and ascites along with jugular venous distention (JVD). She is using some accessory muscles to breathe but is able to speak in full sentences. Her medical history includes diabetes, angina, and hypertension. Medications are a nitroglycerin patch; digoxin, 0.25 mg; and Glucotrol. She is alert and oriented ×4. Skin is pale, warm, and dry. Lung sounds reveal wheezes throughout, with crackles to the midline bilateral. Vital signs are BP, 180/82; P, 150 and irregular; and R, 32. You see the following strip on the monitor:

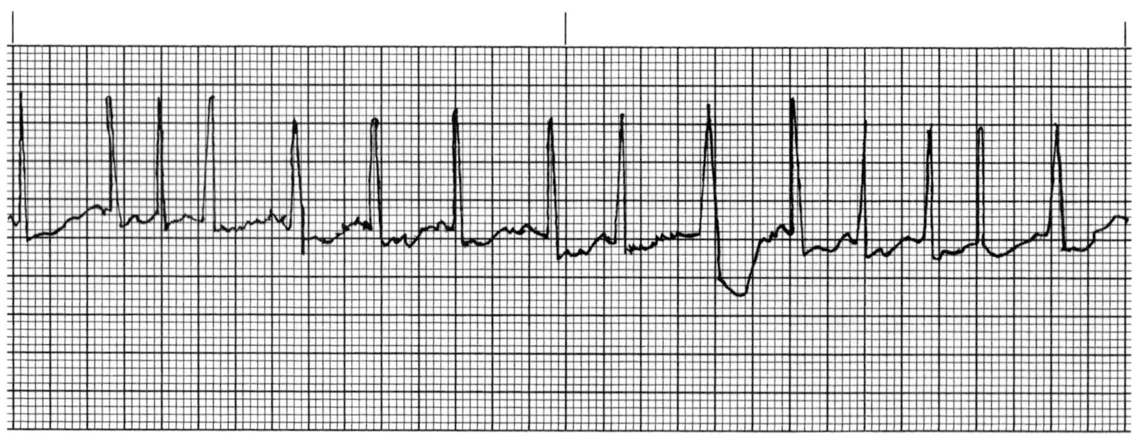

Identify the Rhythm

What is the rate? ____________ What is the rhythm (regular or irregular)? ____________

Is there a P wave before every QRS complex? ____________ Is there a QRS complex after every P wave? ____________

What is the P-R interval? ______________ QRS complex duration? ______________

Interpretation:

____

____

Case 31 Self-Test

In the spaces below give your treatment for the Primary Survey and Secondary Survey, plus the continued care under Oxygen-IV-Monitor-Fluids and Vital Signs. How would you care for this patient, and what orders would you expect from the physician? At the bottom list your potential diagnosis or impression of the patient's problem.

Primary Survey	***Secondary Survey***
A.	A.
B.	B.
C.	C.
D.	D.

Oxygen-IV-Monitor-Fluids: ______________________________

____

Vital Signs: ______________________________

____

Your Impression: ______________________________

____

CASE 32

Scenario (Actual EMS Call)

You are called for a 78-year-old female who went out on a very cold winter morning to get her mail, slipped, and fell. She was unable to get up because of right hip pain. The wind chill factor this morning was about 10° below zero, and she was lying there about 2 hours when someone found her. At present her level of consciousness is responsive to painful stimuli only. Her skin is very pale and cold to touch. Capillary refill is more than 5 seconds! Lung sounds are clear. Vital signs are BP, 98/56; P, 104 and irregular; and R, 10. You see the following on the monitor:

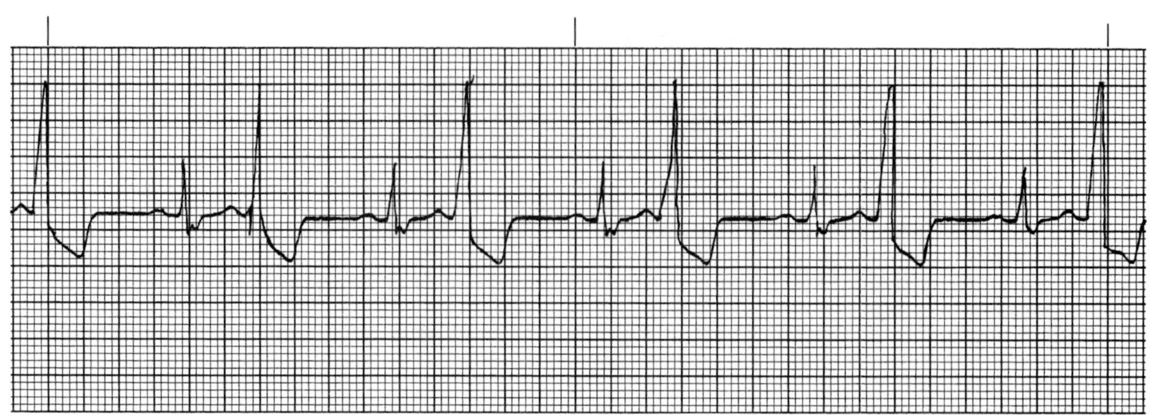

Identify the Rhythm

What is the rate? ______________ What is the rhythm (regular or irregular)? ______________

Is there a P wave before every QRS complex? ______________ Is there a QRS complex after every P wave? ______________

What is the P-R interval? ______________ QRS complex duration? ______________

Interpretation:

____

____

Case 32 Self-Test

In the spaces below give your treatment for the Primary Survey and Secondary Survey, plus the continued care under Oxygen-IV-Monitor-Fluids and Vital Signs. How would you care for this patient, and what orders would you expect from the physician? At the bottom list your potential diagnosis or impression of the patient's problem.

Primary Survey

A.

B.

C.

D.

Secondary Survey

A.

B.

C.

D.

Oxygen-IV-Monitor-Fluids: ____________________

____

Vital Signs: ____________________

____

Your Impression: ____________________

____

CASE 33

Scenario

You are attending a local football game, when a gentleman in his mid-40s collapses in front of you. You check—yes, he is breathing, and yes he does have a pulse. Whew! But there is no one with him to give you any information. Vital signs at present are P, 46 and regular and R, 14. EMS arrives within 3 minutes, and when they connect him to the monitor you see the following rhythm:

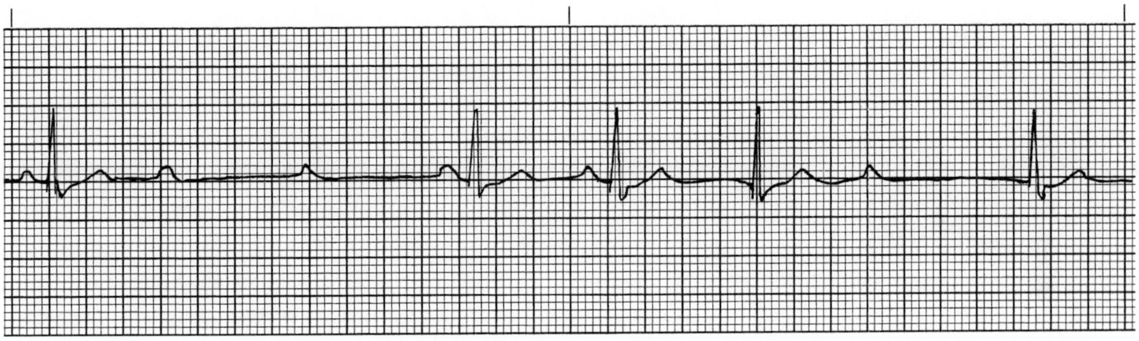

Identify the Rhythm

What is the rate? __________ What is the rhythm (regular or irregular)? __________

Is there a P wave before every QRS complex? __________ Is there a QRS complex after every P wave? __________

What is the P-R interval? __________ QRS complex duration? __________

Interpretation:

____

____

Case 33 Self-Test

In the spaces below give your treatment for the Primary Survey and Secondary Survey, plus the continued care under Oxygen-IV-Monitor-Fluids and Vital Signs. How would you care for this patient, and what orders would you expect from the physician? At the bottom list your potential diagnosis or impression of the patient's problem.

Primary Survey	*Secondary Survey*
A.	A.
B.	B.
C.	C.
D.	D.

Oxygen-IV-Monitor-Fluids: ______________________________

____

Vital Signs: ______________________________

____

Your Impression: ______________________________

____

CASE 34

Scenario

A 78-year-old female comes into the emergency department complaining of being extra tired for the past 1 to 2 weeks. She also states that at times it feels like her heart is beating irregularly. She denies any chest pain, syncope, or difficulty breathing. Her medical history includes coronary artery disease, angina, and high blood pressure. She is alert and oriented ×4 at present. Her skin is pink, warm, and dry. Vital signs are BP, 128/70; P, 96 and irregular; and R, 18. You see the following on the monitor:

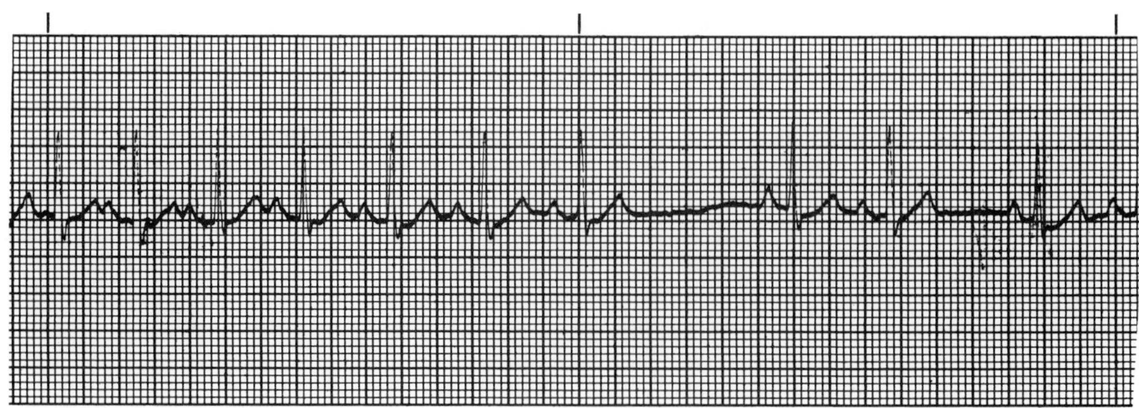

Identify the Rhythm

What is the rate? ____________ What is the rhythm (regular or irregular)? ____________

Is there a P wave before every QRS complex? ____________ Is there a QRS complex after every P wave? ____________

What is the P-R interval? ____________ QRS complex duration? ____________

Interpretation:

____

____

Case 34 Self-Test

In the spaces below give your treatment for the Primary Survey and Secondary Survey, plus the continued care under Oxygen-IV-Monitor-Fluids and Vital Signs. How would you care for this patient, and what orders would you expect from the physician? At the bottom list your potential diagnosis or impression of the patient's problem.

Primary Survey

A.

B.

C.

D.

Secondary Survey

A.

B.

C.

D.

Oxygen-IV-Monitor-Fluids: ____

____

Vital Signs: ____

____

Your Impression: ____

____

CASE 35

Scenario

You are called for a 41-year-old female who is complaining of "heart palpitations." She tells you it began about half an hour ago and is accompanied with weakness. She denies any chest pain, nausea, or shortness of breath. She does have a medical history of cardiac problems, angioplasty, and diabetes. Her medications include nitroglycerin as needed, diltiazem, and NPH insulin, 20 units in the morning and 20 units in the evening. She is alert and oriented ×4, and her skin is pink, warm, and dry. Vital signs are BP, 112/76; P, very weak and rapid; and R, 22. You see the following on the monitor:

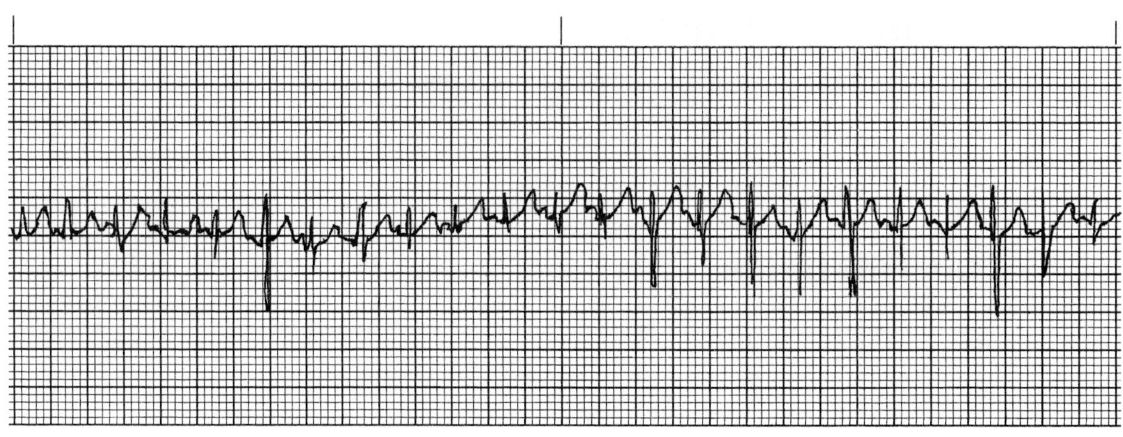

Identify the Rhythm

What is the rate? ____________ What is the rhythm (regular or irregular)? ____________

Is there a P wave before every QRS complex? ____________ Is there a QRS complex after every P wave? ____________

What is the P-R interval? ____________ QRS complex duration? ____________

Interpretation:

____

____

Case 35 Self-Test

In the spaces below give your treatment for the Primary Survey and Secondary Survey, plus the continued care under Oxygen-IV-Monitor-Fluids and Vital Signs. How would you care for this patient, and what orders would you expect from the physician? At the bottom list your potential diagnosis or impression of the patient's problem.

Primary Survey

A.

B.

C.

D.

Secondary Survey

A.

B.

C.

D.

Oxygen-IV-Monitor-Fluids: ______________________________

____

Vital Signs: ______________________________

____

Your Impression: ______________________________

____

CASE 36

Scenario (Actual EMS Call)

You are presented with a 58-year-old male with cardiac history and an implanted defibrillator who tells you that his defibrillator has discharged two or three times in the past hour. He was mowing the lawn the first time it discharged, and the jolt sent him to the ground. At present he is alert and oriented ×4. His skin is pink, warm, and dry. Vital signs are BP, 160/100; P, 120 but very irregular; and R, 24. You see the following on the monitor:

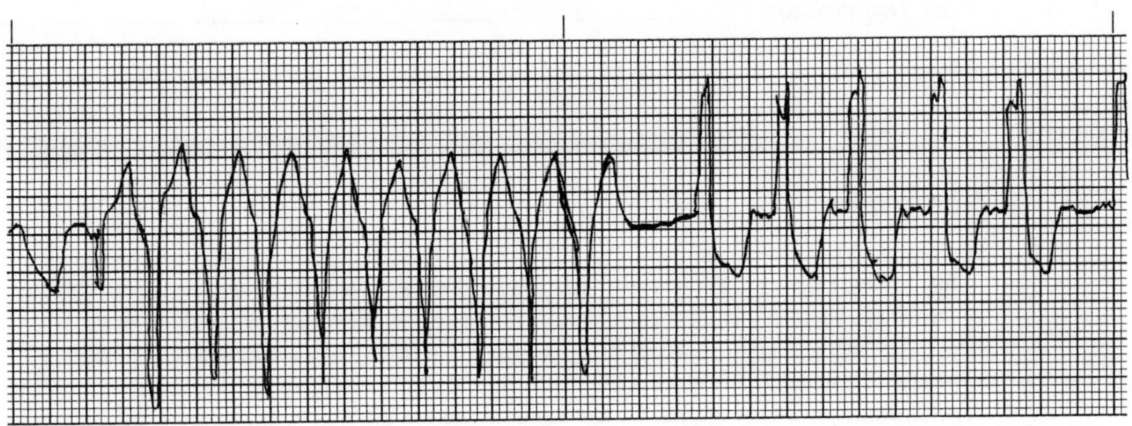

Identify the Rhythm

What is the rate? ____________ What is the rhythm (regular or irregular)? ____________

Is there a P wave before every QRS complex? ____________ Is there a QRS complex after every P wave? ____________

What is the P-R interval? ____________ QRS complex duration? ____________

Interpretation:

____

____

Case 36 Self-Test

In the spaces below give your treatment for the Primary Survey and Secondary Survey, plus the continued care under Oxygen-IV-Monitor-Fluids and Vital Signs. How would you care for this patient, and what orders would you expect from the physician? At the bottom list your potential diagnosis or impression of the patient's problem.

Primary Survey

A.

B.

C.

D.

Secondary Survey

A.

B.

C.

D.

Oxygen-IV-Monitor-Fluids: ____________________

____

Vital Signs: ____________________

____

Your Impression: ____________________

____

CASE 37

Scenario

A 63-year-old male is complaining of an acute onset of left shoulder pain accompanied with numbness and tingling in the left arm, along with shortness of breath. He denies nausea, dizziness, or weakness. He tells you this began about 4 hours ago and he took Advil with no relief. He also denies any medical history except for gout. He is not taking any medications at present. He is alert and oriented ×4. His skin is pink, warm, and dry. Vital signs are BP, 114/60; P, 40 and regular; R, 26; and Sao_2 = 97%. On the monitor you see the following:

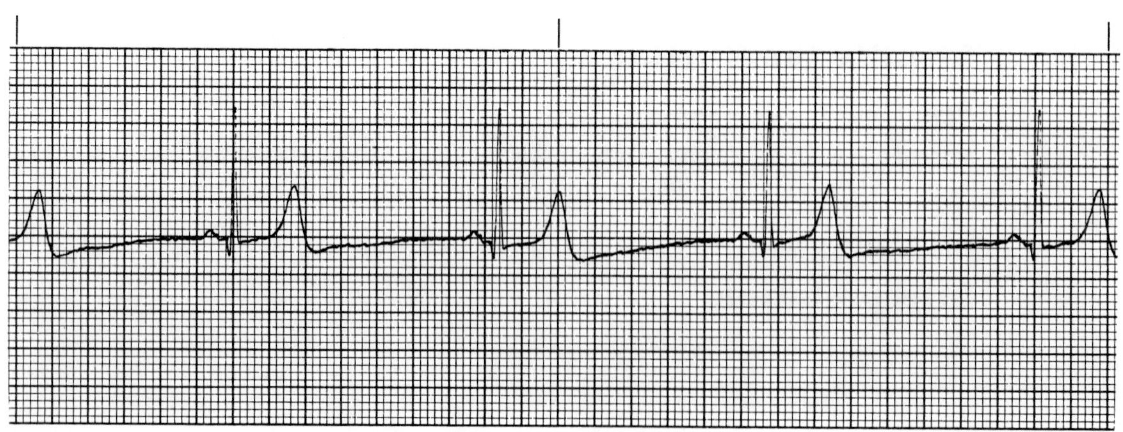

Identify the Rhythm

What is the rate? ____________ What is the rhythm (regular or irregular)? ____________

Is there a P wave before every QRS complex? ____________ Is there a QRS complex after every P wave? ____________

What is the P-R interval? ______________ QRS complex duration? ______________

Interpretation:

____

____

Case 37 Self-Test

In the spaces below give your treatment for the Primary Survey and Secondary Survey, plus the continued care under Oxygen-IV-Monitor-Fluids and Vital Signs. How would you care for this patient, and what orders would you expect from the physician? At the bottom list your potential diagnosis or impression of the patient's problem.

Primary Survey	*Secondary Survey*
A.	A.
B.	B.
C.	C.
D.	D.

Oxygen-IV-Monitor-Fluids: ____

____

Vital Signs: ____

____

Your Impression: ____

____

CASE 38

Scenario

An 18-year-old jogger is brought into the emergency department after running a 10-km marathon. He is complaining of abdominal cramps and light-headedness. He has no medical history and is not taking any medications. He is alert and oriented ×4. His skin is tan, cool, and moist. A finger-stick with the glucometer reveals a blood sugar level of 110. Vital signs are BP, 100/56; P, 92 and irregular; and R, 20. You see the following on the monitor:

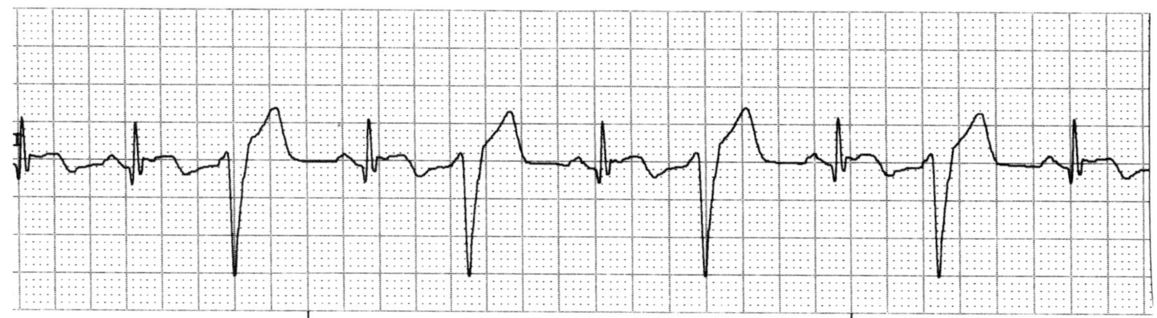

Identify the Rhythm

What is the rate? ____________ What is the rhythm (regular or irregular)? ____________

Is there a P wave before every QRS complex? ____________ Is there a QRS complex after every P wave? ____________

What is the P-R interval? ____________ QRS complex duration? ____________

Interpretation:

____

____

Case 38 Self-Test

In the spaces below give your treatment for the Primary Survey and Secondary Survey, plus the continued care under Oxygen-IV-Monitor-Fluids and Vital Signs. How would you care for this patient, and what orders would you expect from the physician? At the bottom list your potential diagnosis or impression of the patient's problem.

Primary Survey

A.

B.

C.

D.

Secondary Survey

A.

B.

C.

D.

Oxygen-IV-Monitor-Fluids: ____

____

Vital Signs: ____

____

Your Impression: ____

____

CASE 39

Scenario

Treat the patient, not the monitor

A 61-year-old female is your patient. She came into the emergency department complaining of severe chest pain. She rates it as a 10 on a 1 to 10 scale and says it radiates to her left arm. She is also complaining of dizziness and shortness of breath. Her only medical history is cataract surgery and a pulmonary embolism 5 years ago. She is not taking any medications. She is alert and oriented ×4; skin is pink, warm, and dry. Her vital signs when she came in were BP, 118/78; P, 68; and R, 26. You are closely watching the monitor and everything is going great when her granddaughter, age 6, asks, "Why can't I wake my Grandma up?" The monitor is showing the following:

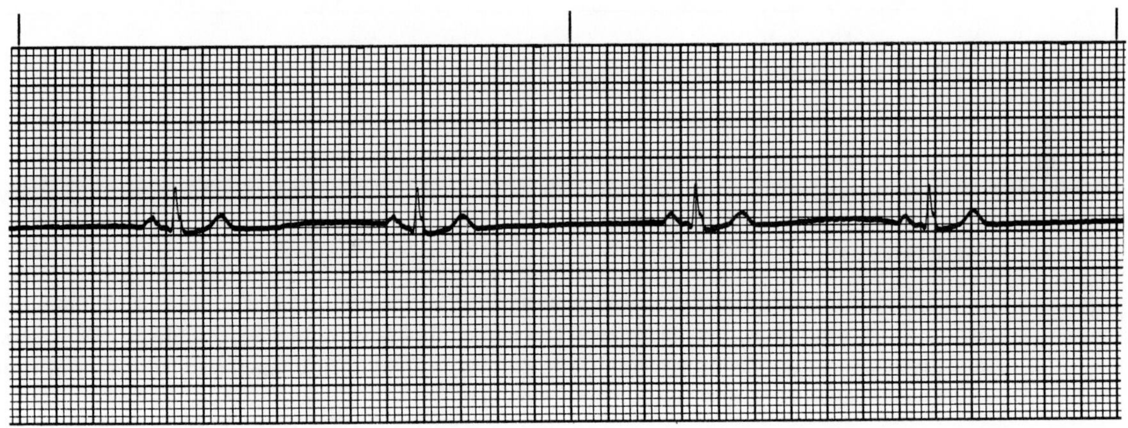

Identify the Rhythm

What is the rate? ____________ What is the rhythm (regular or irregular)? ____________

Is there a P wave before every QRS complex? ____________ Is there a QRS complex after every P wave? ____________

What is the P-R interval? ______________ QRS complex duration? ______________

Interpretation:

____

____

Case 39 Self-Test

In the spaces below give your treatment for the Primary Survey and Secondary Survey, plus the continued care under Oxygen-IV-Monitor-Fluids and Vital Signs. How would you care for this patient, and what orders would you expect from the physician? At the bottom list your potential diagnosis or impression of the patient's problem.

Primary Survey

A.

B.

C.

D.

Secondary Survey

A.

B.

C.

D.

Oxygen-IV-Monitor-Fluids: ________________________________

____

Vital Signs: ________________________________

____

Your Impression: ________________________________

____

CASE 40

Scenario

You are presented with a 71-year-old male in full cardiac arrest. He was down 1 to 2 minutes before CPR was initiated on the scene. The paramedics have intubated, established IV access, and given the appropriate drug therapy. The rhythm changed as he came through the door of your emergency department, and you see the following:

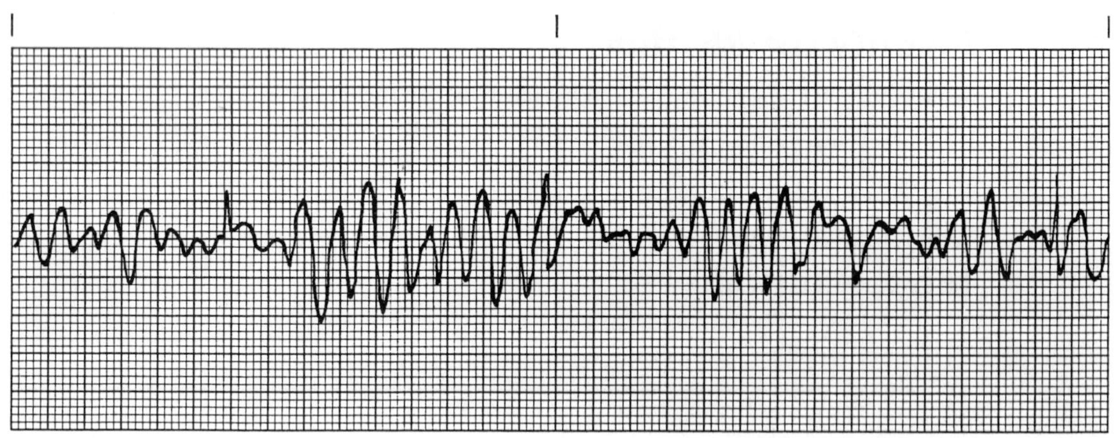

Identify the Rhythm

What is the rate? ______________ What is the rhythm (regular or irregular)? ______________

Is there a P wave before every QRS complex? ______________ Is there a QRS complex after every P wave? ______________

What is the P-R interval? ______________ QRS complex duration? ______________

Interpretation:

____

____

You have shocked the patient at 200 J, 300 J, and 360 J and continued giving the epinephrine every 3 minutes. The ET tube appears to be in place, and the IV is well established. Your physician orders amiodarone 300-mg IV bolus to be given. Just as you finish administering the amiodarone, you look up at the monitor and see the following:

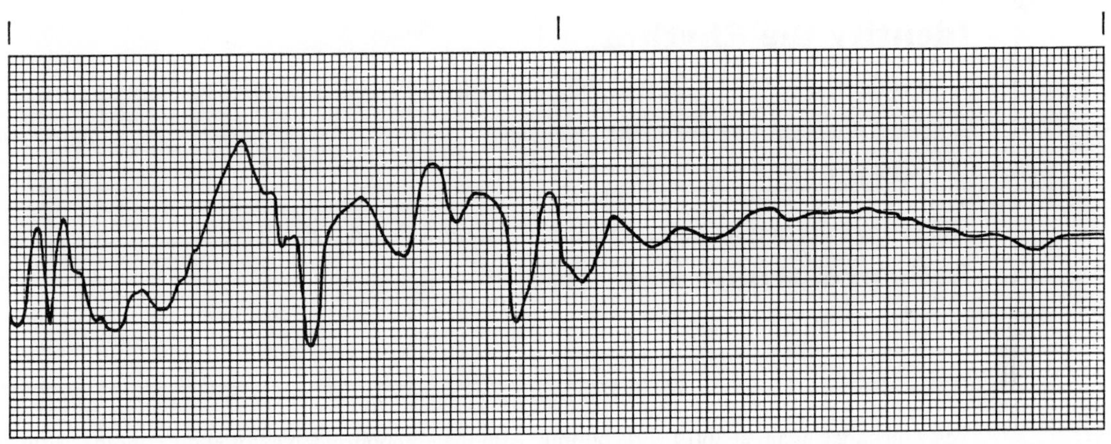

Identify the Rhythm

What is the rate? ______________ What is the rhythm (regular or irregular)? ______________

Is there a P wave before every QRS complex? ______________ Is there a QRS complex after every P wave? ______________

What is the P-R interval? ______________ QRS complex duration? ______________

Interpretation:

____

____

Now the patient is going into asystole. You are continuing with the epinephrine every 3 minutes. Also, you have given atropine 1-mg IV push. You are preparing the transcutaneous pacer because the patient has been in asystole less than 10 minutes, when you suddenly see the following:

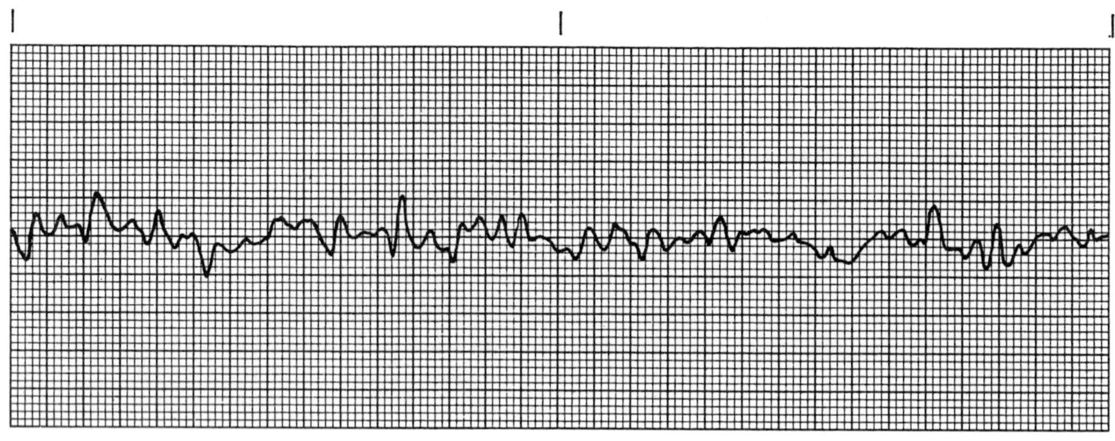

Identify the Rhythm

What is the rate? ____________ What is the rhythm (regular or irregular)? ____________

Is there a P wave before every QRS complex? ____________ Is there a QRS complex after every P wave? ____________

What is the P-R interval? ____________ QRS complex duration? ____________

Interpretation:

____

____

Yes, you shock again at 360 J and continue with the epinephrine. Next you give another bolus of amiodarone: 150-mg IV bolus followed by 20-ml normal saline flush. You use the *drug—shock—drug—shock* method. There still is no pulse, and you are getting ready to shock again when you notice the following:

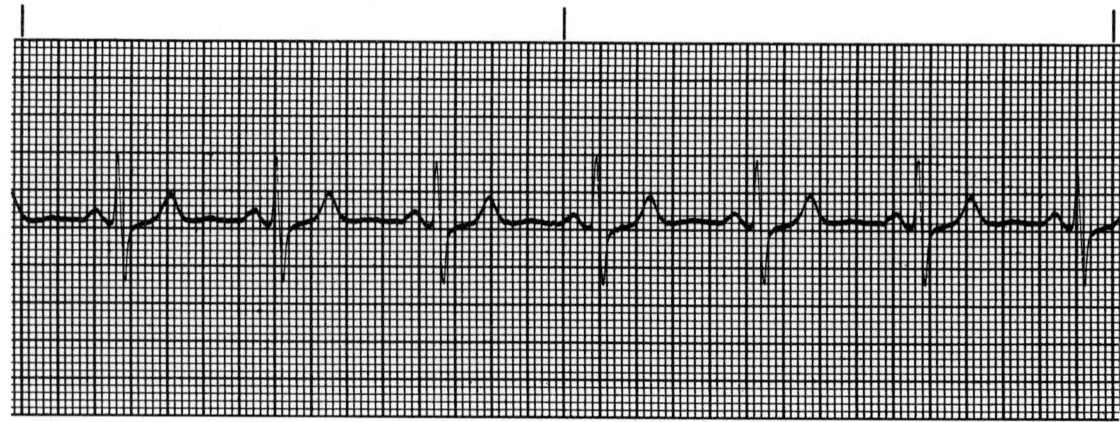

Identify the Rhythm

What is the rate? ____________ What is the rhythm (regular or irregular)? ____________

Is there a P wave before every QRS complex? ____________ Is there a QRS complex after every P wave? ____________

What is the P-R interval? ________________ QRS complex duration? ______________

Interpretation:

____

____

Now that you are over the surprise, does the patient have a pulse? Is the patient breathing? Is there a blood pressure? Yes, there is a pulse, and no the patient is not breathing! So you continue to provide artificial respirations. Yes, there is a low blood pressure. The artificial ventilations are continued, and chest compressions are stopped. You are in the process of hanging a dopamine drip, when the rhythm changes again.

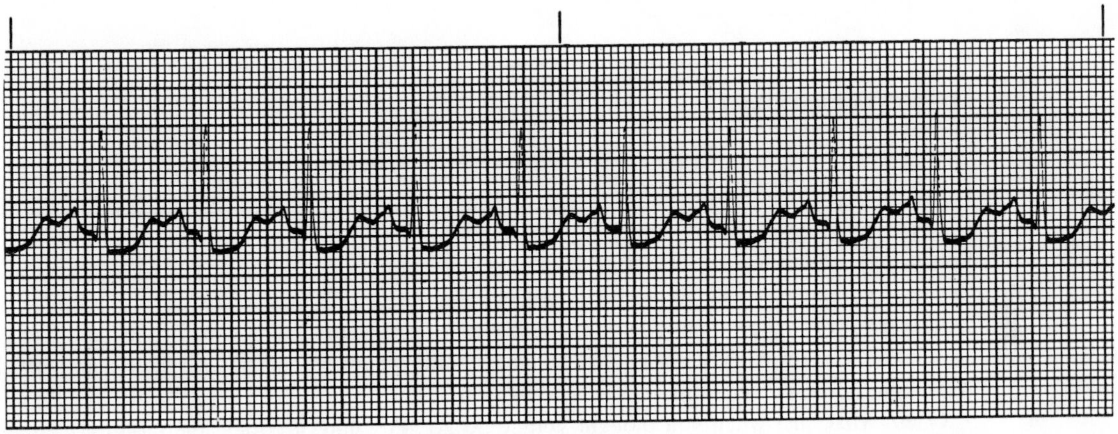

Identify the Rhythm

What is the rate? ____________ What is the rhythm (regular or irregular)? ____________

Is there a P wave before every QRS complex? ____________ Is there a QRS complex after every P wave? ____________

What is the P-R interval? ________________ QRS complex duration? ______________

Interpretation:

____

____

All right, things are looking good! You can take a deep breath now and relax a little. However, do not relax too much; take another look at that monitor!

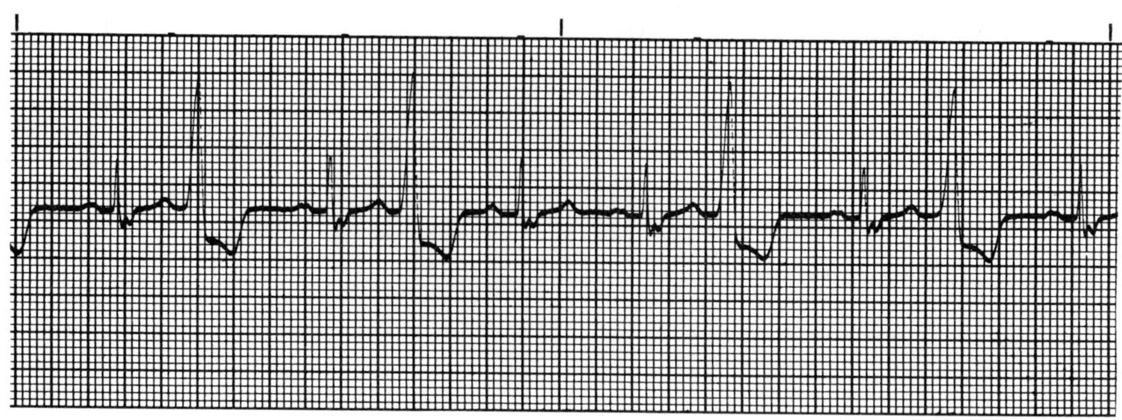

Identify the Rhythm

What is the rate? ____________ What is the rhythm (regular or irregular)? ____________

Is there a P wave before every QRS complex? ____________ Is there a QRS complex after every P wave? ____________

What is the P-R interval? ____________ QRS complex duration? ____________

Interpretation:

____

____

Now things are not too bad. Continue with the dopamine drip starting at 5- to 10-mcg/kg and titrating to effect. Because you seem to have an abundance of PVCs at this time, you might try another bolus (150 mg) of amiodarone. The last thing you want right now is for the patient to go back into V fib. Yes, he still has a pulse and he is being well oxygenated with the ET and BVM. Well, I guess you can call this code a success.

Guess what, just when you thought you could go get a cup of coffee, the monitor changed again. There is no pulse at this time!

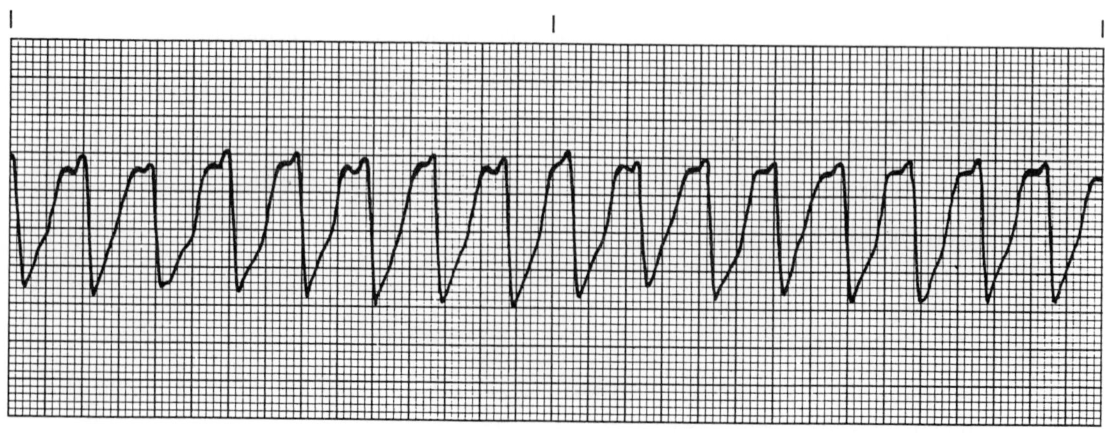

Identify the Rhythm

What is the rate? ______________ What is the rhythm (regular or irregular)? ______________

Is there a P wave before every QRS complex? ______________ Is there a QRS complex after every P wave? ______________

What is the P-R interval? ______________ QRS complex duration? ______________

Interpretation:

____

____

Oh my goodness, where did you leave off? Oh yes, epinephrine was being given every 3 minutes, and you had done the last shock at 360 J. This time you simply continue with a shock at 360 J, begin CPR again, and continue the epinephrine at 1-mg IV push every 3 minutes. Just as you are getting ready to shock again (you are getting tired), the family arrives and states that this patient has terminal cancer and is a DNR (do not resuscitate). You are getting ready to stop all further efforts when you look at the monitor and see the following:

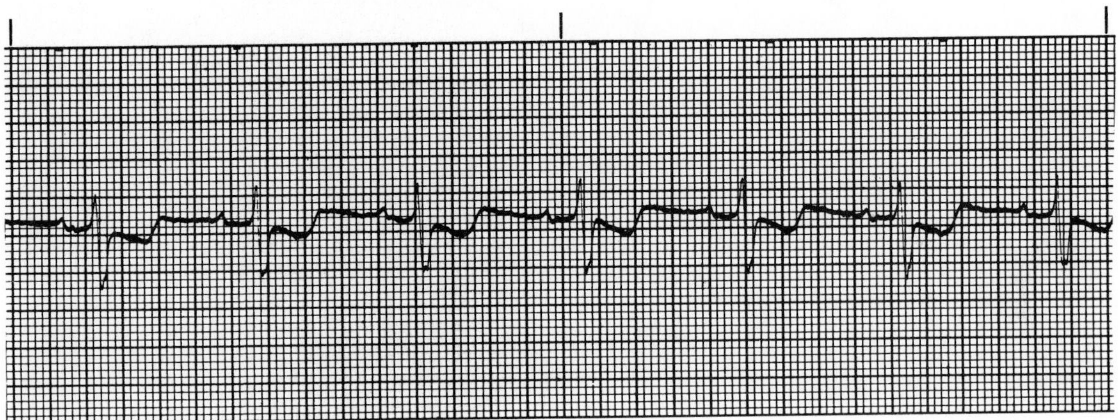

Identify the Rhythm

What is the rate? ______________ What is the rhythm (regular or irregular)? ______________

Is there a P wave before every QRS complex? ______________ Is there a QRS complex after every P wave? ______________

What is the P-R interval? ______________ QRS complex duration? ______________

Interpretation:

____

____

This scenario is not far from true life. You must be on your toes, know your ACLS protocols, and be able to identify rhythms. A patient undergoing cardiac arrest can certainly go from one rhythm into another very rapidly. You must be alert and know what drugs to use and when not to use them. There will be times when the rhythms change so fast that you literally do not have time to draw up and push the drugs. Your quick actions, expert knowledge, and ability to keep a sense of organization at a time when there is only chaos are what will save the patient.

Now, in this case, because the patient is already intubated, it will be a decision for the family to make as to whether they want the ET tube pulled, especially because now there is a normal sinus rhythm. These are issues not discussed in this book because they involve hospital policies, in addition to moral and legal issues.

However, you did a great job, if you identified all the rhythms correctly. This can and does happen, so be prepared.

Appendix

Answer Key

CHAPTER 1 SELF-TEST

1. d—In the mediastinum or middle of the thorax
2. False
3. True
4. d—Pumps oxygenated blood to the lungs where it picks up oxygen
5. c—Double-walled sac enclosing and protecting the heart
6. b—Epicardium, myocardium, and endocardium
7. (1) Vena cava, (2) right atrium, (3) right ventricle, (4) pulmonary artery, (5) lungs, (6) pulmonary vein, (7) left atrium, (8) left ventricle, (9) aorta
8. True
9. (1) Reduce friction between the layers, (2) hold the heart securely in place in the mediastinum, (3) protect the heart from bacteria
10. Myocardium
11. True
12. (1) Posterior descending artery and (2) right margin or acute marginal artery
13. (1) Left anterior descending artery and (2) left circumflex artery
14. b—Starling's law
15. True
16. Tricuspid and mitral valves
17. Tricuspid, pulmonic, mitral or bicuspid, aortic
18. False
19. d—Passive
20. True
21. Parasympathetic

22. Bicuspid
23. Norepinephrine
24. Stroke volume × heart rate
25. True
26. Sympathetic and parasympathetic nervous system
27. Automaticity: b—the ability of specialized cells in the conduction system to initiate an electrical impulse spontaneously
    Excitability: d—the ability of the cardiac cells to respond to an electrical impulse
    Conductivity: a—the ability to transmit an impulse from one cardiac cell to another
    Contractility: c—when the cardiac cells are able to contract after receiving a stimulus
28. b—Right atrium
29. a—Semilunar valves

CHAPTER 2 SELF-TEST

1. c—Pumps blood to the lungs and circulatory system
2. a—Contracts and the chambers empty
3. Negatively
4. True
5. Electrical
6. SA node, internodal pathways, AV node, AV junction, bundle of His, right and left bundle branches, Purkinje fibers
7. False
8. False
9. True
10. False
11. Contractility
12. a—Automatcity
13. Conductivity = M
    Contractility = M
    Automaticity = E
    Excitability = E
14. c—Sodium moves into the cell rapidly, while calcium moves in slowly and potassium begins to leave the cell.
15. True
16. True
17. Negative, positive

18. True

19. True

20. True

21. a—SA node

22. False

23. Einthoven's triangle

24. c—From the right arm to the left leg

25. Upward

26. True

27. Common causes of ECG interference:
    Muscle tremor
    Patient movement
    Excessive chest hair
    Loose electrodes
    Improper grounding
    60-cycle interference
    Electrodes placed over bony prominences, skin folds, breast tissue, or scar tissue

28. Time, voltage

29. b—0.04 second

30. 6 seconds

31. Depolarization

32. c—P-R interval

33. 0.12 to 0.20 second

34. c—0.04 to 0.10 second

35. Repolarization

36. Seven steps for determining an ECG rhythm:
    Determine the rate
    Determine the rhythm (regular or irregular)
    Evaluate the P waves for size, shape, and duration
    Evaluate the P-R interval and duration
    Evaluate the QRS complex. Is it wide or narrow? Is it of normal duration? Is it elevated or depressed?
    Is there a P wave before every QRS complex? Is there a QRS complex after every P wave?
    Evaluate the T wave

37. Automaticity: d—ability to initiate electrical impulses in the pacemaker cells
    Conductivity: b—transmits electrical impulses from one cell to another
    Excitability: a—cardiac cells have the ability to respond to an outside stimulus
    Contractility: c—causes cardiac cells to contract or shorten

38. d—60
39. d—All of the above

CHAPTER 3 SELF-TEST

1. SA node. The SA node is the primary pacemaker in the right atrium, 60 to 100 beats per minute.
2. 64 P waves per minute. In a sinus rhythm there is always a P wave for every QRS complex.
3. Least negative. During the resting phase of the depolarization-repolarization cycle, the SA node has the least negative charge.
4. False. Sinus bradycardia has an intrinsic rate of 40 to 60 beats per minute.
5. False. Sinus rhythms usually have the pacer site originating at the SA node.
6. b. Sinus bradycardia may be normal in a young athletic-type person or may be serious in a person with heart disease and needs immediate attention.
7. 60 to 100 beats per minute: d—normal sinus rhythm
   Less than 60 beats per minute: e—sinus bradycardia
   101 to 180 beats per minute: b—sinus tachycardia
   a—Sinus arrhythmia is a normal variant that occurs with respirations and the changes of intrathoracic pressure
   f—Sick sinus syndrome is basically either a sinus node dysfunction or the failure of an escape pacemaker
   c—Sinus arrest is failure of SA node to initiate an impulse resulting in the absence of P waves, QRS complexes, and T waves
8. True. If it is a sinus rhythm, it has a P wave, a QRS complex, and a T wave.
9. Cardiac compromise with sinus bradycardia may be caused by the following:
   Drugs such as beta blockers, anticholinesterase, digitalis, and morphine
   Myocardial infarction, which may increase vagal tone
   Patients with hyperkalemia, patients with intracranial pressure
   Vomiting, a bowel movement, or any other act of vagal stimulation
   Patients with sick sinus syndrome
   Athletes, because their hearts are well-conditioned, allowing them to maintain the stroke volume with reduced effort
10. SA node. In sinus arrest the failure of the SA node to initiate an impulse results in the absence of a P wave, a QRS complex, and a T wave.
11. d. Any sinus rhythm usually has a P-R interval of 0.12 to 0.20 second.
12. True. Sinus tachycardia is usually without symptoms.
13. c. Sinus tachycardia has an intrinsic rate of 101 to 180 beats per minute.
14. d. Absence of P wave, QRS complex, and T wave
15. False. This is an irregular rhythm because you are missing an entire P-QRS-T complex.
16. d. A sick sinus syndrome may also be known as:
    Tachy-bradycardic syndrome

Brady-tachycardic syndrome
Sick sinus syndrome
Sinus arrhythmia

CHAPTER 3 ECG PRACTICE STRIPS

Figure 3-1 Normal sinus rhythm
Regular
Rate: 68
P-R interval = 0.19 second
QRS complex = 0.06 second
Is there a P wave *before* every QRS complex? Yes
Is there a QRS complex *after* every P wave? Yes

Figure 3-2 Normal sinus rhythm
Regular
Rate: 77
P-R interval = 0.16 second
QRS complex = 0.08 second
Is there a P wave *before* every QRS complex? Yes
Is there a QRS complex *after* every P wave? Yes

Figure 3-3 Sinus tachycardia
Regular
Rate: 125
P-R interval = 0.16 second
QRS complex = 0.07 second
Is there a P wave *before* every QRS complex? Yes
Is there a QRS complex *after* every P wave? Yes

Figure 3-4 Sinus arrest
Underlying rhythm is regular
Rate: 83 (underlying rhythm)
P-R interval = 0.20 second
QRS complex = 0.08 second
Is there a P wave *before* every QRS complex? Yes
Is there a QRS complex *after* every P wave? Yes
You have a long pause where approximately four normal beats should have been

Figure 3-5 Sinus bradycardia
Regular
Rate: 42
P-R interval = 0.16 second
QRS complex = 0.06 second
Is there a P wave *before* every QRS complex? Yes
Is there a QRS complex *after* every P wave? Yes

Figure 3-6 Sinus tachycardia
Regular

Rate: 150
P-R interval = 0.14 second
QRS complex = 0.05 second
Is there a P wave *before* every QRS complex? Yes
Is there a QRS complex *after* every P wave? Yes

Figure 3-7 Normal sinus rhythm
Regular
Rate: 65
P-R interval = 0.16 second
QRS complex = 0.06 second
Is there a P wave *before* every QRS complex? Yes
Is there a QRS complex *after* every P wave? Yes

Figure 3-8 Sinus bradycardia
Regular
Rate: 54
P-R interval = 0.20 second
QRS complex = 0.07 second
Is there a P wave *before* every QRS complex? Yes
Is there a QRS complex *after* every P wave? Yes

Figure 3-9 Normal sinus rhythm
Regular
Rate: 75
P-R interval = 0.20 second
QRS complex = 0.08 second
Is there a P wave *before* every QRS complex? Yes
Is there a QRS complex *after* every P wave? Yes

Figure 3-10 Normal sinus rhythm
Regular
Rate: 68
P-R interval = 0.19 second
QRS complex = 0.06 second
Is there a P wave *before* every QRS complex? Yes
Is there a QRS complex *after* every P wave? Yes

Figure 3-11 Normal sinus rhythm
Regular
Rate: 88
P-R interval = 0.18 second
QRS complex = 0.06 second
Is there a P wave *before* every QRS complex? Yes
Is there a QRS complex *after* every P wave? Yes

Figure 3-12 Sinus tachycardia
Regular
Rate: 104

P-R interval = 0.20 second
QRS complex = 0.05 second
Is there a P wave *before* every QRS complex? Yes
Is there a QRS complex *after* every P wave? Yes

Figure 3-13 Sinus tachycardia
Regular
Rate: 115
P-R interval = 0.16 second
QRS complex = 0.06 second
Is there a P wave *before* every QRS complex? Yes
Is there a QRS complex *after* every P wave? Yes

Figure 3-14 Sinus bradycardia
Regular
Rate: 47
P-R interval = 0.16 second
QRS complex = 0.05 second
Is there a P wave *before* every QRS complex? Yes
Is there a QRS complex *after* every P wave? Yes

Figure 3-15 Sinus bradycardia
Regular
Rate: 42
P-R interval = 0.16 second
QRS complex = 0.06 second
Is there a P wave *before* every QRS complex? Yes
Is there a QRS complex *after* every P wave? Yes

CHAPTER 3, CASE 1

Scenario

This rhythm is a **normal sinus rhythm** at a rate of 75 beats per minute
Rhythm = regular; P-R interval = 0.19 second; QRS complex = 0.07 second
Is there a P wave *before* every QRS? Yes
Is there a QRS complex *after* every P wave? Yes

Primary Survey

The airway is open, the patient is breathing without difficulty, and neither chest compressions nor defibrillation is needed.

Secondary Survey

Airway: adequate
Breathing: apply oxygen, obtain a pulse oximetry
Circulation: cardiac monitor, IV access, 12-lead ECG, initial vital signs
Impression: possible acute myocardial infarction

Oxygen-IV-Monitor-Fluids

Continue the oxygen, cardiac monitoring; no fluids are needed. Obtain a chest x-ray; get the initial lab work to include complete blood cell count (CBC), chemistry, and cardiac enzymes
Sublingual nitroglycerin would be in order to see if the chest pain could be relieved
Hang any needed drips such as nitroglycerin, heparin, thrombolytics

Vital Signs

Ongoing vital signs; monitor heart rate, blood pressure, respirations, and temperature

Rationale

Any patient with chest pain, especially older than 30 years, must be suspected of having an MI until proven otherwise. This patient is having midsternal chest pain along with several associated cardiac symptoms (e.g., the pain radiates to the left arm, the pain occurred while he was at rest, and the patient was diaphoretic). In addition, he rated the pain as a 7 on the 1 to 10 scale (10 being the worst pain he ever felt). Also to consider is the fact chest pain may be caused by many other medical problems, such as muscle strain, pleurisy, pneumonia, bronchitis, and pericarditis. Even though the rhythm is normal sinus, the patient could still be having an MI. Approximately 50% of all patients with MIs have a normal ECG initially. An MI will remain on top of the list of suspected problems because of the sudden onset. He will need a complete workup and most likely a couple of days in the CCU for observation.

CHAPTER 3, CASE 2

Scenario

This rhythm is a **sinus bradycardia** at a rate of 52 beats per minute
Rhythm = regular; P-R interval = 0.16 second; QRS complex = 0.05 second
Is there a P wave *before* every QRS complex? Yes
Is there a QRS complex *after* every P wave? Yes

Primary Survey

The airway is open, the patient is breathing without difficulty, and neither chest compression nor defibrillation is needed.

Secondary Survey

Airway: adequate
Breathing: apply oxygen; obtain a pulse oximetry
Circulation: cardiac monitor, IV access, 12-lead ECG, initial vital signs
Impression: rule out a possible MI

Oxygen-IV-Monitor-Fluids

Continue the oxygen, cardiac monitoring, obtain blood for lab work. Are fluids needed? Probably not until he has had a complete workup.

Vital Signs

Ongoing vital signs; monitor the heart rate and check the blood pressure every 5 minutes; check respirations and temperature

Rationale

Because the patient is age 50, plus the associated symptoms along with the low pulse rate, the patient is placed in the risk category for a possible MI. You are just being cautious by giving him oxygen, monitoring his ECG rhythm, and obtaining IV access, just in case he needs drug therapy. He could very well be experiencing cardiac problems. The symptoms mentioned are most likely due to the sore throat and possible ear infection. His exercising (jogging 5 days a week) would explain the sinus bradycardia. This is normal in athletic-type patients.

CHAPTER 3, CASE 3

Scenario

This rhythm is a **symptomatic sinus bradycardia** at a rate of 42 beats per minute
Rhythm = regular; P-R interval = 0.20 second; QRS complex = 0.06 second
Is there a P wave *before* every QRS complex? Yes
Is there a QRS complex *after* every P wave? Yes

Primary Survey

The airway is open and the patient is breathing without difficulty; no chest compression or defibrillation is needed.

Secondary Survey

Airway: adequate
Breathing: apply oxygen; obtain a pulse oximetry
Circulation: cardiac monitor, IV access, 12-lead ECG, initial vital signs
Impression: workup for a probable MI

Oxygen-IV-Monitor-Fluids

Continue the oxygen, cardiac monitoring, obtain blood for lab work including cardiac enzymes. Are fluids needed? Yes, because he is very symptomatic, but make sure the lungs are clear first. Administer atropine 0.5- to 1-mg IV push, which you may repeat every 3 to 5 minutes up to a total of 0.04 mg/kg. Have the temporary pacer ready just in case the atropine does not increase the rate. You may have to hang dopamine if the blood pressure drops.

Vital Signs

Ongoing vital signs; monitor the heart rate and check the blood pressure every 5 minutes; check respirations and temperature

Rationale

In this case your actions need to be quick, because this patient may very well go into cardiac arrest because his pulse already dropped from 78 beats per minute to 38 to 40 beats per minute. Any patient who has bradycardia accompanied with chest pain and associated symptoms is probably having an MI. With symptomatic bradycardia, atropine is the first drug of choice along with a fluid challenge as long as the lungs are clear. If the blood pressure is under 100 systolic, consider dopamine and definitely consider transcutaneous pacing to increase the heart rate. By increasing the heart rate, you increase the cardiac output.

CHAPTER 3, CASE 4

Scenario

This rhythm is a **sinus tachycardia** at a rate of 136 beats per minute
Rhythm = regular; P-R interval = 0.16 second; QRS = 0.06 second
Is there a P wave *before* every QRS complex? Yes
Is there a QRS complex *after* every P wave? Yes

Primary Survey

The airway is open and the patient is breathing without difficulty; no chest compressions or defibrillation is needed.

Secondary Survey

Airway: adequate
Breathing: apply oxygen; obtain a pulse oximetry
Circulation: cardiac monitor, IV access, 12-lead ECG, initial vital signs
Impression: probable dehydration

Oxygen-IV-Monitor-Fluids

Continue the oxygen, cardiac monitoring, obtain blood for lab work. Are fluids needed? Yes, because she appears to be dehydrated, but make sure the lungs are clear first.

Vital Signs

Ongoing vital signs, monitor the heart rate, the blood pressure, respirations, and temperature

Rationale

The patient has sinus tachycardia because of the fever and possible dehydration. Oxygen always helps. She needs fluid replacement for the questionable dehydration. She also needs cardiac monitoring because of her age. It never hurts to place the patient on the monitor. At times the monitor gives you clues that you might have otherwise missed.

CHAPTER 3, CASE 5

Scenario

This rhythm is a **sinus arrest** at a rate of 55 beats per minute (the underlying rhythm is 68-70 beats per minute)
Rhythm = irregular; P-R interval = 0.20 second; QRS complex = 0.06 second
Is there a P wave *before* every QRS complex? Yes
Is there a QRS complex *after* every P wave? Yes
There is a completely dropped P-QRS-T, leaving a pause where the dropped beat should have occurred.

Primary Survey

The airway is open, the patient is breathing without difficulty, and neither chest compressions nor defibrillation is needed.

Secondary Survey

Airway: adequate
Breathing: apply oxygen; obtain a pulse oximetry
Circulation: cardiac monitor, IV access, 12-lead ECG, initial vital signs
Impression: possible cardiac disease

Oxygen-IV-Monitor-Fluids

Continue the oxygen, cardiac monitoring, obtain blood for lab work. Are fluids needed? No, not at this time because his vital signs are normal.

Vital Signs

Ongoing vital signs; monitor the heart rate and check the blood pressure every 5 minutes; check respirations and temperature

Rationale

The patient is having periods of sinus arrest, which caused the dizziness and eventually led to the syncope. If any further problems develop, atropine would be the drug of choice. If the sinus arrest does not resolve after the atropine is given, then consider the transcutaneous pacemaker. Sinus arrest is the failure of the SA node to initiate an impulse and can lead to cardiac arrest.

CHAPTER 4 SELF-TEST

1. Altered automaticity
2. d—PAC stands for premature atrial contraction
3. Syncope, hypotension, dizziness, or altered level of consciousness are all possible signs and symptoms of decreased cardiac output

4. c—The rate for supraventricular tachycardia or PAT is 150 to 250 beats per minute
5. Normal sinus rhythm: c—60 to 100 beats per minute
   Atrial flutter: b—atrial rate 250 to 400 beats per minute
   Atrial fibrillation: d—atrial rate greater than 350, ventricular rate less than 150 beats per minute
   SVT: a—150 to 250 beats per minute
   Sinus bradycardia: f—less than 60 beats per minute
   Sinus tachycardia: e—101 to 150 beats per minute
6. True—A premature beat is one that occurs early before the next expected beat
7. Noncompensatory
8. Compensatory
9. a—PAT starts and stops suddenly
10. False—Atrial flutter does not have the same atrial and ventricular rates; there is a usually a 2:1, 3:1, or 4:1 conduction rate
11. True—Atrial fibrillation is termed either *grossly irregular* or *irregularly irregular*
12. c—The P-R interval of an atrial fibrillation is not measurable
13. True—The accessory pathway of conduction between the atria and ventricles that normally closes after birth in Wolff-Parkinson-White syndrome remains open

CHAPTER 4 ECG PRACTICE STRIPS

Figure 4-1 Rapid atrial fibrillation
Irregular
Rate: approximately 120
P-R interval = absent, chaotic baseline
QRS complex = 0.06 second
Is there a P wave *before* every QRS complex ? No
Is there a QRS complex *after* every P wave? No

Figure 4-2 Wandering atrial pacemaker
Regular
Rate: 60
P-R interval = 0.16 second
QRS complex = 0.10 second
Is there a P wave *before* every QRS complex ? Yes
Is there a QRS complex *after* every P wave? Yes

Figure 4-3 Atrial flutter
Regular
Rate: atrial = 280; ventricular = 97
P-R interval = absent
QRS complex = 0.10 second
Is there a P wave *before* every QRS complex? Yes
Is there a QRS complex *after* every P wave? No
Note: this has a 3:1 atrial-ventricular conduction with one of the P waves falling on the T wave

Figure 4-4 Atrial tachycardia
Regular
Rate: 250
P-R interval = 0.04 second where present
QRS complex = 0.04 second
Is there a P wave *before* every QRS complex? Yes
Is there a QRS complex *after* every P wave? Yes
P waves are present, but some are buried in the preceding T wave because the rhythm is fast

Figure 4-5 Atrial fibrillation
Irregular
Rate: 50
P-R interval = absent
QRS complex = 0.05 second
Is there a P wave *before* every QRS complex? There are no discernable P waves

Figure 4-6 Sinus rhythm with PACs
Irregular
Rate: 100
P-R interval = 0.16 second
QRS complex = 0.08 second
Is there a P wave *before* every QRS complex ? Yes
Is there a QRS complex *after* every P wave? Yes

Figure 4-7 Atrial flutter
Irregular
Rate: 57
P-R interval = absent
QRS complex = 0.06 second
No discernable P waves, this has a 4:1 atrial-ventricular conduction

Figure 4-8 Atrial fibrillation
Irregular
Rate: 60
P-R interval = absent
QRS complex = 0.10 second
Is there a P wave *before* every QRS complex? There are no discernable P waves

Figure 4-9 Atrial tachycardia
Regular
Rate: 172
P-R interval = varies from 0.08 to 0.12 second
QRS complex = 0.05 second
Is there a P wave *before* every QRS complex? Yes
Is there a QRS complex *after* every P wave? Yes

Figure 4-10 Atrial fibrillation
Irregular
Rate: 114

P-R interval = absent
QRS complex = 0.06 second
Is there a P wave *before* every QRS complex? There are no discernable P waves

Figure 4-11 Atrial flutter
Irregular
Rate: 88
P-R interval = absent
QRS complex = 0.06 second
No discernable P waves are present; there is a 4:1 and 5:1 atrial-ventricular conduction

Figure 4-12 Atrial fibrillation
Irregular
Rate: 50
P-R interval = absent
QRS complex = 0.06 second
Is there a P wave *before* every QRS complex? There are no discernable P waves

Figure 4-13 Atrial tachycardia
Regular
Rate: 158
P-R interval = 0.12 second
QRS complex = 0.08 second
Is there a P wave *before* every QRS complex? Yes
Is there a QRS complex *after* every P wave? Yes

Figure 4-14 Atrial fibrillation
Irregular
Rate: 68
P-R interval = absent
QRS complex = 0.05 second
Is there a P wave *before* every QRS complex? There are no discernable P waves

Figure 4-15 Atrial fibrillation
Irregular
Rate: 88
P-R interval = absent
QRS complex = 0.06 second
Is there a P wave *before* every QRS complex? There are no discernable P waves

CHAPTER 4, CASE 1

Scenario

This rhythm is an **atrial flutter** at a rate of 158 beats per minute
Rhythm = regular; P-R interval = not measurable; QRS complex = 0.06 second
Is there a P wave *before* every QRS complex? There are no discernable P waves

Primary Survey

The airway is open, the patient is breathing without difficulty, and neither chest compressions nor defibrillation is needed.

Secondary Survey

Airway: adequate
Breathing: apply oxygen; obtain a pulse oximetry and an arterial blood gas
Circulation: cardiac monitor, IV access, 12-lead ECG, initial vital signs
Impression: rule out a possible MI; decreased cardiac output due to the atrial flutter

Oxygen-IV-Monitor-Fluids

Continue the oxygen, cardiac monitoring, obtain blood for lab work. Are fluids needed? No, not at this time because his vital signs are stable. Repeat the labs and cardiac enzymes every 8 hours. Consider the possibility of the physician ordering amiodarone, diltiazem, ibutilide, or beta blockers such as esmolol or metoprolol.

Vital Signs

Ongoing vital signs; monitor the heart rate and check the blood pressure every 15 minutes; check respirations and temperature

Rationale

Because the patient is diabetic, the patient is more prone to cardiac disease. As one of the physicians I work with once told me, "Always consider diabetics 20 years older than their actual age and you will have a more accurate picture of their health status." He could be having a "silent MI" because he is in atrial flutter with no chest pain but has all the associated symptoms.

CHAPTER 4, CASE 2

Scenario

This rhythm is **atrial fibrillation** at a rate of 104 beats per minute
Rhythm = irregular; P-R interval = not measurable; QRS complex = 0.10 second

Primary Survey

The airway is open, the patient is breathing with some difficulty, and neither chest compressions nor defibrillation is needed.

Secondary Survey

Airway: adequate
Breathing: apply oxygen, obtain pulse oximetry and an arterial blood gas, and order a respiratory albuterol treatment
Circulation: cardiac monitor, IV access, initial vital signs, 12-lead ECG
Impression: congestive heart failure and COPD, rule out any cardiac involvement

Oxygen-IV-Monitor-Fluids

Continue the oxygen, cardiac monitoring, and obtain needed lab work. Is fluid needed? No, absolutely not; she has enough fluid in her lungs. In fact, Lasix might be ordered to alleviate the fluid problem.

Vital Signs

Ongoing vital signs; monitor the heart rate and check the blood pressure every 15 to 30 minutes; check respirations and temperature

Rationale

Vital signs are stable, and the atrial fibrillation is controlled. Her main problem seems to be respiratory. With her history of CHF and COPD, she probably needs some additional Proventil treatments at the hospital, and it appears she is having a fluid buildup due to CHF and may also need some additional Lasix. Continue to observe the respiratory status so she does not go into respiratory failure and require intubation.

CHAPTER 4, CASE 3

Scenario

This rhythm has a **premature atrial contraction** with a rate of 95 beats per minute
Rhythm = irregular; P-R interval = 0.16 second; QRS complex = 0.04 second

Primary Survey

The airway is open, breathing is adequate, and no chest compressions are needed. No defibrillation is needed.

Secondary Survey

Airway: adequate
Breathing: apply oxygen; obtain pulse oximetry
Circulation: cardiac monitor, IV access, initial vital signs, 12-lead ECG
Impression: stress-related PACs, benign in nature

Oxygen-IV-Monitor-Fluids

Continue the oxygen, cardiac monitoring and obtain needed lab work. Is fluid needed? No, not at this time.

Vital Signs

Ongoing vital signs; monitor the heart rate and check the blood pressure every 10 to 15 minutes; check respirations and temperature

Rationale

Vital signs are stable; the premature contractions are most likely benign and due to the overexertion and added stress she has recently been under. Oxygen is a given in any episode of syncope. Place her on the cardiac monitor to observe for any cardiac abnormalities. Prepare IV access, just in case drug therapy or fluids are needed. After she arrives at the hospital and has undergone a complete workup, simply observe for a while before releasing her home.

CHAPTER 4, CASE 4

Scenario

This rhythm is a **supraventricular tachycardia** at a rate of 228 beats per minute
Rhythm = regular; P-R interval = absent; QRS complex = 0.04 second
Is there a P wave before every QRS complex? There are no P waves

Primary Survey

The airway is open, the patient is breathing, and neither chest compressions nor defibrillation is needed.

Secondary Survey

Airway: adequate
Breathing: apply oxygen; obtain pulse oximetry
Circulation: cardiac monitor IV access, initial vital signs, 12-lead ECG
Impression: decreased cardiac output due to the SVT

Oxygen-IV-Monitor-Fluids

Continue the oxygen, cardiac monitoring, and obtain needed lab work. Is fluid needed? Yes, with a large-bore IV. Prepare for immediate cardioversion, making sure you have Versed or Valium, or some type of benzodiazepine available for hypnotic effects before cardioversion.

Vital Signs

Continue ongoing vital signs; monitor the heart rate and check the blood pressure every 5 minutes; check respirations and temperature. Monitor the respiratory status closely if you give Versed or Valium.

Rationale

The monitor is showing an SVT at a rate of 228 beats per minute, so rapid it is compromising her cardiac output. The heart rate is so fast that the ventricles are not able to completely fill with blood during each cardiac contraction. Cardiac output is decreased; therefore there is a decreased supply of oxygen to the brain and peripheral circulatory system. Some may try adenosine first, but adenosine has a brief, hypotensive effect. Because this patient is already hypotensive, cardioversion would most likely be the best treatment.

CHAPTER 4, CASE 5

Scenario

This rhythm is **supraventricular tachycardia** at a rate of 214 beats per minute
Rhythm = regular; P-R interval = absent; QRS complex = 0.06 second
There are no P waves present.

Primary Survey

The airway is open, the patient is breathing, and neither chest compressions nor defibrillation is needed.

Secondary Survey

Airway: adequate, because she is talking without difficulty
Breathing: apply oxygen 2 to 3 L via the nasal cannula; obtain pulse oximetry
Circulation: cardiac monitor, IV access with large-bore IV, initial vital signs, 12-lead ECG
Impression: decreased cardiac output due to the atrial tachycardia

Oxygen-IV-Monitor-Fluids

Continue the oxygen, cardiac monitoring, and obtain needed lab work. Is fluid needed? Yes, because the blood pressure is low and the pulse extremely rapid. Prepare for immediate cardioversion. Before cardioverting, give conscious sedation medication, such as Versed, Valium, or fentanyl IV.

Vital Signs

Continue ongoing vital signs; monitor the heart rate, check the blood pressure every 5 minutes, respiration and temperature. If conscious sedation medications are given, monitor the respiratory status closely.

Rationale

The monitor is showing a rapid atrial tachycardia at a rate of 214 beats per minute. This is compromising her cardiac output. The heart is beating so fast that the ventricles are not completely filling with blood or emptying properly. Therefore there is a decreased supply of oxygen to the brain and peripheral circulatory system. The patient is definitely unstable and needs immediate cardioversion. The cardioversion should convert the rhythm back into a sinus rhythm. Always monitor the patient closely while the patient is under conscious sedation. Drug therapy, if considered, might include amiodarone, ibutilide, adenosine, or diltiazem, but most likely the physician will want to cardiovert.

CHAPTER 5 SELF-TEST

1. 40 to 60 beats per minute. A junctional rhythm has an intrinsic rate of 40 to 60 beats per minute.
2. Regular. A junctional rhythm usually has a regular R-R rhythm.

3. True. A rhythm with PJCs has an R-R interval that is regular except for an early complex.

4. Junctional tissue. In junctional rhythms the pacemaker site is at the AV node or below. Rhythms that originate in the AV node arise from the tissue between the lower node and the bundle of His.

5. 0.12 second. The P-R interval of a junctional rhythm is less than 0.12 second. A normal P-R interval in sinus rhythm is 0.12 to 0.20 second. A junctional rhythm has a shorter P-R interval because the pacemaker site is at the AV node, is at the AV junction, or is lower in the electrical conduction system.

6. Ischemia, insult to SA node or AV junction, hypoxemia, digitalis toxicity

7. Seldom. A rhythm with PJCs seldom produces symptoms.

8. 60 to 100 beats per minute. When you have a sinus rhythm with PJCs, the rate of the underlying rhythm is usually 60 to 100 beats per minute.

9. Retrograde conduction. Retrograde conduction through the atria causes an inverted P wave in a junctional rhythm in lead II.

10. Accelerated junctional rhythm. A junctional rhythm with a rate of 60 to 100 beats per minute is known as an *accelerated junctional rhythm*.

11. Junctional tachycardia. A junctional rhythm with a rate of 101 to 180 beats per minute is known as *junctional tachycardia*.

12. Escape. In a junctional rhythm also known as *junctional escape rhythm*, the SA node fails to fire intermittently, and the junctional tissue takes over the pacer site as a protective mechanism.

13. 40 to 60 beats per minute. A junctional escape rhythm is usually found to have an R-R rate of 40 to 60 beats per minute.

14. Junctional tachycardia. Ventricular fibrillation or ventricular tachycardia may result from a junctional tachycardia.

15. Inverted P wave preceding the QRS complex, inverted P wave hidden in the QRS complex, inverted P wave after the QRS complex.

    If the inverted P wave precedes the QRS complex, then you must determine if it is an atrial or junctional rhythm. The clue to this is the duration of the P-R interval. If the impulse originated in the atria, it would take the normal sequence of 0.12 to 0.2 second to travel through the node and the ventricles. However, if the P-R interval is less than 0.12 second, then the rhythm must have originated in the AV junction.

CHAPTER 5 ECG PRACTICE STRIPS

Figure 5-1 Accelerated junctional rhythm
Regular
Rate: 80 beats per minute
P-R interval = absent
QRS complex = 0.06 second
There are no P waves present

Figure 5-2 Accelerated junctional rhythm
Regular
Rate: 76 beats per minute
P-R interval = P waves are inverted with a P-R interval of 0.08 second
QRS complex = 0.08 second
Is there a P wave *before* every QRS complex? Yes
Is there a QRS complex *after* every P wave? Yes

Figure 5-3 Junctional rhythm
Regular
Rate: 57
P-R interval = absent
QRS complex = 0.04 second
There are no P waves present

Figure 5-4 Junctional tachycardia
Regular
Rate: 136
P-R interval = absent
QRS complex = 0.05 second
There are no P waves present

Figure 5-5 Accelerated junctional rhythm
Slightly irregular
Rate: 60
P-R interval = absent
QRS complex = 0.10 second
There are no P waves present

Figure 5-6 Junctional rhythm
Regular
Rate: 51
P-R interval = absent
QRS complex = 0.04 second
There are no P waves present

Figure 5-7 Junctional Rhythm
Regular
Rate: 46
P-R interval = 0.08 second
QRS complex = 0.06 second
Is there a P wave *before* every QRS complex? Yes
Is there a QRS complex *after* every P wave? Yes

Figure 5-8 Accelerated junctional rhythm
Regular
Rate: 72
P-R interval = absent

QRS complex = 0.06 second
There are no P waves present

Figure 5-9 Junctional tachycardia
Regular
Rate: 150
P-R interval = varies, 0.06 second, where present
QRS complex = 0.06 second
Is there a P wave *before* every QRS complex? No
Is there a QRS complex *after* every P wave? Yes
Note the P waves in the first, third, fourth, fifth, eighth, eleventh, twelfth, and thirteenth beats

Figure 5-10 Junctional escape rhythm
Regular
Rate: 56
P-R interval = absent
QRS complex = 0.12 second, slightly wide with an intraventricular conduction delay
There are no P waves present

Figure 5-11 Junctional tachycardia
Regular
Rate: 150
P-R interval = absent
QRS complex = 0.07 second
There are no P waves present

Figure 5-12 Junctional escape rhythm with artifact
Irregular
Rate: 54
P-R interval = absent
QRS complex = 0.10 second
There are no P waves present

Figure 5-13 Sinus rhythm with one PJC
Regular: underlying rhythm
Rate: 83
P-R interval = 0.18 second, underlying rhythm
QRS complex = 0.05 second
Is there a P wave *before* every QRS complex? No
Is there a QRS complex *after* every P wave? Yes

Figure 5-14 Junctional rhythm
Regular
Rate: 58
P-R interval = absent, P waves are after the QRS complex
QRS complex = 0.04 second
The P waves fall after the QRS complex

Figure 5-15 Accelerated junctional rhythm
Irregular
Rate: 81
P-R interval = 0.16 where present; the P waves are inverted at the first and fifth beats
QRS complex = 0.06 second
Is there a P wave *before* every QRS complex ? Yes
Is there a QRS complex *after* every P wave? Yes

CHAPTER 5, CASE 1

Scenario

This rhythm is a stable **junctional rhythm** at a rate of 52 beats per minute
Rhythm = regular, but there are no P waves present before each QRS complex; P-R interval = none; QRS complex = 0.10 second
Is there a P wave before every QRS complex? There are no discernable P waves

Primary Survey

The airway is open, breathing is adequate, and no chest compressions are needed because the patient is oriented and alert. No defibrillation is needed.

Secondary Survey

Airway: adequate
Breathing: apply oxygen at 2 L per minute via nasal cannula; obtain pulse oximetry
Circulation: cardiac monitor, IV access, initial vital signs, 12-lead ECG
Impression: possible flu symptoms

Oxygen-IV-Monitor-Fluids

Continue the oxygen and monitoring, and obtain blood for lab work. Is fluid needed? Yes. It would be a good idea to have a bag of normal saline (NS) infusing at a keep-open rate.

Vital Signs

Ongoing vital signs; monitor the heart rate, blood pressure, pulse, and respirations

Rationale

Vital signs are stable and the monitor is showing a junctional rhythm, but the patient seems to be compensating very well for the slow heart rate. The vomiting may have caused the junctional rhythm, which induces a vagal reflex. Vagal reflexes slow the heart rate by activating the parasympathetic nervous system. He is not showing signs of decreased cardiac output. The junctional rhythm may also be connected with the rheumatic fever he had as a child.

IV fluids would be helpful because he lost a considerable amount of fluid from the vomiting, and at this point he is unable to keep any fluids down. Observe the patient, monitor his ECG rhythm, and follow the doctor's orders for IV fluids and antiemetic medications.

CHAPTER 5, CASE 2

Scenario

This rhythm is a stable **accelerated junctional rhythm** at a rate of 72 beats per minute
Rhythm = regular, but there are no P waves present before each QRS complex; P-R interval = none; QRS complex = 0.08 second

Primary Survey

The airway is open, breathing is adequate, and no chest compressions are needed because the patient is oriented and alert. No defibrillation is needed.

Secondary Survey

Airway: adequate
Breathing: apply oxygen at 2 to 3 L per minute via nasal cannula; obtain pulse oximetry
Circulation: cardiac monitor, IV access, initial vital signs, 12-lead ECG
Impression: rule out possible cardiac involvement

Oxygen-IV-Monitor-Fluids

Continue the oxygen and monitoring, and obtain blood for lab work. Is fluid needed? No, not at this time. Vital signs are borderline but still stable.

Vital Signs

Ongoing vital signs; monitor the heart rate, blood pressure, pulse, and respirations

Rationale

Vital signs are stable, but the patient needs to be monitored until the ECG, lab work, and chest x-ray are done and the doctor can evaluate the results. Chances are it is stress related and due to an excess of caffeine. The epigastric distress is most likely due to the stress and the excessive amount of caffeine.

CHAPTER 5, CASE 3

Scenario

This rhythm is a stable **accelerated junctional** at a rate of 93 beats per minute
Rhythm = regular, there are inverted P waves before the QRS complex; P-R interval = 0.16 second, with inverted P waves; QRS complex = 0.06 second
Is there a P wave *before* every QRS complex? Yes
Is there a QRS complex *after* every P wave? Yes

Primary Survey

The airway is open, breathing is adequate, and no chest compressions are needed because the patient is awake and alert. No defibrillation is needed.

Secondary Survey

Airway: adequate
Breathing: apply oxygen at 2 to 3 L per minute via nasal cannula; obtain pulse oximetry
Circulation: cardiac monitor, IV access, initial vital signs, 12-lead ECG
Impression: rule out a possible MI, rule out cardiac contusion from the seat belt

Oxygen-IV-Monitor-Fluids

Continue the oxygen and monitoring, and obtain blood for lab work. Is fluid needed? No, not at this time. Anticipate giving nitroglycerin to see if it alleviates the chest pressure.

Vital Signs

Ongoing vital signs; monitor the heart rate, blood pressure, pulse, and respirations

Rationale

Vital signs are stable. The patient could very well be having an MI because she has had chest pressure for the past several days and felt faint just before the accident. Cardiac enzyme lab work, plus the 12-lead ECG, may give you the answer. Also, she could have a cardiac contusion, but cardiac must always be ruled out first. X-rays to clear the cervical spine (C-spine) and of the right forearm are needed as well as a chest x-ray. She will probably be monitored in the CCU for a day or so if an MI diagnosis is not made in the emergency department.

CHAPTER 5, CASE 4

Scenario

This rhythm is a **junctional tachycardia** at a rate of 142 beats per minute
Rhythm = regular, but there are no P waves before the QRS complex; P-R interval = none; QRS complex = 0.05 second

Primary Survey

The airway is open, breathing is adequate, and no chest compressions are needed because the patient is awake and alert. No defibrillation is needed.

Secondary Survey

Airway: adequate
Breathing: apply oxygen at 2 to 3 L per minute via nasal cannula; obtain pulse oximetry
Circulation: cardiac monitor, IV access, initial vital signs, 12-lead ECG
Impression: rule out possible cardiac problems; may be diabetes related

Oxygen-IV-Monitor-Fluids

Continue the oxygen and monitoring, and obtain blood for lab work. Is fluid needed? Yes. It would be a good idea to have a bag of NS hanging at a keep-open rate.

Vital Signs

Ongoing vital signs; monitor the heart rate, blood pressure, pulse, and respirations

Rationale

Vital signs are stable, but the blood pressure is high and you are concerned because the patient is disoriented. She is taking Lanoxin regularly but cannot remember if she has taken her medications over the past few days, so the digoxin level may be elevated and causing the junctional tachycardia. The heart rate should not be 142 beats per minute. A cardiac workup with lab work is in order to find out what the problem is. The blood glucose level is elevated and needs to be controlled. This may have been the cause for the disorientation.

CHAPTER 5, CASE 5

Scenario

This rhythm is a stable **accelerated junctional rhythm** at a rate of 75 beats per minute
Rhythm = regular; P-R interval = 0.06 second, P waves are inverted; QRS complex = 0.08 second
Is there a P wave *before* every QRS complex? Yes
Is there a QRS complex *after* every P wave? Yes

Primary Survey

The airway is open, breathing is adequate, and no chest compressions are needed because the patient is awake and alert. No defibrillation is needed.

Secondary Survey

Airway: adequate
Breathing: apply oxygen; obtain pulse oximetry
Circulation: cardiac monitor, IV access, initial vital signs, 12-lead ECG
Impression: rule out possible MI

Oxygen-IV-Monitor-Fluids

Continue the oxygen and monitoring, and obtain blood for lab work. Is fluid needed? No, not at this time.

Vital Signs

Ongoing vital signs; monitor the heart rate, blood pressure, pulse, and respirations

Rationale

Vital signs are stable. With the chest pain, shortness of breath, and nausea, he is a prime candidate for a potential acute MI. If he is indeed having an MI, this could be the reason for the accelerated junctional rhythm. He will certainly need a complete cardiac workup with the anticipation of giving nitroglycerin, thrombolytics, and morphine to relieve the pain. Close observation and monitoring for any changes are musts.

CHAPTER 6 SELF-TEST

1. a—The P-R interval is greater than 0.20 second
2. Mobitz I, second-degree AV block type I, Wenckebach
3. True
4. First-degree AV block: c—The P-R interval is longer than normal or greater than 0.20 second
   Mobitz I: a—The P-R interval becomes progressively longer until th QRS complex is dropped
   Mobitz II: d—Atrial rate is greater than the ventricular rate depending on the conduction, which may be 2:1, 3:1, or 4:1
   Third-degree AV block: b—The atria and ventricles are functioning independently of each other. There is no relationship between the P waves and the QRS complexes.
5. False
6. Mobitz II, second-degree type II
7. c—The atrial rate will be faster than the vetnricular rate, resulting in a 2:1, 3:1, or 4:1 conduction
8. True
9. True
10. Faster. The atrial rate of a third-degree AV block is faster than the ventricular rate
11. True
12. Bundle of His or bundle branches

CHAPTER 6 ECG PRACTICE STRIPS

Figure 6-1 Third-degree AV block
Rhythm: regular
Rate: atrial = 70 beats per minute; ventricular = 45 beats per minute
P-R interval = absent
QRS complex = 0.10 second
Is there a P wave *before* every QRS complex? No
Is there a QRS complex *after* every P wave? No

Figure 6-2 Second-degree, Mobitz I AV block
Rhythm: irregular
Rate: atrial = 50; ventricular = 40
P-R interval = varies until absent
QRS complex = 0.08 second
Is there a P wave *before* every QRS complex? Yes
Is there a QRS complex *after* every P wave? No

Figure 6-3 First-degree AV block
Rhythm: slightly irregular
Rate: atrial = 46; ventricular = 46
P-R interval = 0.32 second
QRS complex = 0.10 second

Is there a P wave *before* every QRS complex? Yes
Is there a QRS complex *after* every P wave? Yes

Figure 6-4 Third-degree AV block
Rhythm: irregular
Rate: 36
P-R interval = absent
QRS complex = 0.12 second
No relationship between P waves and QRS complexes

Figure 6-5 Second-degree, type II, AV block
Rhythm: irregular
Rate: atrial = 60; ventricular = 33
P-R interval = absent
QRS complex = 0.08 second
Is there a P wave *before* every QRS complex? Yes
Is there a QRS complex *after* every P wave? No

Figure 6-6 Second-degree Mobitz II AV block
Rhythm: regular
Rate: atrial = 100 beats per minute; ventricular = 48 beats per minute
P-R interval = 0.16 second every other beat
QRS complex: 0.12 second
Is there a P wave *before* every QRS complex? Yes
Is there a QRS complex *after* every P wave? No

Figure 6-7 Third-degree AV block
Rhythm: regular
Rate: atrial = 100; ventricular = 31
P-R interval = not measurable
QRS complex = 0.16 second
Is there a P wave *before* every QRS complex? No
Is there a QRS complex *after* every P wave? No

Figure 6-8 Second-degree, Mobitz II AV block
Rhythm: regular
Rate: atrial = 82; ventricular = 38
P-R interval = 0.24 second where present
QRS complex = 0.08 seconds
Is there a P wave *before* every QRS complex? Yes
Is there a QRS complex *after* every P wave? No

Figure 6-9 Second-degree, Mobitz I AV block
Rhythm: irregular
Rate: atrial = 80; ventricular = approximately 60
P-R interval = longer until dropped
QRS complex = 0.06 second
Is there a P wave *before* every QRS complex? Yes
Is there a QRS complex *after* every P wave? No

Figure 6-10 Second-degree, Mobitz I AV block
Rhythm: irregular
Rate: atrial = 88; ventricular = approximately 50
P-R interval = longer until dropped
QRS complex = 0.12 second
Is there a P wave *before* every QRS complex? Yes
Is there a QRS complex *after* every P wave? No

Figure 6-11 Third-degree AV block
Rhythm: regular
Rate: atrial = 90 beats per minute; ventricular = 34 beats per minute
P-R interval = absent
QRS complex = 0.08 second
Is there a P wave *before* every QRS complex? No
Is there a QRS complex *after* every P wave? No

Figure 6-12 First-degree AV block
Rhythm: regular
Rate: atrial = 68; ventricular rate = 68
P-R interval = 0.28 second
QRS complex = 0.08 second
Is there a P wave *before* every QRS complex? Yes
Is there a QRS complex *after* every P wave? Yes

Figure 6-13 Third-degree AV block
Rhythm: regular
Rate: atrial = approximately 60 beats per minute, some are buried in the T waves; ventricular = 47 beats per minute
P-R interval = absent
QRS complex = varies from 0.08 to 0.10 second
Is there a P wave *before* every QRS complex? No
Is there a QRS complex *after* every P wave? No

Figure 6-14 Second-degree type II AV block
Rhythm: regular
Rate: atrial = 90; ventricular = 40 beats per minute
P-R interval = not measurable
QRS complex = 0.08 second
Is there a P wave *before* every QRS complex? Yes
Is there a QRS complex *after* every P wave? No

Figure 6-15 First-degree AV block
Rhythm: regular
Rate: atrial = 60; ventricular = 60
P-R interval = 0.32 second
QRS complex = 0.06 second
Is there a P wave *before* every QRS complex? Yes
Is there a QRS complex *after* every P wave? Yes

CHAPTER 6, CASE 1

Scenario

This rhythm is a **first-degree AV heart block** with a rate of 62 beats per minute. The rhythm is regular; there are P waves before the QRS complex. The P-R interval is 0.26 second, with a QRS duration of 0.16 second.
Is there a P wave *before* every QRS complex? Yes
Is there a QRS complex *after* every P wave? Yes

Primary Survey

The airway is open, breathing is adequate, and no chest compressions are needed because the patient is awake and alert. No defibrillation is needed.

Secondary Survey

Airway: adequate
Breathing: apply oxygen 2 to 3 L via nasal cannula
Circulation: cardiac monitor, IV access, initial vital signs, repeat pulse oximetry
Impression: rule out a possible MI

Oxygen-IV-Monitor-Fluids

Continue the oxygen, cardiac monitoring, and obtain needed lab work. Is fluid needed? No, not at this time.

Vital Signs

Continue ongoing vital signs; monitor the heart rate, blood pressure, pulse, and respirations

Rationale

Treatment would include a complete workup for a possible MI. The doctor is likely to order nitroglycerin to obtain a pain-free status, along with one baby aspirin. Next would be morphine if the nitroglycerin did not relieve the pain. Morphine also reduces anxiety. Be prepared to begin an infusion of tissue-type plasminogen activator (tPA), Retavase, or glycoprotein IIb/IIIa inhibitors (GPIIb/IIIa) if ordered. Also, heparin, a nitroglycerin drip, and beta blockers may be ordered if the indications are an MI. This patient is in a first-degree block, which indicates a delay at the AV node or Purkinje system. It depends on the length of the P-R interval if this block is slight, moderate, or severe in nature. This patient is having chest pain that has lasted longer than 20 minutes along with associated risk factors (e.g., hypertension, male sex, angina). These are all good indicators of a probable MI. The aspirin is given as an antiplatelet agent. It interferes with platelet aggregation and helps to keep the blood thin. The 12-lead ECG and cardiac enzymes will help to determine if this patient is having an MI. If an MI is present, the tPA, reteplase (r-PA), or GPIIb/IIIb is administered to dissolve the clots, or the physician may order the patient to the cardiac catheterization lab. The patient must be monitored closely while in your care.

CHAPTER 6, CASE 2

Scenario

This rhythm is a **second-degree type I, or Mobitz I AV block** with an atrial rate of 80 beats per minute and a ventricular rate of 52 beats per minute. The rhythm is regular, but the impulse is delayed and partially blocked at the bundle branches.
P-R interval = absent; QRS complex = 0.12 second
Is there a P wave *before* every QRS complex? Yes
Is there a QRS complex *after* every P wave? No

Primary Survey

The airway is open, breathing is adequate, and no chest compressions are needed because the patient is awake and alert. No defibrillation is needed.

Secondary Survey

Airway: adequate
Breathing: apply oxygen at 10 to 15 L per minute via nonbreather mask; obtain pulse oximetry
Circulation: cardiac monitor, IV access, initial vital signs, 12-lead ECG
Impression: rule out possible MI, pericarditis, myocarditis, or endocarditis

Oxygen-IV-Monitor-Fluids

Continue the oxygen and monitoring, and obtain blood for lab work. Is fluid needed? Yes, because the vital signs are showing signs of hypotension. Give atropine 0.5 to 1.0 mg IV. You may give every 3 to 5 minutes as needed, not to exceed total dose of 0.04 mg/kg. Also consider transcutaneous pacing to increase the heart rate.

Vital Signs

Ongoing vital signs; monitor the heart rate, blood pressure, pulse, and respirations

Rationale

Vital signs are unstable. The cardiac output is being compromised. A second-degree type II AV block is usually more serious than a type I. Because of her age, and signs and symptoms, the patient must be worked up for a possible MI. Also consider the fact she was worked up 6 months ago for myocarditis, which is known to be a provoking factor for a type II AV block and may possibly be the reason for this patient's problems.

The first and foremost consideration is to increase the heart rate to allow for better perfusion by increasing the cardiac output. The next consideration would be to treat the probable myocarditis after the MI has been ruled out.

CHAPTER 6, CASE 3

Scenario

This rhythm is a **second-degree type I, AV block** with an atrial rate of 80 beats per minute and a ventricular rate of 72 beats per minute. The P-R interval becomes progressively longer until a

QRS complex is dropped completely. This is a partial AV block in which the impulse originates at the SA node but is delayed and partially blocked in the bundle branches.
Is there a P wave *before* every QRS complex? No
Is there a QRS complex *after* every P wave? No

Primary Survey

The airway is open, breathing is adequate, and no chest compressions are needed because the patient is awake and alert. No defibrillation is needed.

Secondary Survey

Airway: adequate
Breathing: apply oxygen at 2 L per minute via nasal cannula; obtain pulse oximetry
Circulation: cardiac monitor, IV access, initial vital signs, 12-lead ECG
Impression: rule out a possible MI or complications from previous surgery

Oxygen-IV-Monitor-Fluids

Continue the oxygen and monitoring, and obtain blood for lab work. Is fluid needed? Yes, at a keep-open rate because the vital signs are stable at present.

Vital Signs

Ongoing vital signs; monitor the heart rate, blood pressure, pulse, and respirations

Rationale

Vital signs are stable. In this case the AV block is probably caused by the cardiac operation the patient had 3 weeks ago. Monitor carefully because the type I AV block can rapidly progress into a type II AV block that is far more serious. Have the atropine and transcutaneous pacer nearby. The syncope was a warning. Monitor the patient's vital signs and cardiac rhythm frequently.

CHAPTER 6, CASE 4

Scenario

This rhythm is a **third-degree AV heart block** with a ventricular rate of 47 beats per minute and an atrial rate of 140 beats per minute (some are buried in the QRS complexes). Note that there is no relationship between the P waves and the QRS complexes. There is no measurable P-R interval. The QRS measures 0.06 second.
No relationship between P waves and QRS complexes.

Primary Survey

The airway is open, breathing is adequate, and no chest compressions are needed because the patient is awake and alert. No defibrillation is needed.

Secondary Survey

Airway: adequate
Breathing: apply oxygen at 2 to 3 L per minute via nasal cannula; obtain pulse oximetry
Circulation: cardiac monitor, IV access, initial vital signs, 12-lead ECG
Impression: rule out a possible MI or complications from previous surgery

Oxygen-IV-Monitor-Fluids

Continue the oxygen and monitoring, and obtain blood for lab work. Is fluid needed? Yes, at a keep-open rate because the vital signs are borderline stable at present. Consider having the transcutaneous pacer nearby, just in case.

Vital Signs

Ongoing vital signs; monitor the heart rate, blood pressure, pulse, and respirations

Rationale

Vital signs are borderline stable. The patient's valve replacement probably triggered the third-degree heart block. The third-degree block is probably a result of the condition causing the chest pain, not the cause of it. You are going to ask, "Why not atropine to increase the heart rate?" The QRS complex is a wide duration, so the treatment is going to be transcutaneous pacing. Increasing the rate with atropine may actually cause more extensive damage to the heart. The partially or completely occluded vessels could not tolerate the increase in blood flow. Remember: narrow QRS complex = atropine, whereas a wide QRS complex = transcutaneous pacing. In a third-degree block, the atria and ventricles are beating independently of each other. Each is contracting, but there is no correlation between the two. The first and foremost consideration is to increase the heart rate and increase the blood flow thus allowing for better perfusion and cardiac output. Be prepared for transcutaneous pacing and possibly a nitroglycerin drip along with a dopamine drip, which will increase the blood pressure to a more acceptable level.

CHAPTER 6, CASE 5

Scenario

This rhythm is a second-degree AV block, type II or Mobitz II heart block with an atrial rate of 100 beats per minute and a ventricular rate of 47 beats per minute, but there are more P waves than QRS complexes. The P-R interval varies from 0.12 to 0.16 second every other beat. The QRS complex is 0.10 second. This is a 2:1 conduction.
Is there a P wave *before* every QRS complex? Yes
Is there a QRS complex *after* every P wave? No

Primary Survey

The airway is open, breathing is adequate, and no chest compressions are needed. The patient is confused and combative. No defibrillation is needed.

Secondary Survey

Airway: adequate
Breathing: apply oxygen at 10 L per minute via mask; obtain pulse oximetry
Circulation: cardiac monitor, IV access, initial vital signs, 12-lead ECG
Impression: rule out a possible MI

Oxygen-IV-Monitor-Fluids

Continue the oxygen and monitoring, and obtain blood for lab work. Is fluid needed? Yes, at a keep-open rate because the vital signs are borderline stable at present. Have the transcutaneous pacer ready to use, just in case.

Vital Signs

Ongoing vital signs; monitor the heart rate, blood pressure, pulse, and respirations

Rationale

Vital signs are borderline because the pulse is low. The physician may order a nitroglycerin drip to dilate the vessels and reduce the ischemia, may order respiratory treatments to increase the oxygen saturation, and may have the pacemaker ready. The depressed S-T segment is an indication of a probable MI. The physician may order tPA or Retavase, or GP IIb/IIIa inhibitors, or may send the patient to the cardiac catheterization lab. However, the patient's age and illnesses do not make her a good candidate for the cath lab. She will need close observation for some time.

CHAPTER 7 SELF-TEST

1. a—Absent. Ventricular rhythms do not have P waves because the impulse arises below the AV junction.
2. c. The QRS complex is wide and bizarre because depolarization occurs in the ventricles. The normal pathway of conduction throughout the bundle branches is bypassed.
3. b. A ventricular rhythm with PVCs usually has T waves that deflect in the opposite direction of the QRS complex.
4. a. The PVCs produce a "compensatory pause." A compensatory pause is the expected occurrence of the next beat after a premature complex. If you were to measure the R-R interval with calipers, the first beat is normal, the second beat or premature beat occurs early, but the third beat occurs where it is expected.
5. d. PVCs are considered dangerous if:
   - They occur in pairs or couplets
   - There are six or more per minute
   - They are different in shape (multifocal)
   - They fall on the T wave of the preceding beat (R on T)
6. Bigeminy, trigeminy
7. a. Ventricular tachycardia is the occurrence of three or more PVCs in a row with a rate greater than 100 beats per minute.

8. a—101 to 250 beats per minute
9. b. A ventricular rhythm is usually a regular rhythm.
10. e. A patient with ventricular tachycardia may experience all of the above because of resulting hypoxia.
11. d. The Purkinje fibers have an intrinsic firing rate of 20 to 40 beats per minute.
12. c. The QRS complex represents ventricular depolarization as discussed in Chapter 2. The ions move across the cell membrane making the inside of the cell more positive than the outside, allowing for the electrical discharge to cause the ventricles to contract.
13. d—Ventricular relaxtion. Ventricular diastole occurs when the ventricles are relaxed and fill with blood.
14. c. An accelerated idioventricular rhythm usually has a rate of 40 to 100 beats per minute.
15. c. The one characteristic that distinguishes torsades is the "twisting of the points."
16. c. Magnesium sulfate is the drug of choice to correct torsades.
17. d. With ventricular asystole, you will find no electrical activity; thus there is a flat line on the monitor.
18. b. Ventricular fibrillation is a series of chaotic waves.
19. d. The P-R interval of an idioventricular rhythm is not present.
20. c. Escape beats are ventricular complexes that arrive late in the cardiac cycle.
21. c. Escape beats are considered a protective mechanism to prevent extreme slowing of the heart rate or even asystole.
22. R on T

CHAPTER 7 ECG PRACTICE STRIPS

Figure 7-1 The underlying rhythm is a normal sinus rhythm with couplet PVCs
Rate: 84 beats per minute
P-R interval = 0.20 second (sinus rhythm)
QRS complex = 0.05 second
Is there a P wave *before* every QRS complex? No
Is there a QRS complex *after* every P wave? Yes

Figure 7-2 Ventricular tachycardia
Rate: 180 beats per minute
There is no P-R interval
QRS complex is approximately 0.24 second
There are no discernable P waves

Figure 7-3 The underlying rhythm is a sinus rhythm with bigeminy PVCs
Rate: 80 beats per minute
P-R interval (sinus) = 0.20 second
QRS complex = 0.07 second (sinus)
Is there a P wave *before* every QRS complex? No
Is there a QRS complex *after* every P wave? Yes

Figure 7-4 Ventricular fibrillation
No P-R interval and no QRS complex

Figure 7-5 Underlying rhythm is sinus rhythm with bigeminy PVCs
Rate: approximately 90 beats per minute unless the PVCs are not perfusing
P-R interval = 0.16 second
QRS complex = 0.08 second
Is there a P wave *before* every QRS complex? No
Is there a QRS complex *after* every P wave? Yes

Figure 7-6 Ventricular tachycardia
Rate: 175 beats per minute
P-R interval = none
QRS complex = 0.14 second and bizarre

Figure 7-7 Junctional tachycardia with PVCs
Rate: 110 beats per minute if the PVCs are perfusing; if not the rate is 80 beats per minute
P-R interval = absent
QRS complex = 0.06 second
There are no discernable P waves

Figure 7-8 Sinus rhythm with bigeminy PVCs
Rate: 70 beats per minute if the PVCs are perfusing; 40 beats per minute if not perfusing
P-R interval = 0.16 second
QRS complex = 0.07 second
Is there a P wave *before* every QRS complex? No
Is there a QRS complex *after* every P wave? Yes

Figure 7-9 Atrial fibrillation with multifocal PVCs
Rate: 70 beats per minute
P-R interval = none
QRS complex = 0.06 second
There are no discernable P waves

Figure 7-10 Ventricular tachycardia
Rate: 110 beats per minute
P-R interval (sinus) = 0.16 second
QRS complex (sinus) = 0.28 second
Is there a P wave *before* every QRS complex? There are no P waves

Figure 7-11 Sinus rhythm with a PVC
Rate: 65 beats per minute
P-R interval (sinus) = 0.20 second
QRS complex = 0.08 second
Is there a P wave *before* every QRS complex? No
Is there a QRS complex *after* every P wave? Yes

Figure 7-12 Atrial flutter with a run of ventricular tachycardia
Rate: 90 beats per minute

P-R interval = 0.12 where present
QRS complex = 0.08 second
Is there a P wave *before* every QRS complex? Yes
Is there a QRS complex *after* every P wave? No
Atrial flutter has a 3:1 conduction rate

Figure 7-13 Ventricular fibrillation going in to asystole
No rate detectable

Figure 7-14 Sinus rhythm with unifocal PVCs and one pair of couplet PVCs
Rate: 70 beats per minute
P-R interval (sinus) = 0.16 second
QRS complex (sinus) = 0.08 second

Figure 7-15 Ventricular fibrillation
Rate: none, chaotic coarse V-fib
P-R interval = none
QRS complex = none

CHAPTER 7, CASE 1

Scenario

This rhythm is a **ventricular tachycardia**. See Algorithm 7-1 for V-tach treatment.
The rate is 170 and regular. There are no visible P waves, and the QRS duration = 0.16 second.

Primary Survey

Treatment always begins with airway management. Give the patient oxygen, 10 to 15 L per minute via nonrebreather mask. No shock is needed at this time because the vital signs are stable.

Secondary Survey

Airway: continue oxygen.
Breathing: adequate with additional oxygen
Circulation: cardiac monitor, IV access, 12-lead ECG, pulse oximetry
Impression: rule out an MI or potential cardiac problems

Oxygen-IV-Monitor-Fluids

Continue the oxygen, cardiac monitoring, and obtain needed lab work. Is fluid needed? Yes, to infuse the drugs. Antiarrhythmics would include a choice of any of the following: amiodarone 150 mg IV over 10 minutes, procainamide 20 to 30 mg/min IV infusion up to a total dose of 17 mg/kg, lidocaine 75 to 100 mg (1.0-1.5 mg/kg), and beta blockers such as esmolol (0.5 mg/kg over 1 minute IV bolus), atenolol (5 mg over 5 minutes), or metoprolol (5 mg over 2-5 minutes). Of course, cardioversion is always a choice of treatment.

Vital Signs

Continue checking for a rhythm change and checking for a pulse. Once the rhythm has converted, closely observe to ensure the patient does not return to V-tach. Obtain a history, perform a physical examination, and get a chest x-ray (at the hospital).

Rationale

The patient is experiencing ventricular tachycardia, but at the present moment she is stable (as noted by the paramedic) with the previous vital signs. There is no sign of her cardiac output being compromised because she is alert and oriented, plus her skin is pink, warm, and dry. However, ventricular tachycardia is a potentially dangerous rhythm and must be treated rapidly.

Ventricular tachycardia arises from the ventricles, so there is no atrial activity at all and may unexpectedly progress into ventricular fibrillation. The antiarrhythmic drugs must be given quickly, and you must always be anticipating a cardiac arrest. The drugs given raise the fibrillation threshold decreasing the occurrence of ventricular fibrillation. If cardioversion is in order, the patient who is awake must first be sedated with Valium, Versed, fentanyl, or whatever drug you use for conscious sedation. Always keep patients informed of what you are doing, because there may be a momentary change in their perfusion status when they convert, leaving them suddenly weak and dizzy. If you keep patients informed, this will allow you to gain their trust. Never give the patient any unexpected surprises.

CHAPTER 7, CASE 2

Scenario

This rhythm is a **ventricular fibrillation**

Primary Survey

Maintain the airway with an oropharyngeal airway (OPA) and then defibrillate at 200 J, 200 to 300 J, and then 360 J, checking the monitor for a rhythm change and checking for a pulse after each shock. Begin chest compressions.

Secondary Survey

Airway: endotracheal intubation as soon as possible to ensure an adequate airway

Breathing: use the bag-valve-mask (BVM), additional oxygen, and ET tube to provide respirations for the patient

Circulation: cardiac monitor, IV access, and appropriate drug therapy, which in this case would be epinephrine, 1:10,000, 1 mg every 3 to 5 minutes or vasopressin 40 U IV. The epinephrine can be repeated 1 mg every 3 to 5 minutes during the arrest. Vasopressin is a one-time dose only. Next would be amiodarone, 300 mg IV. If the V-fib continues, you may consider a second dose of amiodarone of 150- to 300-mg IV. You could use the lidocaine 1- to 1.5-mg/kg IV push, but this is not used much anymore. After the amiodarone consider magnesium sulfate, 1 to 2 g IV. Also consider procainamide at 20 to 30 mg per minute with a maximum dose of 17 mg/kg. By this time in the arrest you might consider sodium bicarbonate, 1-mEq/kg IV bolus.

Impression: cardiac arrest, rule out an MI

Oxygen-IV-Monitor-Fluids

Continue the oxygen, cardiac monitoring, and obtain needed lab work. Is fluid needed? Yes, to infuse the drugs at a rapid rate.

Vital Signs

Continue checking for a rhythm change and checking for a pulse. Obtain a history from the family if possible.

Rationale

Always, always check for responsiveness, call for help, then *airway, breathing, circulation* and *defibrillation* (if needed). The quicker the electricity is delivered the greater the chance for survival. I cannot emphasize this enough! In the V-fib protocol, you would shock, shock, and shock immediately, checking the monitor and pulse in between shocks. If there were a change, you would want to know it as soon as possible. The one thing that will most likely save this patient is defibrillation, not the drug therapy. Pharmacologic therapy will certainly help, but it is the electricity that will convert the rhythm back into a normal one.

CHAPTER 7, CASE 3

Scenario

This rhythm is **asystole**

Primary Survey

Maintain the airway with an OPA and begin CPR. Confirm the rhythm in two different leads on the monitor.

Secondary Survey

Airway: endotracheal intubation as soon as possible to ensure an adequate airway
Breathing: use the BVM, along with additional oxygen and ET tube to provide respirations for the patient
Circulation: cardiac monitor, IV access. Consider immediate transcutaneous pacing if within the first 10 minutes of arrest. Appropriate drug therapy, which in this case would be vasopressin 40-U IV bolus or epinephrine, 1:10,000, 1-mg IV every 3 to 5 minutes during the arrest. Then administer atropine 1-mg IV push. This may be repeated every 3 to 5 minutes of the arrest until a total maximum dose of 0.04 mg/kg is given. Next consider the possible causes for the asystole. After all efforts have been done, consider termination if there is no change in the rhythm.
Impression: cardiac arrest

Oxygen-IV-Monitor-Fluids

Continue CPR, cardiac monitoring. Is fluid needed? Yes, to rapidly infuse the drugs being given. Continue the oxygen, cardiac monitoring, and obtain needed lab work. Is fluid needed? Yes, to infuse the drugs at a rapid rate.

Vital Signs

Continue to check for a rhythm change and obtain a history from the family if possible.

Rationale

Always, always check for responsiveness, call for help, then *airway, breathing, circulation* and *defibrillation* (if needed). In this case, defibrillation is not needed, so you can advance on to intubation and IV access. In the asystole protocol, you want to consider the possible causes such as acidosis, hypoxia, hypokalemia, hyperkalemia, drug overdose, or hypothermia. These are conditions in which you may be able to correct and reverse the asystole into a manageable rhythm. For transcutaneous pacing to be effective, it must be performed early in the arrest situation and simultaneously with drugs. If the patient remains in asystole after successful intubation and medication therapy and you cannot identify any reasonable causes for the arrest, then consider termination.

CHAPTER 7, CASE 4

Scenario

This rhythm is **pulseless electrical activity**. There is no pulse and no blood pressure. You have electrical activity but no mechanical activity, no contracting of the heart.

Primary Survey

Maintain the airway with an OPA and begin CPR. Is defibrillation needed? No, not at this time.

Secondary Survey

Airway: endotracheal intubation as soon as possible to ensure an adequate airway
Breathing: use the BVM, with supplemental oxygen, and ET tube to provide the respirations for the patient
Circulation: cardiac monitor, IV access, and appropriate drug therapy, which in this case would be vasopressin 40-U IV bolus, one dose, or epinephrine, 1:10,000, 1 mg IV every 3 to 5 minutes during the arrest. Then if the monitor is showing a rate less than 60 beats per minute, administer atropine 1-mg IV push. This may be repeated every 3 to 5 minutes of the arrest until a total maximum dose of 0.04 mg/kg is given. Next consider the possible causes for PEA (e.g., hypovolemia, hypoxia, drug overdose, massive acute myocardial infarction, acidosis, or hyperkalemia).
Impression: cardiac arrest, rule out the possible causes just listed

Oxygen-IV-Monitor-Fluids

Continue the oxygen, cardiac monitoring, and obtain needed lab work. Is fluid needed? Yes, to infuse the drugs at a rapid rate.

Vital Signs

Continue to check for rhythm change and obtain history from the family if possible.

Rationale

Always **A-B-C-D** (primary survey) followed by **A-B-C-D** (secondary survey). In pulseless electrical activity protocol, you need to consider the possible causes mentioned earlier. You might try using a Doppler ultrasound to see if indeed the patient does have a weak pulse that you are unable to detect. Also recheck the placement of the endotracheal tube to ensure the patient is receiving proper oxygenation. If acidosis is suspected, try sodium bicarbonate 1-mEq/kg IV. If any of the mentioned causes can be reversed, then the patient may convert to a sinus rhythm with pulses and a blood pressure. It certainly warrants your close attention to every clue to arrive at a possible cause for the arrest.

CHAPTER 8 SELF-TEST

1. a—Transcutaneous. A transcutaneous pacer has the electrode located on the skin of the chest wall and back. The electrical stimulation travels through the skin and muscle to the heart. It is a quick way to stimulate the heart without doing an invasive procedure.
2. d. A transvenous pacer has the tip of the electrode located in the right atrium, right ventricle, or both.
3. c. A pacemaker that has the electrode implanted within either the venous system or the epicardium is a permanent pacemaker.
4. c. The pulse generator is the power source that contains the battery and the controls that operate and regulate the pacemaker.
5. True. The electrode tip may be placed in any of the three layers of the heart.
6. True. The exposed portion of the pacing wire or lead is the electrode tip, which comes in direct contact with the heart, and provides electrical stimulus to cause the heart to contract.
7. a. A pacing lead with one exposed tip is unipolar, whereas a lead with two exposed tips is bipolar.
8. True. The unipolar lead produces larger ECG spikes because of the distance it travels between the positive and negative poles.
9. False. The unipolar system is more susceptible to inference than the bipolar system.
10. False. Electrical impulses travel from the positive towards the negative pole.
11. Milliamperes (mA)
12. a. A fixed-rate pacer fires or discharges continuously at a preset rate.
13. True. The first letter of the coding system indicates which chamber of the heart is being paced.
14. False. The fourth letter of the coding system indicates the programmable functions of the pacemaker.
15. c. The *S* stands for shock
16. b—*A* = atrial pacing, *A* = atrial sensing, *I* = inhibits pacing
17. c. The AV sequential pacer has one lead placed in the right atrium and the other placed in the right ventricle.

18. Three indications for transcutaneous pacing:
    Significant bradycardia unresponsive to atropine
    Asystole of less than 10 minutes' duration
    It is used as a temporary measure until a permanent pacer can be implanted
    It is used as emergency action in complete heart blocks

19. Three contraindications of transcutaneous pacing are
    Chest trauma
    Flail chest
    Hypothermia
    Pediatric patients weighing less than 15 kg

20. Five indications for transvenous pacing include the following:
    Unstable bradycardia accompanied with chest pain, hypotension, or pulmonary edema
    Complete AV block
    Symptomatic second-degree AV blocks
    Symptomatic sick sinus syndrome
    Permanent pacemaker failure
    Symptomatic atrial fibrillation with a slow ventricular rate
    Bradycardias with escape rhythms not responding to drug therapy
    To override pacing of tachycardias not responding to drug therapy

21. Failure to pace: c—this occurs when the pacemaker fails to discharge an electrical impulse or when it fails to deliver the correct number of impulses per minute.
    Failure to capture: a—this is the inability of the pacemaker stimulus to depolarize the myocardium and allow for ventricular contraction.
    Failure to sense: d—this occurs when the pacemaker fails to recognize myocardial depolarization.
    Oversensing: b—this occurs when there is an inappropriate sensing of electrical signals.

22. Two complications of transcutaneous pacing:
    Pain from electrical stimulation
    Tissue damage
    Failure to recognize that the pacer is not capturing

23. Five complications of transvenous pacing:
    Pneumothorax
    Bleeding, infection
    Myocardial infarction
    Electrode displacement
    Hematoma at insertion site
    Perforation of right ventricle
    Perforation of right vena cava
    Cardiac dysrhythmias
    Pneumothorax

24. Serious permanent pacemaker implantation procedure complications:
    Air embolism
    Cardiac dysrhythmias
    Pneumothorax
    Bleeding

25. Long-term complications of a permanent pacemaker:
    Congestive heart failure
    Pacemaker-induced dysrhythmias
    Infection
    Perforation of right ventricle
    Electrode displacement

CHAPTER 8 ECG PRACTICE STRIPS

Figure 8-1 Atrial fibrillation with ventricular paced beats
Rhythm = irregular
Rate = 70 beats per minute
P-R interval = absent
QRS complex = 0.08 second
Ventricular pacer

Figure 8-2 Ventricular paced rhythm
Rhythm = regular
Rate = 72 beats per minute
P-R interval = absent
QRS complex = 0.13 second
Ventricular pacer

Figure 8-3 Ventricular paced rhythm
Rhythm = regular
Rate = 78 beats per minute
P-R interval = absent
QRS complex = 0.12 second
Ventricular pacer

Figure 8-4 First-degree AV heart block with three ventricular paced beats
Rate = 80 beats per minute
P-R interval = 0.26 second
QRS complex = 0.12 second (sinus beats) and 0.12 second (paced beats)
Ventricular pacer for three beats then sinus rhythm

Figure 8-5 Ventricular paced rhythm
Rhythm = regular
Rate = 72 beats per minute
P-R interval = absent
QRS complex = 0.12 second
Ventricular pacer

Figure 8-6 AV sequential pacemaker rhythm
Rhythm = irregular
Rate = 65 beats per minute
P-R interval = 0.16 second with atrial pacing
QRS complex = 0.16 second
First two beats are A-V pacer, third and fourth are ventricular pacer, fifth is A-V pacer, sixth is ventricular pacer, and seventh is A-V pacer

Figure 8-7 First-degree AV heart block and one paced beat
Rhythm = slightly irregular
Rate = 86 beats per minute
P-R interval = 0.28 second
QRS complex = 0.10 second

Figure 8-8 AV sequential paced rhythm
Rhythm = regular
Rate = 62 beats per minute
P-R interval = absent
QRS complex = 0.16 second
A-V pacing

Figure 8-9 Ventricular paced rhythm
Rhythm = regular
Rate = 90 beats per minute
P-R interval = 0.20 second
QRS complex = 0.16 second

Figure 8-10 AV sequential paced rhythm
Rhythm = regular
Rate = 64 beats per minute
P-R interval = absent
QRS complex = 0.14 second

Figure 8-11 AV sequential paced rhythm
Rhythm = irregular
Rate = 70 beats per minute
P-R interval = 0.16, ventricular paced beats
QRS complex = 0.16 second
The first, third, and sixth are ventricular paced, whereas the second, fourth, and fifth are AV paced

Figure 8-12 Ventricular paced rhythm
Rhythm = regular
Rate = 72 beats per minute
P-R interval = absent
QRS complex = 0.12 second

Figure 8-13 AV sequential paced rhythm
Rhythm = irregular
Rate = 80 beats per minute
P-R interval = 0.20 second where present
QRS complex = 0.15 second
Fourth and ninth beats are AV paced; rest are ventricular paced

Figure 8-14 AV sequential paced rhythm with two ectopic beats
Rhythm = irregular
Rate = 60 beats per minute
P-R interval = absent

QRS complex = 0.12 second
Fourth and seventh are ectopic beats; also appears to have failure to capture after the first paced beat

Figure 8-15 Ventricular paced rhythm
Rhythm = regular
Rate = 78 beats per minute
P-R interval = absent
QRS complex = 0.16 second

CHAPTER 8, CASE 1

Scenario

This rhythm is a **pacemaker, failure to capture** rhythm with a rate of 45 beats per minute
Rhythm = irregular; there are no P waves, but there are pacer spikes. The QRS complex is 0.20 second

Primary Survey

The airway is open, the breathing is adequate, and no chest compressions are needed because the patient is awake and alert. No defibrillation is needed.

Secondary Survey

Airway: adequate
Breathing: apply oxygen 2 to 3 L via nasal cannula
Circulation: cardiac monitor, IV access, 12-lead ECG, pulse oximetry
Impression: rule out a possible pacemaker malfunction

Oxygen-IV-Monitor-Fluids

Continue the oxygen, monitor the heart rate, obtain needed lab work. Are fluids needed? Yes, because he is hypotensive.

Vital Signs

Continue ongoing vital signs, monitor the heart rate, blood pressure, pulse, and respirations; obtain a history, perform a physical examination, and get a chest x-ray

Rationale

Oxygen is the first intervention. When you find that the pacemaker is not functioning properly, you may as well begin preparing this patient for surgery. The patient is showing signs of decreased cardiac output with fatigue, nausea, and sweating for no apparent reason. In addition, the blood pressure seems unusually low for someone with hypertension. The ECG strip is showing bradycardia due to the failure of the pacemaker to capture and fire. Possible reasons for this include (1) the pacemaker voltage is too low, (2) the electrode tip is out of position, (3) a lead wire is broken, and (4) edema or scar tissue has formed at the electrode tip. The tip may need to be repositioned, the voltage may need to be increased, the lead wire may need to be replaced, or the battery in the pacemaker may need to be replaced. Failure to capture is indicated by ECG pacemaker spikes that are *not* followed by P waves (if an atrial pacer) or QRS complexes (if a ventricular pacer). One simple intervention you may try is to reposition the patient on his left side. This may move the catheter tip back into place. The chest x-ray may help determine if the electrode wire is broken.

CHAPTER 8, CASE 2

Scenario

This rhythm is a **pacemaker rhythm, failure to capture** with a rate of 50 beats per minute. The rhythm is irregular. There are no P waves present, just pacer spikes. There is a pacemaker spike before the QRS complex. The QRS complex is 0.16 second.

Primary Survey

The airway is open, breathing is adequate, and no chest compressions are needed. No defibrillation is needed.

Secondary Survey

Airway: adequate
Breathing: apply oxygen 2 to 3 L per minute via nasal cannula
Circulation: cardiac monitor, IV access, 12-lead ECG, pulse oximetry
Impression: rule out a possible MI or pacemaker problems

Oxygen-IV-Monitor-Fluids

Continue the oxygen, cardiac monitoring, and obtain needed lab work. Is fluid needed? No, because the patient has no complaints at present.

Vital Signs

Continue ongoing vital signs; monitor the cardiac rhythm. Perform a physical examination, obtain a complete history, and get a chest x-ray.

Rationale

When you see pacemaker spikes that are not followed by P waves (atrial pacer) or QRS complexes (ventricular pacer), most likely there is a problem with the pacemaker. Because he told you that battery was changed 2 months ago, it is unlikely the battery is at fault. However, because he was wearing a seat belt and was in an accident last evening, there is a possibility that the pressure from the seat belt on the chest caused the electrode tip to be displaced. Another thought is that the lead wire was broken or myocardial perforation was caused from the sudden pressure on the chest from the seat belt in the motor vehicle accident. His chest x-ray may give you the answer. Be prepared to get him ready for the operating room (OR) so he may have another pacemaker inserted.

CHAPTER 8, CASE 3

Scenario

This rhythm is an **AV sequential pacemaker rhythm, with two PVCs, failure to sense**. The underlying rhythm is sinus at a rate of 80 beats per minute. The rhythm is irregular. The QRS complex is 0.16 second. There are two P waves present because of atrial pacing.

Primary Survey

The airway is open, breathing is adequate, and no chest compressions are needed. No defibrillation is needed.

Secondary Survey

Airway: adequate
Breathing: apply oxygen 2 to 3 L per minute via nasal cannula
Circulation: cardiac monitor, IV access, 12-lead ECG, pulse oximetry
Impression: rule out a possible MI or pacemaker problems

Oxygen-IV-Monitor-Fluids

Continue the oxygen, cardiac monitoring, and obtain needed lab work. Is fluid needed? Yes, because he is slightly hypotensive.

Vital Signs

Continue ongoing vital signs; monitor the cardiac rhythm. Perform a physical examination, obtain a complete history, and get a chest x-ray.

Rationale

There could be any number of reasons for this patient's hypotension. He has a pacemaker, which may have malfunctioned, or he could be having cardiac problems. The diabetes may have produced a low blood glucose level, or he may have a gastrointestinal bleed. Thus a full workup is indicated, and treatment initially would be with fluid replacement as long as the lungs are clear. You certainly must be concerned with the fact he had a 2-minute episode of syncope; therefore close observation is essential.

CHAPTER 8, CASE 4

Scenario

This rhythm is a **pacemaker rhythm, failure to sense** with a rate of 72 beats per minute. The rhythm is irregular. The QRS complex is 0.16 second.

Primary Survey

The airway is open, breathing is adequate, and no chest compressions are needed. No defibrillation is needed.

Secondary Survey

Airway: adequate
Breathing: apply oxygen 2 to 3 L per minute via nasal cannula
Circulation: cardiac monitor, IV access,12-lead ECG, pulse oximetry
Impression: rule out a possible MI or pacemaker malfunction

Oxygen-IV-Monitor-Fluids

Continue the oxygen, cardiac monitoring, and obtain needed lab work. Is fluid needed? No, not at this time.

Vital Signs

Continue ongoing vital signs; monitor the cardiac rhythm. Do a physical examination, obtain a complete history, and get a chest x-ray.

Rationale

Failure to sense is a cause for concern. The pacer spikes may fall on the T waves and cause ventricular fibrillation or tachycardia. Most likely there is a problem with the pacemaker. Failure to sense can occur for several reasons, which include the following:

- Battery is dead
- Electrode tip is out of position
- The lead wire is broken
- Increased sensing threshold from edema or scar tissue is at the electrode tip

Your next step would be to prepare him for the OR in case he needs his pacemaker battery or lead wire replaced, or the electrode needs to be repositioned. In the meantime you can place him on his left side, which may correct the problem temporarily.

CHAPTER 9 ECG PRACTICE STRIPS

Figure 9-1 Sinus rhythm with one ectopic beat
Irregular
Rate: 42 beats per minute except for ectopic beat
P-R interval = 0.20 second
QRS complex = 0.10 second
Is there a P wave *before* every QRS complex? No
Is there a QRS complex *after* every P wave? Yes

Figure 9-2 Junctional rhythm
Regular
Rate: 55 beats per minute
P-R interval = absent
QRS complex = 0.06 second
Is there a P wave *before* every QRS complex? There are no P waves

Figure 9-3 Atrial fibrillation
Irregular

Rate: 40 beats per minute
P-R interval = absent
QRS complex = 0.05 second
There are no discernable P waves

Figure 9-4 Sinus arrhythmia
Irregular
Rate: 71 beats per minute
P-R interval = 0.16 second
QRS complex = 0.08 second
Is there a P wave *before* every QRS complex? Yes
Is there a QRS complex *after* every P wave? Yes

Figure 9-5 Sinus bradycardia with first-degree AV block
Regular
Rate: 50 beats per minute
P-R interval = 0.32 second
QRS complex = 0.10 second
Is there a P wave *before* every QRS complex? Yes
Is there a QRS complex *after* every P wave? Yes

Figure 9-6 Atrial fibrillation with one PVC and artifact
Irregular
Rate: 52 beats per minute
P-R interval = absent
QRS complex = 0.06 second
There are no discernable P waves

Figure 9-7 Sinus tachycardia
Regular
Rate: 140 beats per minute
P-R interval = 0.16 second
QRS complex = 0.08 second
Is there a P wave *before* every QRS complex? Yes
Is there a QRS complex *after* every P wave? Yes

Figure 9-8 Atrial tachycardia
Regular
Rate: 178 beats per minute
P-R interval = 0.10 second (shortened)
QRS complex = 0.05 second
Is there a P wave *before* every QRS complex? Yes
Is there a QRS complex *after* every P wave? Yes

Figure 9-9 Normal sinus rhythm
Regular
Rate: 90 beats per minute
P-R interval = 0.16 second
QRS complex = 0.04 second

Is there a P wave *before* every QRS complex? Yes
Is there a QRS complex *after* every P wave? Yes

Figure 9-10 Normal sinus rhythm
Regular
Rate: 60 beats per minute
P-R interval = 0.18 second
QRS complex = 0.06 second
Is there a P wave *before* every QRS complex? Yes
Is there a QRS complex *after* every P wave? Yes

Figure 9-11 Ventricular paced rhythm
Regular
Rate: 72 beats per minute
P-R interval = absent
QRS complex = 0.12 second
Is there a P wave *before* every QRS complex? There are no P waves

Figure 9-12 Ventricular fibrillation
Irregular
Rate: none
P-R interval = absent
QRS complex = absent
Is there a P wave *before* every QRS complex? There are no P waves

Figure 9-13 Junctional tachycardia with two atrial beats
Regular
Rate: 130 beats per minute
P-R interval = 0.16 second
QRS complex = 0.08 second
Is there a P wave *before* every QRS complex? No
Is there a QRS complex *after* every P wave? Yes

Figure 9-14 Atrial tachycardia
Irregular
Rate: 200 beats per minute
P-R interval = 0.10 second
QRS complex = varies 0.04 second
Is there a P wave *before* every QRS complex? Yes
Is there a QRS complex *after* every P wave? Yes

Figure 9-15 Rapid atrial fibrillation
lrregular
Rate: 140 beats per minute
P-R interval = absent
QRS complex = 0.07 second
There are no discernable P waves

Figure 9-16 Second-degree AV heart block, Mobitz II
Irregular

Rate: 40 beats per minute
P-R interval = 0.16 second
QRS complex = 0.05 second
Is there a P wave *before* every QRS complex? Yes
Is there a QRS complex *after* every P wave? No

Figure 9-17 Ventricular pacemaker rhythm
Regular
Rate: 72 beats per minute
P-R interval = absent
QRS complex = 0.14 second
Is there a P wave *before* every QRS complex? There are no P waves

Figure 9-18 Normal sinus rhythm
Regular
Rate: 82 beats per minute
P-R interval = 0.16 second
QRS complex = 0.05 second
Is there a P wave *before* every QRS complex? Yes
Is there a QRS complex *after* every P wave? Yes

Figure 9-19 Third-degree AV heart block, two junctional beats and two PVCs
Irregular
Rate: 40 beats per minute
P-R interval = absent
QRS complex = varies 0.06 to 0.22 second
Is there a P wave *before* every QRS complex? No
Is there a QRS complex *after* every P wave? No

Figure 9-20 Sinus rhythm with PACs
Irregular
Rate: 100 beats per minute
P-R interval = normal beats 0.16 second, PACs 0.12 second; second, sixth, and tenth beats are early
QRS complex = 0.05 second
Is there a P wave *before* every QRS complex? Yes
Is there a QRS complex *after* every P wave? Yes

Figure 9-21 Atrial flutter
Irregular
Rate: 100 beats per minute
P-R interval = 0.20 second
QRS complex = 0.06 second
Is there a P wave *before* every QRS complex? Yes
Is there a QRS complex *after* every P wave? Yes

Figure 9-22 Sinus tachycardia
Regular
Rate: 120 beats per minute
P-R interval = 0.16 second

QRS complex = 0.06 second
Is there a P wave *before* every QRS complex? Yes
Is there a QRS complex *after* every P wave? Yes

Figure 9-23 Supraventricular tachycardia (SVT)
Regular
Rate: 170 beats per minute
P-R interval = absent
QRS complex = 0.07 second
Is there a P wave *before* every QRS complex? There are no P waves

Figure 9-24 Sinus arrhythmia with a run of ventricular tachycardia
Irregular
Rate underlying rhythm 110 beats per minute
P-R interval = 0.16 second where present
QRS complex = 0.12 second, wide
Is there a P wave *before* every QRS complex? No
Is there a QRS complex *after* every P wave? No
Some P waves are buried in preceding T waves

Figure 9-25 Junctional rhythm with wide conduction, or idioventricular rhythm
Regular
Rate: 50 beats per minute
P-R interval = absent
QRS complex = 0.16 second
Is there a P wave *before* every QRS complex? There are no P waves

Figure 9-26 Atrial fibrillation
Irregular
Rate: 92 beats per minute
P-R interval = absent
QRS complex = 0.08 second
There are no discernable P waves

Figure 9-27 Junctional rhythm
Regular
Rate: 52 beats per minute
P-R interval = absent
QRS complex = 0.10 second
Is there a P wave *before* every QRS complex? There are no P waves

Figure 9-28 Sinus bradycardia
Regular
Rate: 56 beats per minute
P-R interval = 0.16 second
QRS complex = 0.04 second
Is there a P wave *before* every QRS complex? Yes
Is there a QRS complex *after* every P wave? Yes

Figure 9-29 Third-degree AV heart block
Irregular
Rate: 26 beats per minute
P-R interval = absent
QRS complex = 0.12 second
Is there a P wave *before* every QRS complex? No
Is there a QRS complex *after* every P wave? No
There is no relationship between the P waves and the QRS complexes

Figure 9-30 Normal sinus rhythm
Regular
Rate: 74 beats per minute
P-R interval = 0.16 second
QRS complex = 0.08 second
Is there a P wave *before* every QRS complex? Yes
Is there a QRS complex *after* every P wave? Yes

Figure 9-31 Sinus tachycardia
Regular
Rate: 102 beats per minute
P-R interval = 0.16 second
QRS complex = 0.10 second
Is there a P wave *before* every QRS complex? yes
Is there a QRS complex *after* every P wave? Yes

Figure 9-32 Atrial flutter
Regular
Rate: atrial rate, 360 beats per minutes; ventricular rate, 90 beats per minute
P-R interval = absent
QRS complex = 0.12 second, wide connection
4:1 conduction rate; there are four P waves for each QRS complex

Figure 9-33 Supraventricular tachycardia (SVT)
Regular
Rate: 150 beats per minute
P-R interval = absent
QRS complex = 0.06 second
Is there a P wave *before* every QRS complex? There are no P waves

Figure 9-34 Atrial fibrillation
Irregular
Rate: 116 beats per minute
P-R interval = absent
QRS complex = 0.06 second
There are no discernable P waves

Figure 9-35 Supraventricular tachycardia (SVT), with artifact
Regular
Rate: 187 beats per minute

P-R interval = absent
QRS complex = 0.04 second
Is there a P wave *before* every QRS complex? There are no P waves

Figure 9-36 Junctional tachycardia
Irregular
Rate: 100 beats per minute
P-R interval = 0.08 second where present
QRS complex = 0.06 second
Some P waves are inverted, some are absent; P waves are present in first, sixth, seventh, and ninth beats

Figure 9-37 Ventricular escape rhythm with one paced beat
Regular
Rate: 75 beats per minute
P-R interval = absent
QRS complex = 0.12 second
Is there a P wave *before* every QRS complex? There are no P waves

Figure 9-38 Sinus tachycardia
Irregular
Rate: 105 beats per minute
P-R interval = 0.14 second
QRS complex = 0.05 second
Is there a P wave *before* every QRS complex? Yes
Is there a QRS complex *after* every P wave? Yes

Figure 9-39 Sinus tachycardia
Regular
Rate: 115 beats per minute
P-R interval = 0.20 second
QRS complex = 0.08 second
Is there a P wave *before* every QRS complex? Yes
Is there a QRS complex *after* every P wave? Yes

Figure 9-40 Atrial fibrillation with bigeminy PVCs
Irregular
Rate: 130 beats per minutes
P-R interval = absent
QRS complex = varies 0.06 to 0.12 second
There are no discernable P waves

Figure 9-41 Idioventricular rhythm
Irregular
Rate: 28 beats per minute
P-R interval = absent
QRS complex = 0.10 second
Is there a P wave *before* every QRS complex? There are no P waves
"Dying heart"

Figure 9-42 Supraventricular tachycardia or ventricular tachycardia
Regular
Rate: 180 beats per minute
P-R interval = absent
QRS complex = 0.14 second
Is there a P wave *before* every QRS complex? There are no P waves

Figure 9-43 Sinus bradycardia
Regular
Rate: 54 beats per minute
P-R interval = 0.19 second
QRS complex = 0.07 second
Is there a P wave *before* every QRS complex? Yes
Is there a QRS complex *after* every P wave? Yes

Figure 9-44 Sinus bradycardia
Regular
Rate: 40 beats per minute
P-R interval = 0.16 second
QRS complex = 0.06 second
Is there a P wave *before* every QRS complex? Yes
Is there a QRS complex *after* every P wave? Yes

Figure 9-45 Atrial fibrillation
Irregular
Rate: 90 beats per minute
P-R interval = absent
QRS complex = 0.08 second
There are no discernable P waves

Figure 9-46 Atrial tachycardia with sinus arrest
Irregular
Rate: 130 beats per minute
P-R interval = 0.08 second, where visible
QRS complex = 0.08 second
Some of the P waves are buried in the preceding T waves

Figure 9-47 Sinus arrhythmia with run of ventricular tachycardia
Irregular
Rate: underlying rhythm, 100 beats per minute
P-R interval = 0.20 second where present
QRS complex = 0.10 second
Is there a P wave *before* every QRS complex? No
Is there a QRS complex *after* every P wave? Yes

Figure 9-48 Atrial tachycardia
Regular
Rate: 162 beats per minute
P-R interval = 0.08 second where present

QRS complex = 0.04 second
Not all P waves are visible; some are buried in preceding T waves

Figure 9-49 Second-degree AV heart block, Wenckebach or Mobitz I
Irregular
Rate: 49 beats per minute
P-R interval = varies, longer until QRS complex is dropped
QRS complex = 0.12 second
Is there a P wave *before* every QRS complex? Yes
Is there a QRS complex *after* every P wave? No

Figure 9-50 Third-degree AV heart block
Irregular
Rate: 28 beats per minute
P-R interval = absent
QRS complex = 0.15 second
Is there a P wave *before* every QRS complex? No
Is there a QRS complex *after* every P wave? No

Figure 9-51 AV sequential pacemaker with ventricular escape beats
Irregular
Rate: 68 beats per minute (approximate)
P-R interval = absent
QRS complex = 0.12 second
Second, third, fifth, and sixth are paced beats; first, fourth, and seventh are ventricular beats

Figure 9-52 Normal sinus rhythm with one PAC
Irregular
Rate: 62 beats per minute
P-R interval = 0.20 second, where present
QRS complex = 0.08 second
Is there a P wave *before* every QRS complex? No
Is there a QRS complex *after* every P wave? Yes

Figure 9-53 Sinus tachycardia
Regular
Rate: 110 beats per minute
P-R interval = 0.12 second
QRS complex = 0.08 second
Is there a P wave *before* every QRS complex? Yes
Is there a QRS complex *after* every P wave? Yes

Figure 9-54 Normal sinus rhythm
Regular
Rate: 85 beats per minute
P-R interval = 0.12 second
QRS complex = 0.10 second
Is there a P wave *before* every QRS complex? Yes
Is there a QRS complex *after* every P wave? Yes

Figure 9-55 Sinus tachycardia
Regular
Rate: 116 beats per minute
P-R interval = 0.16 second
QRS complex = 0.06 second
Is there a P wave *before* every QRS complex? Yes
Is there a QRS complex *after* every P wave? Yes

Figure 9-56 Accelerated junctional rhythm with one PVC
Irregular
Rate: 68 beats per minute
P-R interval = absent
QRS complex = 0.12 second, wide conduction
Is there a P wave *before* every QRS complex? There are no P waves

Figure 9-57 Sinus arrhythmia with one PAC
Irregular
Rate: 52 beats per minute
P-R interval = 0.16 second
QRS complex = 0.12 second, wide conduction
Is there a P wave *before* every QRS complex? No
Is there a QRS complex *after* every P wave? Yes

Figure 9-58 Sinus rhythm with multifocal PVCs
Irregular
Rate: 60 beats per minute
P-R interval = 0.16 second
QRS complex = 0.08 second
Is there a P wave *before* every QRS complex? No
Is there a QRS complex *after* every P wave? Yes

Figure 9-59 Idioventricular rhythm
Irregular
Rate: 29 beats per minute
P-R interval = absent
QRS complex = 0.12 second
Is there a P wave *before* every QRS complex? There are no P waves

Figure 9-60 Normal sinus rhythm
Regular
Rate: 70 beats per minute
P-R interval = 0.16 second
QRS complex = 0.04 second
Is there a P wave *before* every QRS complex? Yes
Is there a QRS complex *after* every P wave? Yes

Figure 9-61 Normal sinus rhythm
Regular
Rate: 90 beats per minute

P-R interval = 0.16 second
QRS complex = 0.08 second
Is there a P wave *before* every QRS complex? Yes
Is there a QRS complex *after* every P wave? Yes

Figure 9-62 Atrial fibrillation
Irregular
Rate: 140 beats per minute
P-R interval = absent
QRS complex = 0.04 second
There are no discernable P waves

Figure 9-63 Sinus arrest
Irregular
Rate: 54 beats per minute
P-R interval = 0.16 second
QRS complex = 0.06 second
Is there a P wave *before* every QRS complex? Yes
Is there a QRS complex *after* every P wave? Yes
However, to find a long pause where the entire P-QRS-T complex is absent (there are two complete P-QRS-T complexes that are absent), use the calipers and measure where the next expected beats should be present

Figure 9-64 Sinus arrhythmia
Irregular
Rate: 64 beats per minute
P-R interval = 0.14 second
QRS complex = 0.07 second
Is there a P wave *before* every QRS complex? Yes
Is there a QRS complex *after* every P wave? Yes

Figure 9-65 Ventricular tachycardia
Fairly regular
Rate: 120 beats per minute
P-R interval = absent
QRS complex = 0.36 second, wide conduction
Is there a P wave *before* every QRS complex? There are no P waves

Figure 9-66 Atrial fibrillation
Irregular
Rate: 110 beats per minute
P-R interval = absent
QRS complex = 0.04 second
There are no discernable P waves

Figure 9-67 Sinus tachycardia
Regular
Rate: 124 beats per minute
P-R interval = 0.14 second

QRS complex = 0.05 second
Is there a P wave *before* every QRS complex? Yes
Is there a QRS complex *after* every P wave? Yes

Figure 9-68 Atrial fibrillation with couplet PVCs
Irregular
Rate: varies from 130 to 140 beats per minute
P-R interval = absent
QRS complex = 0.12 second, wide conduction
There are no discernable P waves

Figure 9-69 Normal sinus rhythm
Regular
Rate: 68 beats per minute
P-R interval = 0.14 second
QRS complex = 0.05 second
Is there a P wave *before* every QRS complex? Yes
Is there a QRS complex *after* every P wave? Yes

Figure 9-70 Normal sinus rhythm with one PVC
Irregular
Rate: 75 beats per minute
P-R interval = 0.16 second
QRS complex = 0.06 second
Is there a P wave *before* every QRS complex? No
Is there a QRS complex *after* every P wave? Yes

Figure 9-71 Atrial fibrillation
Irregular
Rate: 75 beats per minute
P-R interval = absent
QRS complex = 0.08 second
There are no discernable P waves

Figure 9-72 Junctional rhythm with trigeminy PVCs
Irregular
Rate: 64 beats per minute
P-R interval = inverted, 0.12 second
QRS complex = 0.06 second
Is there a P wave *before* every QRS complex? No
Is there a QRS complex *after* every P wave? Yes

Figure 9-73 Sinus tachycardia with artifact
Regular
Rate: 150 beats per minute
P-R interval = 0.16 second
QRS complex = 0.04 second
Is there a P wave *before* every QRS complex? Yes
Is there a QRS complex *after* every P wave? Yes

Figure 9-74 Sinus arrhythmia with artifact
Irregular
Rate: 90 beats per minute
P-R interval = 0.20 second
QRS complex = 0.06 second
Is there a P wave *before* every QRS complex? Yes
Is there a QRS complex *after* every P wave? Yes

Figure 9-75 Normal sinus rhythm with one atrial beat (no P wave visible)
Regular
Rate: 100 beats per minute
P-R interval = 0.16 second
QRS complex = 0.10 second
Is there a P wave *before* every QRS complex? No
Is there a QRS complex *after* every P wave? No

Figure 9-76 Sinus tachycardia
Regular
Rate: 122 beats per minute
P-R interval = 0.14 second, P wave falls on previous T wave
QRS complex = 0.06 second
Is there a P wave *before* every QRS complex? Yes
Is there a QRS complex *after* every P wave? Yes

Figure 9-77 Sinus rhythm with one PJC
Irregular
Rate: varies approximately 80 beats per minute
P-R interval = 0.16 second
QRS complex = 0.10 second
Is there a P wave *before* every QRS complex? Yes
Is there a QRS complex *after* every P wave? Yes
The fifth beat has an inverted P wave

Figure 9-78 Atrial flutter
Regular
Rate: 60 beats per minute
P-R interval = 0.20 second, where present
QRS complex = 0.12 second, wide conduction
Is there a P wave *before* every QRS complex? Yes
Is there a QRS complex *after* every P wave? No

Figure 9-79 Ventricular tachycardia
Regular
Rate: 230 beats per minute
P-R interval = absent
QRS complex = 0.16 second
Is there a P wave *before* every QRS complex? There are no P waves

Figure 9-80 Normal sinus rhythm with first-degree AV block
Regular
Rate: 104 beats per minute
P-R interval = 0.34 second
QRS complex = 0.04 second
Is there a P wave *before* every QRS complex? Yes
Is there a QRS complex *after* every P wave? Yes

Figure 9-81 Normal sinus rhythm with artifact
Regular
Rate: 50 beats per minute
P-R interval = 0.20 second
QRS complex = 0.08 second
Is there a P wave *before* every QRS complex? Yes
Is there a QRS complex *after* every P wave? Yes

Figure 9-82 Accelerated junctional rhythm
Regular
Rate: 100 beats per minute
P-R interval = absent
QRS complex = 0.12 second, wide conduction
Is there a P wave *before* every QRS complex? There are no P waves

Figure 9-83 Sinus rhythm with multifocal PVCs
Irregular
Rate: approximately 80 beats per minute
P-R interval = 0.14 second
QRS complex = 0.06 second
Is there a P wave *before* every QRS complex? No
Is there a QRS complex *after* every P wave? Yes

Figure 9-84 Atrial flutter
Irregular
Rate: approximately 80 beats per minute
P-R interval = absent
QRS complex = 0.06 second
Is there a P wave *before* every QRS complex? Yes
Is there a QRS complex *after* every P wave? No
This has 2:1, 3:1, and 4:1 conduction

Figure 9-85 Normal sinus rhythm with PACs
Irregular
Rate: 56 beats per minute
P-R interval = 0.19 second
QRS complex = 0.08 second
Is there a P wave *before* every QRS complex? Yes
Is there a QRS complex *after* every P wave? Yes

Figure 9-86 Sinus rhythm with couplet PVCs
Irregular
Rate: 55 beats per minute
P-R interval = 0.20 second
QRS complex = 0.10 second
Is there a P wave *before* every QRS complex? No
Is there a QRS complex *after* every P wave? Yes

Figure 9-87 Junctional rhythm with PVCs
Irregular
Rate: 75 beats per minute, varies
P-R interval = absent
QRS complex = 0.06 second
Is there a P wave *before* every QRS complex? There are no P waves

Figure 9-88 Normal sinus rhythm with artifact
Regular
Rate: 92 beats per minute
P-R interval = 0.16 second
QRS complex = 0.07 second
Is there a P wave *before* every QRS complex? Yes
Is there a QRS complex *after* every P wave? Yes

Figure 9-89 Normal sinus rhythm
Regular
Rate: 74 beats per minute
P-R interval = 0.20 second
QRS complex = 0.04 second
Is there a P wave *before* every QRS complex? Yes
Is there a QRS complex *after* every P wave? Yes

Figure 9-90 Sinus bradycardia
Regular
Rate: 53 beats per minute
P-R interval = 0.20 second
QRS complex = 0.06 second
Is there a P wave *before* every QRS complex? Yes
Is there a QRS complex *after* every P wave? Yes

Figure 9-91 Sinus tachycardia with PVCs
Irregular
Rate: 115 beats per minute
P-R interval = 0.16 second
QRS complex = 0.06 second
Is there a P wave *before* every QRS complex? No
Is there a QRS complex *after* every P wave? Yes

Figure 9-92 Sinus rhythm with first-degree AV block and one PVC
Irregular

Rate: 50 beats per minutes except for ectopic beat
P-R interval = 0.32 second
QRS complex = 0.10 second
Is there a P wave *before* every QRS complex? No
Is there a QRS complex *after* every P wave? Yes

Figure 9-93 Ventricular pacemaker rhythm
Regular
Rate: 75 beats per minute
P-R interval = absent
QRS complex = 0.12 second
Is there a P wave *before* every QRS complex? No
Is there a QRS complex *after* every P wave? Yes

Figure 9-94 Junctional tachycardia
Irregular
Rate: 112 beats per minute
P-R interval = absent
QRS complex = 0.06 second
Is there a P wave *before* every QRS complex? There are no P waves

Figure 9-95 Accelerated idioventricular rhythm
Regular
Rate: 48 beats per minute
P-R interval = absent
QRS complex = 0.12 second
Is there a P wave *before* every QRS complex? There are no P waves

Figure 9-96 Sinus tachycardia with intraventricular conduction deficit
Regular
Rate: 130 beats per minute
P-R interval = varies 0.12 to 0.16 second
QRS complex = 0.10 second
Is there a P wave *before* every QRS complex? Yes
Is there a QRS complex *after* every P wave? Yes

Figure 9-97 Sinus arrhythmia with peaked T waves
Irregular
Rate: 86 beats per minute
P-R interval = 0.16 second
QRS complex = 0.08 second
Is there a P wave *before* every QRS complex? Yes
Is there a QRS complex *after* every P wave? Yes

Figure 9-98 Idioventricular with PVCs
Irregular
Rate: 25 beats per minute
P-R interval = absent

QRS complex = 0.12 second
Is there a P wave *before* every QRS complex? There are no P waves

Figure 9-99 Third-deree AV heart block
Regular
Rate: 30 beats per minute
P-R interval = absent
QRS complex = 0.16 second
There is no relationship between the P waves and QRS complexes

Figure 9-100 Sinus arrhythmia
Irregular
Rate: 43 beats per minute
P-R interval = 0.12 second
QRS complex = 0.008 second
Is there a P wave *before* every QRS complex? Yes
Is there a QRS complex *after* every P wave? Yes

Figure 9-101 Slow junctional escape rhythm
Regular
Rate: 30 beats per minute
P-R interval = absent
QRS complex = 0.10 second
Is there a P wave *before* every QRS complex? There are no P waves

Figure 9-102 Junctional rhythm
Regular
Rate: 52 beats per minute
P-R interval = 0.16 second, inverted P waves
QRS complex = 0.08 second
Is there a P wave *before* every QRS complex? Yes
Is there a QRS complex *after* every P wave? Yes

Figure 9-103 Normal sinus rhythm with one PVC
Irregular
Rate: 94 beats per minute
P-R interval = 0.12 second
QRS complex = 0.05 second
Is there a P wave *before* every QRS complex? No
Is there a QRS complex *after* every P wave? Yes

Figure 9-104 Rapid atrial fibrillation
Irregular
Rate: 115 beats per minute
P-R interval = 0.16 second, where present
QRS complex = 0.08 second
Most P waves are not measurable

Figure 9-105 Junctional rhythm (wide conduction), or idioventricular with one PJC
Irregular
Rate: 60 beats per minute
P-R interval = absent
QRS complex = 0.14 second, wide conduction
P waves are absent, except for one inverted P wave after PJC

Figure 9-106 First-degree AV heart block
Regular
Rate: 66 beats per minute
P-R interval = 0.28 second
QRS complex = 0.12 second
Is there a P wave *before* every QRS complex? Yes
Is there a QRS complex *after* every P wave? Yes

Figure 9-107 Sinus bradycardia
Regular
Rate: 34 beats per minute
P-R interval = 0.20 second
QRS complex = 0.06 second
Is there a P wave *before* every QRS complex? Yes
Is there a QRS complex *after* every P wave? Yes

Figure 9-108 Atrial fibrillation
Irregular
Rate: 50 beats per minute
P-R interval = absent
QRS complex = 0.05 second
There are no discernable P waves

Figure 9-109 Atrial fibrillation with multifocal PVCs
Irregular
Rate: 90 beats per minute
P-R interval = varies
QRS complex = 0.10 second
There are no discernable P waves

Figure 9-110 Normal sinus rhythm
Regular
Rate: 86 beats per minute
P-R interval = 0.19 second
QRS complex = 0.08 second
Is there a P wave *before* every QRS complex? Yes
Is there a QRS complex *after* every P wave? Yes

Figure 9-111 Sinus rhythm with bigeminy PJCs
Irregular
Rate: 90 beats per minute (counting PJCs as perfusing)
P-R interval = varies 0.12 to 0.18 second

QRS complex = 0.06 second
Is there a P wave *before* every QRS complex? No
Is there a QRS complex *after* every P wave? Yes

Figure 9-112 Second-degree AV heart block, Mobitz I (Wenckebach)
Irregular
Rate: 60 beats per minute
P-R interval = increasingly longer until dropped
QRS complex = 0.06 second
Is there a P wave *before* every QRS complex? Yes
Is there a QRS complex *after* every P wave? No

Figure 9-113 First-degree AV heart block
Regular
Rate: 66 beats per minute
P-R interval = 0.28 second
QRS complex = 0.08 second
Is there a P wave *before* every QRS complex? Yes
Is there a QRS complex *after* every P wave? Yes

Figure 9-114 Third-degree AV heart block
Irregular
Rate: less than 20 beats per minute
P-R interval = absent
QRS complex = 0.06 second in one beat only
There is no relationship between the P waves and QRS complexes; atrial rate of 80 beats per minute, ventricular rate of less than 20 beats per minute

Figure 9-115 Rapid atrial fibrillation
Irregular
Rate: 130 beats per minute
P-R interval = absent
QRS complex = 0.05 second
There are no discernable P waves

Figure 9-116 Sinus bradycardia
Regular
Rate: 50 beats per minute
P-R interval = 0.20 second
QRS complex = 0.05 second
Is there a P wave *before* every QRS complex? Yes
Is there a QRS complex *after* every P wave? Yes

Figure 9-117 Normal sinus rhythm with artifact
Regular
Rate: 75 beats per minute
P-R interval = 0.20 second
QRS complex = 0.08 second
Is there a P wave *before* every QRS complex? Yes
Is there a QRS complex *after* every P wave? Yes

Figure 9-118 Sinus rhythm with bigeminy PVCs
Irregular
Rate: 80 beats per minute (counting PVCs)
P-R interval = 0.12 second
QRS complex = 0.08 second
Is there a P wave *before* every QRS complex? No
Is there a QRS complex *after* every P wave? Yes

Figure 9-119 Rapid atrial fibrillation
Irregular
Rate: 130 beats per minute
P-R interval = absent
QRS complex = 0.08 second
There are no discernable P waves

Figure 9-120 Normal sinus rhythm with unifocal couplet PVCs
Irregular
Rate: underlying rhythm = 78 beats per minute
P-R interval = 0.20 second
QRS complex = 0.06 second
Is there a P wave *before* every QRS complex? No
Is there a QRS complex *after* every P wave? Yes

Figure 9-121 Idioventricular rhythm
Irregular
Rate: 30 beats per minute
P-R interval = absent
QRS complex = 0.08 second
Is there a P wave *before* every QRS complex? There are no P waves

Figure 9-122 Second-degree AV heart block, Wenckebach (Mobitz I)
Irregular
Rate: 50 beats per minute
P-R interval = absent
QRS complex = 0.12 second
P-R interval becomes longer until finally a QRS complex is dropped

Figure 9-123 Supraventricular tachycardia (SVT)
Regular
Rate: 200 beats per minute
P-R interval = absent
QRS complex = 0.07 second
Is there a P wave *before* every QRS complex? There are no P waves

Figure 9-124 Sinus tachycardia with PACs
Irregular
Rate: 130 beats per minute
P-R interval = 0.12 second
QRS complex = 0.06 second

Is there a P wave *before* every QRS complex? No
Is there a QRS complex *after* every P wave? Yes

Figure 9-125 Normal sinus rhythm with artifact
Regular
Rate: 64 beats per minute
P-R interval = 0.16 second
QRS complex = 0.05 second
Is there a P wave *before* every QRS complex? Yes
Is there a QRS complex *after* every P wave? Yes

Figure 9-126 Sinus arrhythmia
Irregular
Rate: 70 beats per minutes, varies
P-R interval = 0.11 second
QRS complex = 0.08 second
Is there a P wave *before* every QRS complex? Yes
Is there a QRS complex *after* every P wave? Yes

Figure 9-127 Atrial fibrillation
Irregular
Rate: 120 beats per minute
P-R interval = absent
QRS complex = 0.04 second
There are no discernable P waves

Figure 9-128 Sinus arrhythmia with PACs changing to first-degree AV block
Irregular
Rate: 90 beats per minute
P-R interval = 0.20 changing to 0.32 second
QRS complex = 0.10 second
Is there a P wave *before* every QRS complex? No
Is there a QRS complex *after* every P wave? Yes

Figure 9-129 Normal sinus rhythm
Regular
Rate: 86 beats per minute
P-R interval = 0.20 second
QRS complex = 0.008 second
Is there a P wave *before* every QRS complex? Yes
Is there a QRS complex *after* every P wave? Yes

Figure 9-130 AV sequential pacemaker rhythm, failure to sense, with artifact
Regular
Rate: 72 beats per minute
P-R interval = absent
QRS complex = 0.10 second
Is there a P wave *before* every QRS complex? There are no P waves
There are atrial pacer spikes before the first, third, fifth, and seventh beats; there are ventricular pacer spikes after the second and sixth beats

Figure 9-131 Sinus tachycardia with one ectopic beat, appears to be PAC
Irregular
Rate: 107 beats per minute
P-R interval = 0.18 second
QRS complex = 0.10 second
Is there a P wave *before* every QRS complex? No
Is there a QRS complex *after* every P wave? Yes

Figure 9-132 AV sequential pacemaker rhythm
Irregular
Rate: 70 beats per minute
P-R interval = absent
QRS complex = 0.10 second
Is there a P wave *before* every QRS complex? There are no P waves

Figure 9-133 Normal sinus rhythm
Regular
Rate: 66 beats per minute
P-R interval = 0.17 second
QRS complex = 0.04 second
Is there a P wave *before* every QRS complex? Yes
Is there a QRS complex *after* every P wave? Yes

Figure 9-134 Sinus tachycardia with runs of bigeminy PVCs
Irregular
Rate: 120 beats per minute
P-R interval = varies 0.16 to 0.18 second
QRS complex = 0.08 second
Is there a P wave *before* every QRS complex? No
Is there a QRS complex *after* every P wave? Yes

Figure 9-135 Junctional rhythm with wide conduction or idioventricular rhythm
Regular
Rate: 56 beats per minute
P-R interval = absent
QRS complex = 0.14 second, wide conduction
Is there a P wave *before* every QRS complex? There are no P waves

Figure 9-136 Third-degree AV heart block changing to asystole
Irregular
Rate: initially 50 beats per minute, then zero
P-R interval = absent
QRS complex = 0.09 second
Is there a P wave *before* every QRS complex? There are no P waves

Figure 9-137 Sinus tachycardia
Regular
Rate: 102 beats per minute
P-R interval = 0.16 second

QRS complex = 0.08 second
Is there a P wave *before* every QRS complex? Yes
Is there a QRS complex *after* every P wave? Yes

Figure 9-138 Sinus arrhythmia with artifact
Irregular
Rate: 74 beats per minute
P-R interval = 0.16 second
QRS complex = 0.07 second
Is there a P wave *before* every QRS complex? Yes
Is there a QRS complex *after* every P wave? Yes

Figure 9-139 Sinus bradycardia
Regular
Rate: 51 beats per minute
P-R interval = 0.20 second
QRS complex = 0.08 second
Is there a P wave *before* every QRS complex? Yes
Is there a QRS complex *after* every P wave? Yes

Figure 9-140 AV sequential pacemaker rhythm
Regular
Rate: 64 beats per minute
P-R interval = absent
QRS complex = 0.09 second
Is there a P wave *before* every QRS complex? Yes
Is there a QRS complex *after* every P wave? Yes

Figure 9-141 Supraventricular tachycardia (SVT) or ventricular tachycardia with wide conduction
Regular
Rate: 200 beats per minute
P-R interval = absent
QRS complex = 0.12 second
Is there a P wave *before* every QRS complex? No
There are no P waves present

Figure 9-142 Normal sinus rhythm
Regular
Rate: 80 beats per minute
P-R interval = 0.16 second
QRS complex = 0.04 second
Is there a P wave *before* every QRS complex? Yes
Is there a QRS complex *after* every P wave? Yes

Figure 9-143 Sinus bradycardia with one PVC
Irregular
Rate: 50 beats per minute
P-R interval = 0.14 second
QRS complex = 0.04 second

Is there a P wave *before* every QRS complex? Yes
Is there a QRS complex *after* every P wave? Yes

Figure 9-144 Sinus bradycardia
Regular
Rate: 42 beats per minute
P-R interval = 0.16 second
QRS complex = 0.04 second
Is there a P wave *before* every QRS complex? Yes
Is there a QRS complex *after* every P wave? Yes

Figure 9-145 Second-degree AV heart block, Mobitz II
Regular
Rate: 48 beats per minute
P-R interval = 0.12 second
QRS complex = 0.10 second
Is there a P wave *before* every QRS complex? Yes
Is there a QRS complex *after* every P wave? No

Figure 9-146 Wandering atrial pacemaker rhythm with two PJCs
Irregular
Rate: 124 beats per minute
P-R interval = varies
QRS complex = 0.06 second
Is there a P wave *before* every QRS complex? No
Is there a QRS complex *after* every P wave? No

Figure 9-147 Ventricular pacemaker rhythm
Regular
Rate: 72 beats per minute
P-R interval = absent
QRS complex = 0.12 second
Is there a P wave *before* every QRS complex? No
There are no P waves present

Figure 9-148 Normal sinus rhythm with one PVC
Irregular
Rate: 78 beats per minute
P-R interval = 0.16 second
QRS complex = 0.08 second
Is there a P wave *before* every QRS complex? No
Is there a QRS complex *after* every P wave? Yes

Figure 9-149 First-degree AV heart block with one PJC, changing to accelerated junctional
Irregular
Rate: begins at 75 beats per minute, then changes to approximately 90 beats per minute
P-R interval = 0.36 second in first-degree block
QRS complex = 0.10 second
Is there a P wave *before* every QRS complex? No

Is there a QRS complex *after* every P wave? No
First three beats are sinus, fourth is PJC as P wave is inverted, and the rest are absent

Figure 9-150 Supraventricular tachycardia (SVT) with some atrial beats
Regular
Rate: 200 beats per minute
P-R interval = absent
QRS complex = 0.08 second
There are no discernable P waves

Figure 9-151 Atrial flutter
Irregular
Rate: 90 beats per minute
P-R interval = not measurable
QRS complex = 0.05 second
There is a 2:1 and 4:1 conduction rate; atrial rate = 260 beats per minute, ventricular rate = 90 beats per minute

Figure 9-152 Atrial fibrillation with one PVC
Irregular
Rate: 50 beats per minute
P-R interval = absent
QRS complex = 0.06 second
There are no discernable P waves

Figure 9-153 Sinus tachycardia with sinus arrest
Irregular
Rate: ST = 140 beats per minute, then zero
P-R interval = 0.16 second
QRS complex = 0.06 second
Is there a P wave *before* every QRS complex? Yes
Is there a QRS complex *after* every P wave? Yes

Figure 9-154 Sinus bradycardia
Regular
Rate: 42 beats per minute
P-R interval = 0.17 second
QRS complex = 0.07 second
Is there a P wave *before* every QRS complex? Yes
Is there a QRS complex *after* every P wave? Yes

Figure 9-155 Sinus bradycardia with unifocal PVCs
Irregular
Rate: underlying rhythm is 55 beats per minute
P-R interval = 0.16 second
QRS complex = 0.05 second
Is there a P wave *before* every QRS complex? No
Is there a QRS complex *after* every P wave? Yes

Figure 9-156 Junctional rhythm with one PVC
Irregular
Rate: 60 beats per minute
P-R interval = absent
QRS complex = 0.10 second
Is there a P wave *before* every QRS complex? No
There are no P waves present

Figure 9-157 Second-degree AV heart block, Mobitz I (Wenckebach)
Irregular
Rate: 60 beats per minute
P-R interval = not measurable
QRS complex = 0.06 second
Is there a P wave *before* every QRS complex? Yes
Is there a QRS complex *after* every P wave? No

Figure 9-158 Normal sinus rhythm with artifact
Regular
Rate: 66 beats per minute
P-R interval = 0.20 second
QRS complex = 0.06 second
Is there a P wave *before* every QRS complex? Yes
Is there a QRS complex *after* every P wave? Yes

Figure 9-159 Atrial fibrillation
Irregular
Rate: 56 beats per minute
P-R interval = absent
QRS complex = 0.08 second
There are no discernable P waves

Figure 9-160 Sinus arrhythmia with ventricular tachycardia
Irregular
Rate: underlying rhythm = 120 beats per minute; V-tach = 200 beats per minute
P-R interval = 0.14 second where visible
QRS complex = 0.12 second
Is there a P wave *before* every QRS complex? No
Is there a QRS complex *after* every P wave? Yes

Figure 9-161 Normal sinus rhythm one PAC
Irregular
Rate: 78 beats per minute
P-R interval = 0.16 second
QRS complex = 0.06 second
Is there a P wave *before* every QRS complex? No
Is there a QRS complex *after* every P wave? Yes

Figure 9-162 Sinus rhythm with two paced beats (failure to sense)
Regular

Rate: 72 beats per minute
P-R interval = 0.20 second
QRS complex = 0.08 second
Is there a P wave *before* every QRS complex? No
Is there a QRS complex *after* every P wave? Yes
The first beat has pacer spike after the QRS complex, and the seventh beat has pacer spike before the QRS complex

Figure 9-163 Normal sinus rhythm
Regular
Rate: 78 beats per minute
P-R interval = 0.16 second
QRS complex = 0.04 second
Is there a P wave *before* every QRS complex? Yes
Is there a QRS complex *after* every P wave? Yes

Figure 9-164 Third-degree AV heart block
Regular
Rate: 30 beats per minutes except for ectopic beat
P-R interval = not measurable
QRS complex = 0.14 second
Is there a P wave *before* every QRS complex? No
Is there a QRS complex *after* every P wave? No
Atrial rate = 80 beats per minute and ventricular rate = 30 beats per minute

Figure 9-165 Normal sinus rhythm with unifocal PVCs
Irregular
Rate: 75 beats per minute
P-R interval = 0.20 second
QRS complex = 0.05 second
Is there a P wave *before* every QRS complex? No
Is there a QRS complex *after* every P wave? Yes

Figure 9-166 AV sequential pacemaker rhythm
Regular
Rate: 66 beats per minute
P-R interval = 0.20 second where present (second and fifth beats)
QRS complex = 0.14 second
Is there a P wave *before* every QRS complex? No
Is there a QRS complex *after* every P wave? Yes
The first, third, fourth, and sixth beats are dual paced, whereas the second and fifth beats are ventricular paced

Figure 9-167 Sinus bradycardia
Regular
Rate: 47 beats per minute
P-R interval = 0.16 second
QRS complex = 0.08 second
Is there a P wave *before* every QRS complex? Yes
Is there a QRS complex *after* every P wave? Yes

Figure 9-168 First-degree AV heart block
Irregular
Rate: 58 beats per minute
P-R interval = 0.32 second
QRS complex = 0.16 second, wide conduction
Is there a P wave *before* every QRS complex? Yes
Is there a QRS complex *after* every P wave? Yes

Figure 9-169 Atrial fibrillation
Irregular
Rate: 50 beats per minute
P-R interval = absent
QRS complex = 0.08 second
There are no discernable P waves

Figure 9-170 Junctional escape rhythm
Regular
Rate: 51 beats per minute
P-R interval = 0.20 second, inverted P waves
QRS complex = 0.10 second
Is there a P wave *before* every QRS complex? Yes
Is there a QRS complex *after* every P wave? Yes

Figure 9-171 Second-degree AV heart block, Wenckebach (Mobitz I)
Irregular
Rate: 50 beats per minute
P-R interval = not measurable
QRS complex = 0.10 second
Is there a P wave *before* every QRS complex? No
Is there a QRS complex *after* every P wave? No

Figure 9-172 Sinus rhythm with bigeminy PVCs
Irregular
Rate: underlying rhythm = 50 beats per minute
P-R interval = 0.17 second
QRS complex = 0.07 second
Is there a P wave *before* every QRS complex? No
Is there a QRS complex *after* every P wave? Yes

Figure 9-173 Normal sinus rhythm with one PJC
Irregular
Rate: 70 beats per minute
P-R interval = 0.16 second
QRS complex = 0.09 second
Is there a P wave *before* every QRS complex? Yes
Is there a QRS complex *after* every P wave? Yes
The sixth beat has an inverted P wave and falls early making it a PJC

Figure 9-174 Sinus rhythm with PJCs
Irregular

Rate: 90 beats per minute
P-R interval = 0.20 second
QRS complex = 0.06 second
Is there a P wave *before* every QRS complex? No
Is there a QRS complex *after* every P wave? Yes
The first, fourth, and seventh beats are PJCs

Figure 9-175 Junctional rhythm with unifocal PVCs
Irregular
Rate: 90 beats per minute
P-R interval = absent
QRS complex = 0.08 second, junctional beats
Is there a P wave *before* every QRS complex? No
There are no P waves present

Figure 9-176 Sinus arrhythmia to atrial fibrillation with one ectopic beat
Irregular
Rate: 110 beats per minute
P-R interval = 0.16 second where measurable
QRS complex = 0.07 second
The first three beats appear to be sinus; the rest do not have discernable P waves

Figure 9-177 Accelerated junctional rhythm
Regular
Rate: 68 beats per minute
P-R interval = 0.12 second, P waves inverted
QRS complex = 0.06 second
Is there a P wave *before* every QRS complex? Yes
Is there a QRS complex *after* every P wave? Yes

Figure 9-178 Pacemaker rhythm
Regular
Rate: 60 beats per minute
P-R interval = 0.22 second (atrial pacer)
QRS complex = 0.04 second
Is there a P wave *before* every QRS complex? Yes
Is there a QRS complex *after* every P wave? Yes
Rhythm has atrial pacer spikes but does not appear to have ventricular pacer spikes

Figure 9-179 Sinus rhythm (first and second beats) with ectopic beat changing into junctional rhythm
Irregular
Rate: 80 beats per minute
P-R interval = 0.14 second, where present
QRS complex = 0.08 to 0.10 second
Is there a P wave *before* every QRS complex? No
Is there a QRS complex *after* every P wave? No

Figure 9-180 Junctional tachycardia with artifact
Regular

Rate: 150 beats per minute
P-R interval = varies 0.06 to 0.12 second
QRS complex = 0.06 second
Some of the P waves are difficult to distinguish because of the artifact

Figure 9-181 Sinus bradycardia with artifact
Regular
Rate: 42 beats per minute
P-R interval = 0.18 second
QRS complex = 0.08 second
Is there a P wave *before* every QRS complex? Yes
Is there a QRS complex *after* every P wave? Yes

Figure 9-182 Normal sinus rhythm with one PVC
Irregular
Rate: 72 beats per minute
P-R interval = 0.18 second
QRS complex = 0.08 second
Is there a P wave *before* every QRS complex? No
Is there a QRS complex *after* every P wave? Yes

Figure 9-183 Normal sinus rhythm with a run of ventricular tachycardia
Irregular
Rate: 70 beats per minute
P-R interval = 0.18 second
QRS complex = 0.06 second
Is there a P wave *before* every QRS complex? Yes
Is there a QRS complex *after* every P wave? Yes

Figure 9-184 Atrial fibrillation with one PJC
Irregular
Rate: 60 beats per minute
P-R interval = not measurable
QRS complex = 0.06 second
There are no discernable P waves

Figure 9-185 Normal sinus rhythm
Regular
Rate: 80 beats per minute
P-R interval = 0.20 second
QRS complex = 0.05 second
Is there a P wave *before* every QRS complex? Yes
Is there a QRS complex *after* every P wave? Yes

Figure 9-186 Atrial fibrillation with two PVCs
Irregular
Rate: 80 beats per minute
P-R interval = absent
QRS complex = 0.06 second
There are no discernable P waves

Figure 9-187 Rapid atrial fibrillation with couplet PVCs
Irregular
Rate: 110 beats per minute
P-R interval = absent
QRS complex = 0.08 second
There are no discernable P waves

Figure 9-188 Wandering atrial pacemaker
Regular
Rate: 84 beats per minute
P-R interval = 0.12 to 0.16 second
QRS complex = 0.10 second
Is there a P wave *before* every QRS complex? Yes
Is there a QRS complex *after* every P wave? Yes

Figure 9-189 Sinus rhythm with bigeminy PVCs
Irregular
Rate: 70 beats per minute
P-R interval = 0.20 second where present
QRS complex = 0.10 second
Is there a P wave *before* every QRS complex? No
Is there a QRS complex *after* every P wave? Yes

Figure 9-190 Sinus tachycardia
Regular
Rate: 128 beats per minute
P-R interval = 0.16 second
QRS complex = 0.10 second
Is there a P wave *before* every QRS complex? Yes
Is there a QRS complex *after* every P wave? Yes

Figure 9-191 Atrial flutter with artifact
Regular
Rate: 70 beats per minute
P-R interval = 0.12 second where measurable
QRS complex = 0.08 second
Basically a 4:1 conduction rate; the atrial rate is 270 and the ventricular rate is 70 beats per minute

Figure 9-192 Ventricular aystole with P waves
No regularity
Rate: 0
P-R interval = absent
QRS complex = absent

Figure 9-193 Junctional tachycardia with multifocal PVCs
Irregular
Rate: 115 beats per minute
P-R interval = 0.16 second (P waves inverted)
QRS complex = 0.06 second

Is there a P wave *before* every QRS complex? No
Is there a QRS complex *after* every P wave? Yes

Figure 9-194 Normal sinus rhythm to sinus tachycardia
Irregular
Rate: 100 to 130 beats per minute
P-R interval = 0.16 to 0.12 second
QRS complex = 0.05 second
Is there a P wave *before* every QRS complex? Yes
Is there a QRS complex *after* every P wave? Yes

Figure 9-195 Normal sinus rhythm
Regular
Rate: 80 beats per minute
P-R interval = 0.16 second
QRS complex = 0.04 second
Is there a P wave *before* every QRS complex? Yes
Is there a QRS complex *after* every P wave? Yes

Figure 9-196 Normal sinus rhythm with two PVCs
Irregular
Rate: 75 beats per minute
P-R interval = 0.16 second
QRS complex = 0.04 second (sinus beats)
Is there a P wave *before* every QRS complex? No
Is there a QRS complex *after* every P wave? Yes

Figure 9-197 Sinus tachycardia with two PACs
Irregular
Rate: 104 beats per minute
P-R interval = 0.18 second
QRS complex = 0.12 second, wide conduction
Is there a P wave *before* every QRS complex? Yes
Is there a QRS complex *after* every P wave? Yes

Figure 9-198 Pacemaker rhythm
Regular
Rate: 80 beats per minute
P-R interval = 0.22 second
QRS complex = 0.15 second
Ventricular pacemaker rhythm

Figure 9-199 First-degree AV heart block
Regular
Rate: 76 beats per minute
P-R interval = 0.24 second
QRS complex = 0.08 second
Is there a P wave *before* every QRS complex? Yes
Is there a QRS complex *after* every P wave? Yes

Figure 9-200 Sinus rhythm with unifocal and couplet PVCs
Irregular
Rate: 100 beats per minute
P-R interval = 0.16 second where present
QRS complex = 0.12 second
Is there a P wave *before* every QRS complex? No
Is there a QRS complex *after* every P wave? Yes

CHAPTER 10, CASE 1

Scenario

This rhythm is a **sinus rhythm with PVCs** at a rate of 80 beats per minute
Rhythm = irregular; P-R interval = 0.18 seconds; QRS complex = 0.06 second

Primary Survey

The airway is open, breathing is adequate, and no chest compressions are needed because the patient is awake and alert. No defibrillation is needed.

Secondary Survey

Airway: adequate
Breathing: apply oxygen 2 to 3 L via nasal cannula
Circulation: cardiac monitor, IV access, initial vital signs, repeat pulse oximetry; obtain a 12-lead ECG
Impression: rule out a possible MI

Oxygen-IV-Monitor-Fluids

Continue the oxygen, cardiac monitoring, and obtain needed lab work. Is fluid needed? No, not at this time.

Vital Signs

Continue ongoing vital signs; monitor the heart rate, blood pressure, pulse, and respirations. Obtain a history, do a physical examination, and get a chest x-ray.

Rationale

Treatment would include a complete workup for a possible MI. The dizziness, light-headedness, and syncope are probably due to the fact he is having the PVCs and not all the beats are perfusing. With no cardiac history, what may have caused this? PVCs may be caused by excessive exercise, alcohol, smoking, or caffeine. With the rhythm being symptomatic, an antiarrhythmic agent is the answer to eliminate the ventricular escape activity. The physician may consider one of the following drug therapies: amiodarone, procainamide, lidocaine or beta blockers such as atenolol, esmolol, and metoprolol. Amiodarone has become the drug of choice if cardiac function is impaired and/or the ejection factor is less than 40%. Amiodarone has vasodilator effects and negative inotropic effects.

The syncope was caused by a decrease in cardiac output. He will need a full cardiac workup to eliminate any cardiac problems. Most likely the cause is the smoking and excess caffeine combined with the stress over the past few months.

CHAPTER 10, CASE 2

Scenario

This rhythm is a **ventricular tachycardia** at a rate of 115 beats per minute
Rhythm = regular; P-R interval is absent; QRS complex = 0.24 second, wide and bizarre

Primary Survey

The airway is open, breathing is adequate, and no chest compressions are needed because the patient is awake and alert. No defibrillation is needed at this time because vital signs are stable.

Secondary Survey

Airway: adequate
Breathing: apply oxygen 10 to 15 L via nonrebreather mask
Circulation: cardiac monitor, IV access, initial vital signs, pulse oximetry, 12-lead ECG
Impression: rule out a possible acute myocardial infarction or electrolyte imbalance

Oxygen-IV-Monitor-Fluids

Continue the oxygen, cardiac monitoring, and obtain needed lab work. Is fluid needed? Yes, at a keep-open rate in case the patient needs immediate medications infused. IV medications may include amiodarone, procainamide, or lidocaine.

Vital Signs

Continue ongoing vital signs; monitor the heart rate, blood pressure, pulse and respirations, and pulse oximetry. Obtain a physical examination and chest x-ray.

Rationale

This patient is stable with a good blood pressure and pulse indicating good cardiovascular perfusion. Because the patient is not in immediate danger, drug therapy with an antiarrhythmic agent may be instituted to attempt to convert the rhythm into a normal sinus rhythm (NSR). Such agents include amiodarone 150 mg IV over 10 minutes; procainamide 20 to 30 mg/min IV up to a total dose of 17 mg/kg; or lidocaine 1.0 to 1.5 mg/kg IV bolus slowly. The amiodarone may be repeated twice if needed every 10 to 15 minutes, and the lidocaine may be repeated at a 0.5- to 0.75-mg/kg IV bolus to a total maximum dose of 3 mg/kg. If the patient was unstable and showing signs of poor perfusion, then immediate cardioversion is the treatment of choice. Cardioversion selects when the monitor will discharge, so the electrical charge will not fall on the T wave. Cardioversion would start at 100 J, and may be repeated with 200 J, then 300 J, and then 360 J. Always administer a sedative before cardioversion. Known causes of V-tach include electrolyte imbalances, congestive heart failure, toxicity from medications such as digoxin, and stimulants such as caffeine or alcohol. In this case the patient was given a lidocaine bolus; the lidocaine bolus was repeated with conversion into a normal sinus rhythm.

CHAPTER 10, CASE 3

Scenario

This rhythm is an **atrial tachycardia** at a rate of 176 beats per minute
Rhythm = regular; P-R interval = 0.12 second; QRS complex = 0.04 second

Primary Survey

The airway is open, breathing is adequate, and no chest compressions are needed because the patient is awake and alert. No defibrillation is needed because vital signs are stable.

Secondary Survey

Airway: adequate
Breathing: apply oxygen 2 to 3 L via nasal cannula
Circulation: cardiac monitor, IV access, initial vital signs, pulse oximetry, 12-lead ECG
Impression: rule out possible cardiac problems, flu, and diabetic abnormalities

Oxygen-IV-Monitor-Fluids

Continue the oxygen, cardiac monitoring, and obtain needed lab work. Is fluid needed? Yes, because her skin is pale, cool, and dry. Place the IV at the antecubital site because it is the closest to the heart in anticipation of medications to be given. IV drug therapy may include adenosine 6-mg IV bolus, which may be repeated at 12-mg boluses in 1 to 2 minutes. Other drug therapy may be diltiazem 20-mg IV bolus over 2 minutes or a beta blocker agent such as esmolol, atenolol, or metoprolol. Digoxin also may be considered (0.5 mg IV over 5 minutes). It is a physician's choice as to which of the drug therapies may be used.

Vital Signs

Continue ongoing vital signs; monitor the heart rate, blood pressure, pulse and respirations, and pulse oximetry. Obtain a patient history and get a chest x-ray.

Rationale

The patient may be dehydrated from the present flulike illness and the vomiting over the past 3 days. Although she has kept some fluids down, she may need some fluid replacement. Being a diabetic and not able to eat, she needs finger sticks on a regular basis to ensure normal glucose levels. The tachycardia is probably due to the illness, but definitely needs to be slowed down. At a rate of 176 beats per minute, her cardiac output is decreased and compromising her circulatory status. You might consider giving fluid replacement before the first adenosine bolus, but close observation is necessary.

CHAPTER 10, CASE 4

Scenario

This rhythm is a **sinus bradycardia** rate of 45 beats per minute
Rhythm = regular; P-R interval = 0.14 seconds; QRS complex = 0.08 second

Oxygen-IV-Monitor-Fluids

Continue the oxygen, cardiac monitoring, and obtain needed lab work. Is fluid needed? Yes, because she is so light-headed when she sits up. Be prepared to administer adenosine 6-mg rapid IV push, followed by a 12-mg bolus if needed. A second 12-mg bolus may be given if needed, or drug therapy such as amiodarone 150 mg over 10 minutes or diltiazem 20-mg IV bolus over 2 minutes may be given.

Vital Signs

Continue ongoing vital signs; monitor the heart rate, blood pressure, pulse, and respirations. Obtain a history, do a physical examination, and get a chest x-ray.

Rationale

Oxygen is always the first intervention. Becoming light-headed when sitting tells you the patient is orthostatic positive and cardiac output is decreasing with elevation of the upper body. Give the adenosine to convert the rhythm back into a normal sinus rhythm. You might also try vagal maneuvers to convert the SVT. However, if trying carotid massage, ensure that the patient does not have a carotid bruit first or you may dislodge an embolus and cause a stroke or MI. Also consider digoxin, diltiazem, or beta blockers. If the patient becomes unstable have the equipment ready to cardiovert, starting at 100 J, and continuing with 200 J, then 300 J, and last at 360 J. Cardioversion usually requires a sedative such as Valium, Versed, or fentanyl IV to be given first.

Because the patient is alert and oriented with no signs of chest pain, shortness of breath, low blood pressure or a decreased level of consciousness, she is considered stable. The rapid rhythm caused a brief decrease in her cardiac output, decreasing perfusion to the brain. The end result is syncope! Therefore the first intervention is oxygen, followed by adenosine. Adenosine is an antiarrhythmic agent that can restore normal sinus rhythms by slowing conduction through the AV node and by interrupting reentry pathways through the AV node and junction.

Now you are going to ask, "What causes a sudden supraventricular tachycardia?" In a healthy young person it may be an excessive use of caffeine, other stimulants, hypokalemia, hyperkalemia, physical or psychologic stress, but remember, this rhythm may be a warning of more serious ventricular dysrhythmias to follow. Vagal maneuvers include carotid sinus massage, gag reflex, application of eyeball pressure, or Valsalva maneuver. The other drugs mentioned are antiarrhythmics, which will slow conduction through the AV node.

Remember to look at your monitor before starting the IV. If there is any indication that you will need to push Adenocard (adenosine), then the IV needs to be placed as close to the heart as possible. The half-life of adenosine is 10 seconds, which basically means it has 10 seconds or less to reach its target, the heart. You should also have an IV bag of saline running wide open to speed the drug along its path through the vein.

Once converted the patient will probably be discharged to home and not need to remain in the hospital.

CHAPTER 10, CASE 7

Scenario

This rhythm is a **ventricular fibrillation**. The rhythm is irregular; there are no P waves and QRS complexes.

Primary Survey

The airway is not open, there is no breathing by the patient, and the patient is unresponsive. The first order is to ventilate the lungs along with CPR, and defibrillation is needed as soon as possible. Defibrillate at 200, 200 to 300, and 360 J checking the monitor after each shock. Continue CPR until there is a change in the patient's status or the code is terminated.

Secondary Survey

Airway: inadequate
Breathing: use the BVM to apply manual respirations and do endotracheal intubation
Circulation: cardiac monitor, IV access. Give epinephrine 1 mg IV or vasopressin 40 U IV, a single dose one time only. The epinephrine may be repeated every 3 to 5 minutes while the patient is in arrest. Continue to shock at 360 J after each drug administration as long as the patient remains in ventricular fibrillation. Next is amiodarone 300 mg IV given rapidly, which may be repeated at 150 mg doses × 2 if necessary. Lidocaine or procainamide may be considered. Always shock after each drug is given and check the monitor for a change in the rhythm, checking for a pulse if there is a rhythm change. If there is no change, give magnesium sulfate 1- to 2 g IV and sodium bicarbonate at this time.
Impression: cardiac arrest, with a probable MI

Oxygen-IV-Monitor-Fluids

Continue the oxygen, cardiac monitoring, and obtain needed lab work. Is fluid needed? Yes, fluid is needed, a 20-ml bolus each time to infuse each of the drugs being given.

Vital Signs

Continue to monitor the circulatory status while doing CPR. Especially observe the skin color and pupils (are they constricted or dilated and fixed?).

Obtain a history if possible from the family or bystanders. Get an x-ray when resuscitation is successful to ensure ET tube placement.

Rationale

Always, always—airway, breathing, circulation, and quick-look. The quicker electricity is delivered, the greater the chance for survival. I cannot emphasize this enough. In the V-fib protocol you would shock, shock, shock immediately, checking the monitor and checking for a pulse in between each shock. Then if no change, perform your intubation and establish IV access. Now on to drug therapy. The pattern in V-fib is always ***drug-shock, drug-shock***. Epinephrine is a natural catecholamine, which increases the following: systemic vascular resistance, electrical activity in the myocardium, coronary and cerebral blood flow, strength of myocardial contraction, and automaticity. Amiodarone is an antiarrhythmic agent that has effects that result in decreased number of ventricular events. Amiodarone prolongs the duration of the action potential of cardiac fibers. It also raises the threshold for V-fib and thus reduces the chance for reoccurrence. Next, magnesium sulfate may be considered if hypomagnesemia is suspected. Magnesium sulfate acts as a physiologic calcium channel blocker and blocks neuromuscular transmission by reducing acetylcholine release at the myoneural junction. Also, procainamide suppresses ventricular ectopy and may be effective when other antidysrhythmics are not. Procainamide suppresses

Primary Survey

CPR is in progress; you place the monitor on the patient and see asystole. No defibrillation is needed at this time. Also, do not forget to observe spinal immobilization precautions because this was a trauma.

Secondary Survey

Airway: inadequate, intubate the patient as soon as possible
Breathing: apply oxygen via BVM through the ET tube
Circulation: cardiac monitor, IV access, continue CPR, cardiac monitoring. Fluid is needed to infuse the drugs during the code. If you are considering transcutaneous pacing, do it immediately. Give epinephrine 1-mg IV push. This may be repeated every 3 to 5 minutes during the arrest. Next give atropine 1-mg IV push and repeat every 3 minutes until a total dose of 0.04 mg/kg has been given. Consider sodium bicarbonate 1 mEq/kg.
Impression: consider the possible reasons for the cardiac arrest and determine if any of them can be corrected. Next consider termination of the code.

Rationale

The ice fell, striking him on the head and neck causing severe trauma to the head and neck. End result—respiratory arrest, followed by cardiac arrest. As with any arrest situation, the first concern is CPR. The second concern is "Does the patient need electricity?" The third concern is advanced airway management with endotracheal intubation, followed by IV access (antecubital site) and appropriate drug therapy. Obviously spinal precautions must be taken in case you do manage to resuscitate this patient.

In any arrest situation, you need to be on your toes, and act and think quickly. You need to know your ACLS protocols so you can recite them in your sleep, because a patient's life may depend on *you*!

CHAPTER 10, CASE 27

Scenario

This rhythm is a sinus tachycardia with a rate of 102 beats per minute. The rhythm is regular. There is a P wave before every QRS complex and a QRS complex after every P wave. The P-R interval is 0.18 second, and the QRS is 0.07 second.

Primary Survey

The airway is open, breathing is adequate, and no chest compressions are needed. No defibrillation is needed.

Secondary Survey

Airway: adequate
Breathing: apply oxygen 2 to 3 L via nasal cannula
Circulation: cardiac monitor, IV access, initial vital signs, 12-lead ECG, pulse oximetry
Impression: rule out chest trauma

Oxygen-IV-Monitor-Fluids

Continue the oxygen, cardiac monitoring, and obtain needed lab work. Is fluid needed? No, not at this time.

Vital Signs

Continue ongoing vital signs; monitor the heart rate, blood pressure, pulse, and respirations. Obtain a history, do a physical examinations, and get a chest x-ray.

Rationale

Treatment should begin by checking for any signs of a possible rib fracture, or flail chest, which might produce a pneumothorax. The ECG is a normal sinus rhythm. However, questions should arise in your mind while caring for this patient. Why is she so disoriented? Why did respiratory distress develop? Did she become disoriented and fall out of bed, or did she fall out of bed and strike her head? Does she have a possible transient ischemic attack (TIA) or cerebrovascular accident (CVA) in progress? The blood pressure is slightly on the high side.

Next on the agenda is the lung status. Does she have a fractured rib or several fractured ribs (flail chest)? Are the lung sounds equal on both sides? Is there good air movement? Are there adventitious lung sounds? When you first found her, 2 to 3 L of oxygen was fine, but then the situation changed. Now she needs 10 to 15 L of oxygen via nonrebreather mask.

There are many possible answers to this case, because she may have more than one medical problem.

CHAPTER 10, CASE 28

Scenario

This rhythm is a **rapid atrial fibrillation (uncontrolled)** with a rate of 170 beats per minute. The rhythm is irregular. P waves are absent. The QRS complex is 0.04 second.

Primary Survey

The airway is open, breathing is adequate, and no chest compressions are needed. No defibrillation is needed.

Secondary Survey

Airway: adequate
Breathing: apply oxygen 10 to 15 L via nonrebreather mask
Circulation: cardiac monitor, IV access, initial vital signs, 12-lead ECG, pulse oximetry
Impression: rule out cardiac problems and medication reaction

Oxygen-IV-Monitor-Fluids

Continue the oxygen, cardiac monitoring, and obtain needed lab work. Is fluid needed? Yes, because he is hypotensive.

Venous return: amount of blood returning to the heart from the systemic circulation.

Ventricle: bottom two chambers of the heart; right ventricle and left ventricle.

Ventricular tachycardia: arrhythmia in which the pacemaker site is in the ventricles; has a rate greater than 100 beats per minute.

Wandering atrial pacemaker: arrhythmia in which the pacemaker site is above the AV junction; in the SA node, the atria, or AV junction. This rhythm is diagnosed by having at least three different P waves in the same lead on the ECG.

Waveform: movement away from the isoelectric line or baseline; may be positive if above the line or is negative if below the baseline.

Wolff-Parkinson-White syndrome: arrhythmia with a preexcitation syndrome; this is characterized by a slurred upstroke of the QRS complex and a wide QRS.

Index

A

Figures denoted by *f*; tables denoted by *t*.

B

C

D

P

Q

R

E

F

H

V

W

Make sure you are prepared!

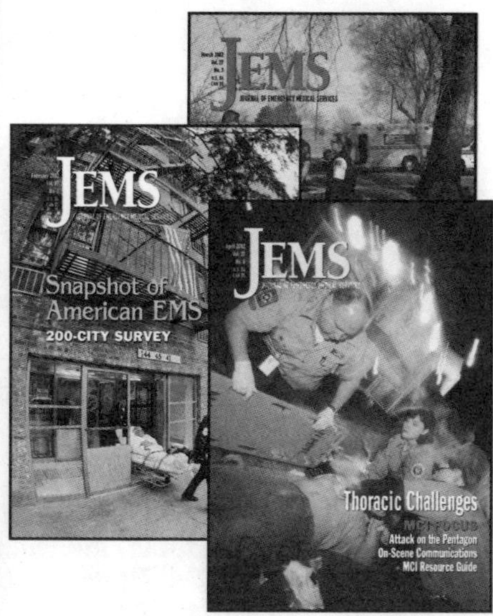

You already know the value of continuing education. Here's your opportunity to supply yourself with articles, columns, and practical tips to continue your education on a monthly basis.

Each month, you'll receive:

☆ Tricks of the Trade
☆ Special reports on major responses
☆ AJ Heightman's insightful Editor's Page
☆ Features on new clinical techniques with full color photos and illustrations
☆ Continuing education articles

...as well as the annual issues: Career Issue, Buyer's Guide, Salary Survey and more!

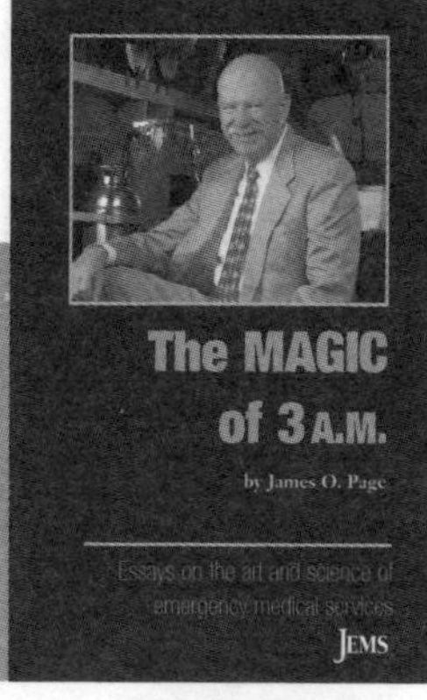

Subscribe today and receive a **FREE BONUS GIFT!**

Plus! ***THE MAGIC OF 3 A.M.*, BY JAMES O. PAGE**

Re-released after being out of print for several years, The Magic of 3 A.M. includes Jim Page's timeless essays on EMS. His words are as meaningful today as they were 20 years ago.

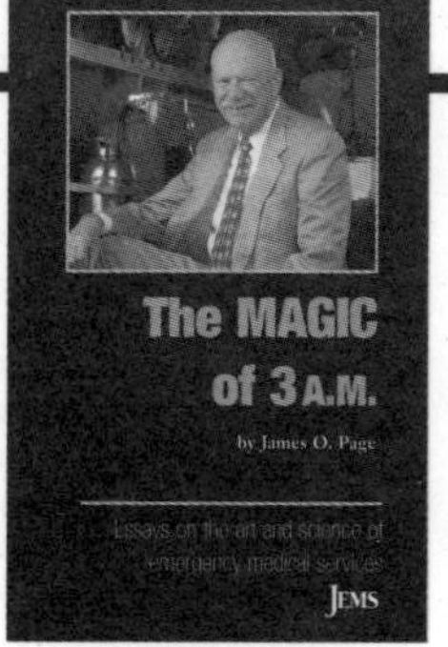

JEMS

The premier professional journal for EMS personnel.

To Subscribe call:
1-888-456-5367
Or Visit the Web
www.jems.com

FREE BONUS GIFT!

❑ **Yes!** I want to stay on top of the latest issues of EMS. Send me 12 issues (one-year) for only $28.97 and my **FREE** copy of ***The Magic of 3 A.M.***

Name ______________________________

Title ____________ Organization ____________

Address ______________________________

City ____________ State ______ Zip ____________

Phone (   ) ____________ Fax (   ) ____________

Email ______________________________

We occasionally send promotions on products and services via email. If you do not wish to receive these messages, please check here ❑

❑ Payment Enclosed ❑ Bill me

Charge my: ❑ Visa ❑ MasterCard ❑ Discover ❑ American Express

Exp. Date ________ Card # ______________________

Signature ______________________________

Occupation/Position:
(Please circle one)
A. Physician
B. Nurse/Inst./Coord.
C. Administrator/Supervisor
D. Paramed./EMT-I/EMT-D
E. EMT (Basic, 1st Resp.)
F. Other (Specify) ________

Employer/Affiliation:
(Please circle one)
1. Hospital
2. Private Ambulance
3. Fire Dept./Rescue Squad
4. Third Serv./Mun. Agency
5. Industrial Commercial
6. Other (Specify) ________

Canada please add $18 per year for postage. All other foreign please add $20 per year for surface mail postage. Add $70 per year for air mail postage. Subscriptions must be paid in U.S. funds. Please allow 6-8 weeks for delivery of first issue. Offer expires 12/31/03

*New subscribers only. Bonus gift will be sent when your payment is received. Subscription price includes shipping & handling of book.

326ZG-2

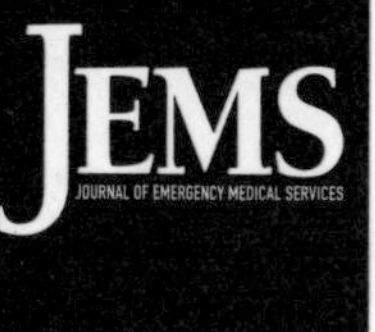